PHILANTHROPY FOR HE

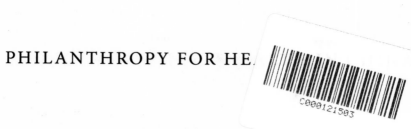

Warren F. Ilchman, Alice Stone Ilchman, and Mary Hale Tolar, editors. *The Lucky Few and the Worthy Many: Scholarship Competitions and the World's Future Leaders*

Thomas H. Jeavons. *When the Bottom Line Is Faithfulness: Management of Christian Service Organizations*

Amy A. Kass, editor. *The Perfect Gift*

Amy A. Kass, editor. *Giving Well, Doing Good: Readings for Thoughtful Philanthropists*

Ellen Condliffe Lagemann, editor. *Philanthropic Foundations: New Scholarship, New Possibilities*

Daniel C. Levy. *To Export Progress: The Golden Age of University Assistance in the Americas*

Mike W. Martin. *Virtuous Giving: Philanthropy, Voluntary Service, and Caring*

Kathleen D. McCarthy, editor. *Women, Philanthropy, and Civil Society*

Marc A. Musick and John Wilson, editors. *Volunteers: A Social Profile*

Mary J. Oates. *The Catholic Philanthropic Tradition in America*

Robert S. Ogilvie. *Voluntarism, Community Life, and the American Ethic*

J. B. Schneewind, editor. *Giving: Western Ideas of Philanthropy*

William H. Schneider, editor. *Rockefeller Philanthropy and Modern Biomedicine: International Initiatives from World War I to the Cold War*

Bradford Smith, Sylvia Shue, Jennifer Lisa Vest, and Joseph Villarreal. *Philanthropy in Communities of Color*

David Horton Smith, Robert A. Stebbins, and Michael A. Dover, editors. *A Dictionary of Nonprofit Terms and Concepts*

David H. Smith. *Entrusted: The Moral Responsibilities of Trusteeship*

David H. Smith, editor. *Good Intentions: Moral Obstacles and Opportunities*

Jon Van Til. *Growing Civil Society: From Nonprofit Sector to Third Space*

Andrea Walton. *Women and Philanthropy in Education*

PHILANTHROPY
FOR HEALTH IN CHINA

Edited by Jennifer Ryan
        Lincoln C. Chen
        Tony Saich

Foreword by Peter Geithner and Wang Zhenyao

Indiana University Press

Bloomington & Indianapolis

This book is a publication of

Indiana University Press
Office of Scholarly Publishing
Herman B Wells Library 350
1320 East 10th Street
Bloomington, Indiana 47405 USA

iupress.indiana.edu

Telephone 800-842-6796
Fax 812-855-7931

Manufactured in the United States of America

Library of Congress Cataloging-in-Publication Data

Philanthropy for health in China / edited by Jennifer
Ryan, Lincoln C. Chen, and Tony Saich.
    p. ; cm. — (Philanthropic and nonprofit studies)
    Includes bibliographical references and index.
    ISBN 978-0-253-01442-9 (cloth : alk. paper) — ISBN 978-0-253-
01450-4 (pbk. : alk. paper) — ISBN 978-0-253-01458-0 (ebook)
    I. Ryan, Jennifer, [date] editor of compilation. II. Chen,
Lincoln C., editor of compilation. III. Saich, Tony, editor of
compilation. IV. Series: Philanthropic and nonprofit studies.
    [DNLM: 1. Delivery of Health Care—economics—China.
2. Gift Giving—China. 3. Delivery of Health Care—history—
China. 4. History, 20th Century—China. 5. History, 21st Century—
China. 6. Organizations, Nonprofit—China. W 84 JC6]
    RA395.C53
    362.10951—dc23

                                                    2014000904

1 2 3 4 5   19 18 17 16 15 14

Contents

Foreword

We are pleased to launch this volume on the frontier challenges of health philanthropy in China. In many respects, this theme has grown in significance. Given the extraordinary growth of China's economy and the consequent accumulation of private wealth, China has achieved the necessary preconditions for the blossoming of private philanthropy.

Also, China has recently embarked on a massive reform of its national health care system to achieve universal coverage with equity. That is a daunting challenge for the most populous country in the world, one which would benefit from the contribution of private philanthropy. National health need and philanthropic opportunity underscore that health philanthropy in China is a highly salient subject matter for both academic study and professional practice.

We have come together to co-organize this volume because of shared vision and experiences. One of us (PG) has devoted nearly four decades to professional philanthropic work in Asia. PG served as the founding resident representative of the Ford Foundation in China starting in 1987, and has continued China engagement over the past 25 years with a host of academic, nongovernmental, and philanthropic organizations. PG also serves as senior advisor for management at the China Medical Board, which provides a direct link to this volume.

Another of us (WZY) is Professor at Beijing Normal University, heading the university's One Foundation Philanthropy Research Institute. Previously, WZY was the director of the Department of Social Welfare and Charity Promotion in the Ministry of Civil Affairs, the principal government regulatory body for nonprofit organizations, including private foundations. WZY is a leader and among the most knowledgeable about the growth and emergence of private philanthropy in China.

Through our longstanding collaborative relationship, we have come together as partners in designing and organizing this volume in celebration of the one hundredth anniversary of the China Medical Board. We commissioned a series of chapters on health philanthropy in China, and the invited contributors shared views in two authors' workshops. The 14 chapters that were produced have been organized around three core themes.

We are thankful to Lincoln Chen, Jennifer Ryan, and Tony Saich, who joined us by undertaking the editorial work. They in turn were greatly assisted by Holly Chang of Golden Bridges, who provided logistical support and facilitated the authors' workshops; and Stephen Ford, Duncan Harte, Sun Taiyi, David Tea, and CMB staff Joshua Bocher and Mariel Reed, in translation, editing, reference checking, and other production work. All of us are proud of this unprecedented volume on the history, development, current status, and future trajectory of health philanthropy in China.

Peter Geithner and Wang Zhenyao
August 8, 2013

PHILANTHROPY FOR HEALTH IN CHINA

Introduction

Philanthropy for Health in China: Distinctive Roots and Future Prospects

Lincoln C. Chen, Jennifer Ryan,
and Tony Saich

Introduction

There is considerable excitement over two recent developments in global philanthropy—the prospect of an explosive growth of new philanthropy in China
and the promise of social impact through investing in global health. China's
spectacular economic growth to become the world's second-largest economy
has been accompanied by enormous accumulation of private wealth. According
to Forbes, between 2002 and 2011, China went from having zero billionaires to
having 115 billionaires, second in number only to the United States. Nor is this
accumulation occurring solely among society's wealthiest: the number of millionaires increased by 1.4 million, and the country's middle class has become the
fastest-expanding in the world. With the accumulation and diffusion of wealth
almost certain to continue and even accelerate, private philanthropy in China
holds great promise for launching a new and exciting era.

The rise of wealth in China is not the sole reason for the growth of philanthropy. A proliferation of NGOs has emerged, showing not only that financial
resources exist, but also that there is the civic desire to deploy private wealth
to aid society via philanthropy. Other factors have also led to an expansion of
philanthropy in China, including government slowly opening up space for private-sector resources to engage in social services and relief efforts as social gaps
become more widely recognized.

In parallel, the field of global health has been dramatically transformed by
major philanthropic investments made by some of the world's largest foundations. The Bill & Melinda Gates Foundation—which has taken a leading role in

the fight against diseases such as HIV and malaria—commands a substantial annual budget comparable to or even greater than that of the World Health Organization, and the Bloomberg Foundation is pioneering public health programs through interventions in tobacco, diet, exercise, and the urban environment. The long-neglected health sector in China has recently gained priority in the national policy agenda. In 2009, the Chinese government launched an ambitious reform of its national health care system. Confronting daunting challenges, China's health system would seem especially ripe for the innovation and experimentation that private philanthropy is uniquely equipped to offer.

These parallel developments in health and philanthropy motivated the China Medical Board (CMB) to sponsor this academic study of the history and future of health philanthropy in China. CMB, a modestly sized but historically rich foundation, was founded in 1914 and endowed as an independent foundation with two separate gifts from the Rockefeller family in 1928 and 1947. Its initial goal was to establish the Peking Union Medical College in Beijing as the flagship of modern medical sciences in China, but over the past three decades CMB has expanded its China partnership to a dozen more Chinese medical universities. Throughout the twentieth century, CMB has been inextricably connected to the two major strands of philanthropy and health in China.

This connectivity will continue into the future; CMB will celebrate its one hundredth anniversary in 2014, embarking at that time on its strategy for the second century. In designing its future work, CMB recognizes that a rapidly changing China is undergoing dynamic health transitions. Many questions naturally arise: Which lessons of the past can inform the future? What are the historical roots of philanthropy in China? What is distinctive about Chinese philanthropy? What is the current status of health philanthropy in China? And what are its future prospects?

To address these questions, CMB invited Peter Geithner and Wang Zhenyao to commission 14 authors to construct a story of health philanthropy in China. The commissioned chapters were shaped during two intensive authors' workshops in China and the United States, featuring contributions from leading historians, social scientists, policymakers, and health and philanthropic professionals. Importantly, the group of contributors reflects the positive partnership among Chinese and foreign authors, academics from diverse disciplines, and intellectuals and philanthropic practitioners. These contributors include distinguished academic scholars and professional leaders in philanthropy, both within China and internationally. Some chapters were originally authored in English, while others were translated from Chinese. Together, they offer the first comprehensive academic study of health philanthropy in China.

We the co-editors assumed the responsibility for editing the individual contributions into a volume which is organized into three sections. The three chapters in part I, "Revitalization after Collapse," describe the closure and reemergence of philanthropy amid a changing regulatory environment and evolving health conditions over the past half-century. The six chapters in part II, "Chinese Roots and Foreign Engagement," examine the cultural roots and the historical blending of Chinese and Western philanthropy, followed by an analysis of the work of American foundations in twentieth-century China. The last three chapters in this section summarize three major internationally driven programs in contemporary China dealing with HIV/AIDS, reproductive health, and tobacco control. The four chapters in part III, "Transitions and Prospects," focus attention on Chinese-led philanthropic projects and their future prospects. The current landscape of the nonprofit sector is dominated by government-organized nongovernmental organizations (GONGOs) that are active in all endeavors, as exemplified by the in-depth case study of the Red Cross Society of China. The rapid emergence of genuinely independent Chinese nonprofit organizations is illustrated by six case studies of newly established foundations, along with an account of the continuation of philanthropic flows from the Chinese diaspora through Hong Kong. Both mainland and diaspora flows illustrate the robust and additional channels of private funding that are opening up. The final chapter presents a powerful case for reforming the sector to realize the full potential of civil society and private philanthropy in China.

Five Major Themes

The chapters in this volume highlight five core themes critical for an informed understanding of health philanthropy in China today: its relationship with the state, its deep historical roots, its distinctiveness in the global context, its growing needs and opportunities, and its future prospects. Four of the themes are discussed here, with the last theme—future prospects—addressed in the concluding section.

A Dynamic Landscape

No one knows precisely the number or type of nonprofit NGOs and private foundations in China, for two major reasons. First, data are scarce or inconsistent and nomenclature is poorly defined. Second, in China as elsewhere, there is great imprecision in the use of such terms as charity, philanthropy, NGOs, foundations, nonprofit organizations, and civil society, with the resulting terminology consisting of countless permutations and combinations thereof.

By far the most important demarcation in China is that of official registration, and even with this classification, two out of the three categories—registration-exempt, registered, and unregistered—are based on exceptions to the rule. Firstly it is important to note that many nonprofit bodies in name are actually large and powerful government-organized nongovernmental organizations (GONGOs) that exist outside the bounds of the registration system itself. These organizations are exempt from registration and receive government funding, special privileges, and access, including the right to publicly fundraise. Indeed, it is estimated that 45 government departments have registered 86 GONGOs as public foundations, which means they can actively raise funds from the public, while many true NGOs, like private foundations and social organizations, cannot.

In terms of officially registered organizations, China had approximately 462,000 registered nonprofits in 2011 according to government statistics from the China Charity Donation Information Center. These organizations are classified into three types. Social organizations (*shehui tuanti*), which are societies or associations (trade, professional, or industrial), constitute roughly half of the nonprofits. The remaining half are people-run non-enterprise organizations (*minban feiqiye danwei*) such as private hospitals, private schools, and some nonprofit organizations. Foundations (*jijinhui*) are the third and final type, numbering about 2,600 in 2011 and constituting less than 0.5 percent of all nonprofit organizations. About half of all foundations are private and half public or state-related.

Unregistered organizations are by far the largest type by sheer number. In 2011 China had an estimated three million unregistered NGOs, or six times the number registered. China's three million independent NGOs—about five out of every six registered nonprofit organizations in China—operate mostly below the government's radar, their lack of registration excluding them from legal guarantees, tax deduction, official seals, and bank accounts. The Chinese government turns a blind eye to these NGOs, following the principle of the "Three No's"—No recognition, No banning, No interference. To circumvent barriers, some nonprofits register—not, strictly speaking, legally—with the State Administration for Industry and Commerce as unprofitable for-profit businesses. Beyond nonprofit organizations there are of course many quasi-government institutions such as universities, scientific academies, research institutes, and sports and cultural bodies.

It should be noted that official registration as a nonprofit is very difficult to obtain, but even if successfully acquired also something of a double-edged sword. On the positive side registration confers legitimacy, recognition, and security, expediting visa approval for staff and enabling organizational participation in banking and official accounting, among other things. Registration also, however, imposes governmental "dual management," with the Ministry of Civil Affairs (MoCA) providing general organizational supervision and another substantive government ministry, assigned based on the nonprofit's focus, providing technical or other specialized supervision. This dual registration imposes extra work and costs on the registered nonprofit by requiring regular reporting, annual audits, and periodic work reviews. The procedure treats the registered entity almost like a department of the government, since ultimately the two ministries are held responsible for its behavior and performance.

Nonprofits can register with different levels of government—i.e., with national, provincial, municipal, or even township officials—but the geographical scope of their work is confined to that of the registering body. Health ranks third among the fields tackled by nonprofits in China, trailing only education and poverty alleviation. There are presently 11,521 registered social organizations and 70 registered foundations working as nonprofits in the health field.

A second major demarcating factor for nonprofits in China is financing, especially qualification for tax exemption. Domestic resource mobilization is one of the privileges of government-organized entities like GONGOs. Philanthropic donations made in China in 2010 reportedly totaled 103 billion RMB and 84 billion RMB in 2011, constituting less than 0.4 percent of GDP—a relatively low level of voluntary giving. These funds go to foundations large and small, from the China Charity Federation, which received 8.6 billion RMB in 2010, to the China Transplant Development Foundation, which received 31,000 RMB in 2010. It has been estimated that more than 90 percent of donations are utilized by fewer than 1 percent of the nonprofit organizations. Only public foundations can accept donations; private foundations cannot. Among public foundations, 95 percent are directly operational; there are only 30 grant-making foundations. These organizations are moreover overwhelmingly domestic in origin. As of 2012, only 18 foreign foundations had successfully registered for work in China. Grassroots NGOs, not surprisingly, are starved for funding.

While their numbers are few, international foundations remain significant players in China. In 2011, the Chinese government estimated that they contributed 12.9 billion RMB, 17 percent of which was earmarked for health activities. This figure may understate the magnitude of international foundations' activities in China. In some instances, international funding goes to parent overseas headquarters and is then perhaps routed informally into China, and is thus not easily counted. This routing may be especially important for nonprofits that have not been able to secure official registration. Finally, UN and international agencies continue their work in China, but their funding volume is declining. International foundations and agencies often work together harmoniously, though tensions occasionally arise when agreements are not fulfilled. An example of disagreement between the government and an international agency was the freezing of contributions from the Global Fund for AIDS, TB, and Malaria, because the Chinese government failed to comply with its stipulation that at least 35 percent of the funds be distributed to NGOs.

Historical Roots

The roots of Chinese philanthropy go back to antiquity, with charity deeply embedded in Confucian, Buddhist, and Daoist ethics. Motivated by a mix of religious inclination, moral obligation, and loyalty to native place, individuals sponsored the building of temples, schools, orphanages, and hospitals; provided relief during famine and in the aftermath of natural disasters; and offered funeral aid to those who could not afford to bury their loved ones. Imperial governments played a role too, administering charity for widows, orphans, the handicapped, and the indigent. From the Song dynasty (960–1279) until the end of imperial rule in 1912, for example, county magistrates commonly sponsored poorhouses and foundling homes, and subsidized burial plots for the state's needy subjects. Occasionally, the government would work with the religious establishment as well: during the Tang dynasty (618–907), government-sponsored Buddhist temples established soup kitchens and medical dispensaries to serve the poor. Outside of government, "charitable estates" held and operated by family lineages aided the poor both within and outside their kinship group, ensuring both corporate cohesion internally and a good reputation externally. Charitable work has been best documented since the Ming dynasty (1368–1644) when *shantang*, or benevolent societies, first emerged. Also known as charitable halls, *shantang* were nongovernmental charitable organizations supported by local elites. They were active in a variety of spheres, from donating coffins and burying the poor to collecting and distributing food. In the Qing dynasty (1644–1912), private charity spread but continued to be generally directed toward one's native place. Wealthy merchants established *shantang* in such cities as Hangzhou, Shanghai, and Tianjin in cooperation with local elites and government, while in Hong Kong, Chinese established the famous Tung Wah Hospital in 1870 and continued to transfer homeward the overseas diaspora's philanthropic remittances.

The nineteenth century saw not only further development of domestic philanthropy but also the parallel development of foreign philanthropy. Initially, such philanthropy was significantly linked with the missionary movement, which prized health work and specifically the establishment of hospitals. Many of China's enduring health legacies were established by such philanthropy. Shanghai's Renji Hospital traces its roots to William Lockhart's 1844 founding of the Chinese Hospital in Shanghai, and Guangzhou's Zhongshan Ophthalmic Center to Peter Parker's 1835 opening of the Canton Ophthalmic Hospital. Over time, and especially during the Republican period (1912–1949), foreign philanthropy steadily expanded and grew increasingly secular. Perhaps the premier achievement of this stage of philanthropic development was the China Medical Board's establishment of the Peking Union Medical College.

China's long history of domestic charitable endeavors and foreign philanthropic involvement has perhaps been obscured by the political vicissitudes of the second half of the twentieth century, which severely impinged on the profile of philanthropy in China. Nonetheless, the pre-1949 history of philanthropy remains significant insofar as it shows how deeply rooted both domestic and foreign approaches to charity are. Although foreign philanthropic organizations were effectively excluded from China during the Mao era, the earlier roots that were laid down have helped to encourage and vitalize the international involvement that has taken place since the Open Door policy reforms, and can been seen in the enduring resonances and the resurgence of Chinese private philanthropy today.

Distinctiveness

There are of course many similarities in philanthropy across different countries—motivation by the wealthy, solicitation of public donations, targeting of charity to the most needy, surges in giving during humanitarian crises, and government control mechanisms designed to regulate such activity. China exhibits all of these common aspects of philanthropy, with health philanthropy in particular noteworthy.

Philanthropy in China is distinctive in several ways, with its development—like that of China's health system—having been significantly impacted by the disruptions of the Mao era. The health system challenges of the present day have been heavily determined by the legacies of that period, as have the path to recovery for private and foreign philanthropy after their elimination, the incipient legislative frameworks for charitable giving, and the state's continued dominance of the sector. These aspects continue to ensure that philanthropy in China has "Chinese characteristics."

The founding of the People's Republic of China witnessed the sudden closure of all private initiatives, NGOs, and philanthropies, as Communist ideology regarded social welfare functions as the responsibility of the state. Domestic civil society and nonprofit organizations, including the traditional *shantang*, were suppressed, while transnational foundations like the Red Cross were absorbed into the state apparatus, and foreign nonprofit groups departed. Space for nonprofit organizations reopened after China embraced market-based economic growth in the post-Mao reform era. By 1984, when the government gave its explicit endorsement during a conference in Fujian, the significance of and need for the contributions of nongovernmental organizations were recognized, inaugurating a legal regime to accommodate the growth and function of the nonprofit sector. This legal regime is still a work in progress.

While few countries have witnessed such dramatic reemergence after complete closure as China has, space for state-sanctioned nonprofit social organizations has been open for only a little more than three decades. The emergence and rise to prominence of such groups was especially pronounced in 2008, when the disastrous Wenchuan earthquake rekindled China's philanthropic spirit by engendering a huge outpouring of donations from the Chinese public for humanitarian aid. Most recently, the 2013 Ya'an earthquake, also in Sichuan, similarly mobilized philanthropy nationwide.

Many governments, central to local, attempt to regulate NGO development. Registration, tax exemption, and reporting requirements, with concomitant tax exemptions, are not uncommon in many countries, especially those with governments concerned with the autonomy of civil society and the potentially undue influence of foreign funding. Government regulations play, however, an especially powerful role in China, and the current legal framework perpetuates a restrictive if evolving political and economic environment. Official registration in particular determines organizations' legitimacy and their capacity to operate in China. As China continues to allow nonprofits to expand their role, the government has begun to shift the balance, opening space for nonprofits to solve social problems while maintaining control over the growth and development of civil organizations that could become a threat to societal control and stability. This has resulted in a governmental preference for service-oriented but not independent or advocacy-based NGOs. This juxtaposition of opening up with tight control very much characterizes the government's political ambivalence concerning philanthropic activity.

In China, the government not only regulates the philanthropic sector but is also itself a major actor, controlling numerous and powerful GONGOs that almost universally dominate their respective fields. These large organizations—among them the Red Cross Society, the China Charity Federation, the All-China Women's Federation, and the Soong Ching Ling Foundation—absorb much of the available public donations. GONGOs also assume societal roles that in other countries may be filled by nongovernmental actors. In health, the China Medical Association is a body that performs many professional functions, including training, forming specialty groups, publishing academic journals, and overseeing professional education; it is, however, a GONGO, and not an independent organization governed by professionals. Grant-making foundations, meanwhile, are few and limited. Of China's 2,600 registered foundations, only 30 are grant-making, with the remainder directly operating foundations. This leaves domestic funding support for genuinely independent NGOs severely limited.

The foreign philanthropic mix in China is unique in that international organizations face many barriers in reaching genuinely private grassroots organizations. Foreign foundations are particularly constrained by regulatory barriers both in sending funds from their own countries and in receiving them in China. In some home-base countries, foreign foundation giving overseas requires assurances that the recipient is a qualified nonprofit organization (i.e., the equivalent of a 501(c) organization in the United States), a status that is not attainable for most unregistered Chinese NGOs. In China, meanwhile, laws and regulations prohibit the receipt of foreign resources pending official approval. These are among the reasons why many foreign foundations have conducted their work through GONGOs (e.g., the Preventive Medicine Association for HIV/AIDS), Chinese universities (e.g., for medical education and research), and even municipal governments (e.g., for pioneering smoke-free zones in the pursuit of tobacco control). This same channeling applies to the work of UN agencies and the World Bank, which must provide their assistance through officially recognized bodies.

Needs and Opportunities

China's health sector faces daunting challenges. Reforms introduced in 2009 are aimed at five pillars of the health care system: universal coverage of health insurance, access to primary care, effective prevention, affordability of essential drugs, and reform in the management of public hospitals. For a society with 1.3 billion people, accomplishing any one of these reforms alone would be a Herculean challenge. Universal health insurance that would provide protection against financial catastrophe due to the costs of treating illness is a complicated problem in a country with enormous geographical and economic diversity. Improving primary care requires convincing doctors to practice in remote rural areas, and the rehabilitation of derelict village and township service facilities. To be effective, preventative care must be revamped to address noncommunicable diseases such as cancer, diabetes, and heart disease, even as China's Center for Disease Control and Prevention remains overwhelmingly an infectious disease control agency. To make essential drugs affordable, China must manage both modern and traditional medicines in a market contested by profit-seeking domestic and international pharmaceutical companies. Finally, Chinese public hospitals are owned by the government but operate like private businesses seeking to maximize income, often by overprescribing medications and diagnostic tests.

To grapple with these challenges, the Chinese government will have to solve difficult and complex problems throughout a vast national system. Filling the gaps, innovation by civil society organizations, and social venture capital of private foundations are needed. Hard-to-reach populations and severely disadvantaged groups need special services that sometimes only a dedicated NGO can effectively provide. Despite the high national priority accorded to the health care sector, the government will not be able to do it all. Most essential will be systemic innovations aimed at crafting effective and efficient health service delivery systems and working toward health equity wherein the poorest members of society are reached. Piloting and local experimentation can test new approaches for subsequent scaling-up by larger systems, and evaluation can inform policymakers on what is working or not, and why. Academic development of health policy and management is also necessary to strengthen the information and knowledge base needed to design, monitor, evaluate, and improve health care systems. Clearly, there are both needs and opportunities for private philanthropy to make a difference in China.

Part Summaries

Part I: Revitalization after Collapse

The three chapters in this section cover the changing philanthropic and health landscape in China over the past half-century.

In chapter 1, Wang Zhenyao and Zhao Yanhui retrace the collapse and revitalization of private philanthropy in China through three phases: closure from 1949 to 1977; reopening from 1978 to 2003; and governmental recognition and support, which has been steadily improving since 2004 but still faces challenges. Policies and regulations that have marked these phases are described and analyzed by Mark Sidel in chapter 2. While the overall trend has been toward liberalization for independent NGOs and foundations, the government appears to be balancing two policy impulses. To keep up with dynamic changes in domestic, diaspora, foreign, private, and corporate giving, the regulatory environment is in a state of change. While government recognizes the positive aspects of civic participation in contributing to social problem-solving, especially in health service delivery, it is only slowly shedding deeply rooted bureaucratic systems that seek to control and constrain civil society. Government hesitancy appears to be based on concerns that genuinely independent civil organizations could challenge political stability.

In chapter 3, Vivian Lin and Bronwyn Carter describe China's changing health problems and health systems. In previous decades, improvements in health in China ran counter to trends in philanthropy. During the planned economy, Communist policies left no room for private initiatives and poverty-linked health problems were tackled by a state-funded and state-operated health system that improved health outcomes despite being rudimentary and underfinanced. With the opening and growth of a market-based economy, the Communist health system was dismantled without a sufficient replacement. Health care became marketized as the rural collective medical scheme and free health care for urban state workers collapsed. At the same time, health conditions changed as poverty-linked diseases were eclipsed by the noncommunicable diseases of affluence. In the past decade, the government has launched an ambitious health system reform that faces daunting challenges—many of which could be helped by health philanthropy. The authors conclude that the need and demand for private philanthropy and civil society capable of complementing the government's efforts in addressing health system challenges and implementing reform is greater than ever.

Part II: Chinese Roots and Foreign Engagement

The six chapters in this section reach back into history and extend into overseas philanthropy to demonstrate both the historical roots of Chinese philanthropy and the longstanding engagement of foreign philanthropy in China.

The deep historical roots of Chinese charity and philanthropy are recounted in chapter 4 by Zhang Xiulan and Zhang Lu. Through the Qing dynasty and Republican period, Chinese philanthropy involved merchants, businessmen, and the state, often through private-public partnerships. The nineteenth century witnessed the arrival of the missionary movement accompanied by Western-style philanthropy. The earliest sustained foreign philanthropic involvement came not from major private foundations but from a wide array of church-sponsored philanthropies. In a "golden era," China experienced some of the twentieth century's greatest philanthropic success stories, among them the building of the Peking Union Medical College, during which Western scientific medicine became a tool of both Chinese and foreign philanthropy. Although both indigenous Chinese and foreign philanthropy were closed during the post-1949 Communist period, the pre-1949 history of philanthropy remains significant, both in its evidence of more deeply rooted Chinese approaches to charity, and in its demonstration of early foreign philanthropic ventures into China. Roots that were laid down before the Mao era have helped to encourage and vitalize the enthusiastic international involvement that has taken place since the economic reforms, as philanthropies such as the China Medical Board returned and were joined by newer arrivals to China such as the Ford Foundation and the Bill & Melinda Gates Foundation.

Chapter 5, by Zi Zhongyun and Mary Brown Bullock, and chapter 6, by Darwin Stapleton, address the purposes, strategies, and activities of American foundations in China. By reviewing the work of the Rockefeller, Ford, and Luce Foundations, as well as that of CMB itself, Zi and Bullock ask why American foundations came to work in China, reviewing their historic cross-cultural engagement. Five motivations are hypothesized: to reform China specifically, to provide assistance to China as a developing country, to promote Chinese-American mutual understanding, to encourage Chinese philanthropy, and to promote sustainable development and thereby advance the cause of world peace and prosperity. In chapter 6, Stapleton examines the strategic content of Rockefeller and CMB philanthropy, focusing on technological innovations and the appeal of scientific solutions—hard technologies like the X-ray, and other technologies such as the facilities design and scientific equipment of PUMC's modern medical campus, insecticides deployed against malaria, hookworm control measures, and the establishment of public health stations where technologies were transferred to the field.

The remaining three chapters are written by practicing foundation officers to describe their own health work, addressing three specific health threats—HIV/AIDS, reproductive health, and tobacco—with global dimensions in which China is a major player. The case studies open up questions concerning the alignment of Chinese priorities with international norms and practices, and hold lessons for approaches to tackling global health problems. Ray Yip of the Bill & Melinda Gates Foundation describes in chapter 7 how foreign foundations and international agencies worked to support China's response to the HIV/AIDS epidemic, transforming official denial into strong action and moving through the three phases of the epidemic: intravenous drug use, blood supply contamination through unsafe plasma collection, and men who have sex with men. Joan Kaufman and her Ford Foundation colleagues describe in chapter 8 the cooperative, constructive, and often sensitive relationships encountered when working in China, especially in light of its highly controversial one-child population policy. Operating at the interface of international standards and domestic groups, the work of Ford and the UNFPA has grappled with a range of sensitive subjects, among them gender equity and human rights, reproductive health care services, sexually transmitted diseases, and sex education for adolescents. Finally, in chapter 9, Jeffrey Koplan and Pamela Redmon of Emory University review foreign philanthropic work on China's devastating tobacco threat. China is the world's largest tobacco manufacturer and cigarette consumer, and has attracted the health investment of two American foundations (Bloomberg and Gates) and the technical contributions of the UN, international NGOs, and universities (including, respectively, WHO, the Campaign for Tobacco-Free Kids, and John Hopkins and Emory Universities). This engagement illustrates the complexity of foreign philanthropy efforts amid the "pushes and pulls" of different state interests within the Chinese government, notably the Ministry of Health's charge to protect public health and the Ministry of Commerce's to advance business and increase revenue.

Part III: Transitions and Prospects

The four chapters in the final section capture the dynamics of contemporary philanthropy by describing the dominance of governmental nonprofit organizations, the evolution of the century-old Red Cross, and the vibrancy of six new startups, concluding with a call for the reform of the philanthropic sector.

The most distinctive feature of Chinese philanthropy is the dominance of GONGOs, as analyzed by Deng Guosheng and Zhao Xiaoping in chapter 10. Since the opening of this space, GONGOs have grown in number, size, and coverage. GONGOs permeate the health sector, including professional associations, advocacy, medical assistance, and disaster relief. They have many advantages over grassroots NGOs and any consideration of independence for NGOs in the future cannot ignore these government-created entities. But GONGOs are also undergoing change as they cooperate more with—and face increased competition from—NGOs. China's premier GONGO is the Red Cross Society of China, which is examined by Caroline Reeves in chapter 11. Founded in 1904, the Red Cross Society has demonstrated enormous agility in adapting to changing circumstances over the past century, evolving from an autonomous and internationally linked NGO, to a unit absorbed into the government, to its current status as a GONGO. Despite regime changes, its size has expanded and its functions have diversified. Notwithstanding a massive drop in donations to the Red Cross between the Wenchuan and Ya'an earthquakes, the organization has weathered recent scandals. In health, the Red Cross Society today works primarily on blood transfusion, tobacco control, and organ transplantation, though it has also served as an incubator for new philanthropic startups such as the Smile Angel Foundation and Jet Li's One Foundation.

The past decade has witnessed the emergence of many genuinely independent NGOs and private foundations. Li Fan in chapter 12 presents six cases of new Chinese foundations that address the special needs of the 83 million disabled persons in China. These cases underscore the motivation of wealthy philanthropists and the social conscience of the donating public. For instance, Faye Wong, a national pop star, created the Smile Angel Foundation to surgically correct cleft palates because her own child suffered from this disability, while Huiping Tian, a mother with an autistic child, started the Beijing Star and Rain Education Institute. Other foundations profiled in the chapter have tackled brittle bone disease and hearing impairment. Strong political support for such work has been mobilized by Deng Pufang, the son of Deng Xiaoping, who himself became disabled due to a broken back during the Cultural Revolution. That diaspora philanthropy also maintains its vibrancy is demonstrated by David Faure's review in chapter 13 of activities in Hong Kong, which underscores such philanthropy's multidimensionality within Hong Kong and the ongoing repatriation of money to home villages. The Tung Wah Hospital and medical schools in Hong Kong are examples of the former, and Sir Run Run Shaw Hospital in Hangzhou and Li Ka-shing's Shantou University Medical School are two examples of the latter. Interestingly, major international NGOs like Oxfam, Médicins Sans Frontières, and Save the Children are successfully raising funds in Hong Kong and using the donated funds for work both in mainland China and elsewhere.

Xu Yongguang in chapter 14 emphasizes that Chinese philanthropy has arrived at a critical juncture. While applauding the opening of space for nonprofit development, Xu argues that it is imperative to accelerate reforms. The monopoly on fundraising by governmental entities should be ended, permitting other organizations that fulfill certain criteria to raise money. Rather than discouraging registration, Xu proposes that legitimization, best practices, and sound operations should be encouraged among nongovernmental NGOs and foundations, while public trust and credibility must be enhanced through greater transparency.

Future Prospects

Looking to the future, health philanthropy in China is experiencing a rapid transition. The current landscape is powerfully dominated by GONGOs and long- and well-established organizations like the Red Cross Society of China and the China Medical Association have demonstrated their resilience in adapting to contextual change. Fresh and new independent civil society groups, NGOs, and foundations are also emerging rapidly. Meanwhile, public giving for emergencies and disasters are robust and diaspora philanthropy from overseas Chinese communities is undiminished.

Given the uncertainties of the present, the best way to peer into the future is to understand the past. Lessons suggest that caution about the future is warranted. China's policies and its regulation of genuinely independent civil society organizations, while changing, have not yet reached a point where civic governance, responsibility, and operations can be easily achieved. At the same time, the large number of unregistered NGOs have made creative adjustments enabling them to work with and around regulatory hurdles. Even registered bodies have the daunting challenge of dual supervision. How the government will streamline its bureaucratic systems and resolve its concerns over the political instability that could arise from independent civil society remains uncertain.

There are, however, many countervailing reasons for optimism. First, since 1984 the trend has been distinctively positive in terms of philanthropies' opening up, approval of registrations, and operational independence. All signs suggest that this trend will continue. Second, this is a time of considerable experimentation by diverse governmental units. Recently, Beijing and Shenzhen governments have been experimenting with a single (not double) registration body, while Guangdong Province has been testing registration at the township (rather than provincial or municipal) level, and Shanghai has started to pilot the outsourcing of social services to NGOs. Fundraising guidelines have been adjusted in Hunan Province, and Yunan Province is modifying its ground rules for receipt of foreign funding. These and other experiments at the local level are all consistent with a movement toward a more open environment. Successful experiments could be scaled up to national policy.

Most importantly, the Chinese public has become much more engaged, demanding greater effectiveness, more transparency, and the control of corruption. Watchdogs and *weibo* messages (the Chinese equivalent of Twitter) are flooding the internet, seeking to expose malfeasance and inform the public about the conduct and performance of governmental and nongovernmental organizations alike. In 2008, the Red Cross received perhaps 90 percent of public donations for the Wenchuan earthquake. Following the Guo Meimei scandal of 2011, which featured a young woman allegedly working at the Red Cross showing off on the internet her luxury car and designer clothing, the Red Cross received less than 50 percent of public donations after the Ya'an earthquake in 2013. Some of the money was channeled instead to the one-hundred-plus NGOs that had publicized their philanthropic work and their transparent reporting on the One Foundation website.

Will China witness a renaissance of private philanthropy? No one can answer this question with certainty, although it is quite plausible that many innovations in philanthropy will emerge in China. More likely is the steady but not spectacular growth and development of private philanthropy in China. This trajectory will be strengthened by the growing infrastructure for and professionalism of philanthropy. Information and knowledge about NGOs and civil society are being generated by universities like the Tsinghua University NGO Research Center and the Peking University NGO Law Research Center, and the networking of foundations is being supported by the likes of the China Foundation Center. Such infrastructure provides the field with information, knowledge, transparency, and sharing of best practices that can strengthen the performance of all organizations. Through training programs, study tours, and networking, there is also a growing cadre of professionals entering the field of philanthropy. Professional staff will bring better planning, strategy development, and program management into improved organizational operating systems. While they are still at an early stage, there is every hope that these developments point to the beginnings of yet another vibrant era of philanthropy in China.

Part I
Revitalization after Collapse

1 The Collapse and Reemergence of Private Philanthropy in China, 1949–2012

Wang Zhenyao and Zhao Yanhui

Introduction

In order to better understand the opportunities and challenges for contemporary health philanthropy in China, this chapter aims to provide a brief overview of the evolving relationship between health care, philanthropy, and the state since the founding of the People's Republic of China in 1949. It first considers the period 1949–1977, which saw the creation of a state health care system, as well as an increasingly antagonistic governmental stance toward philanthropy, which was perceived as antithetical to the socialist project. Next it discusses the rehabilitation of health philanthropy from 1978 to 2003. This period was characterized by the recognition that health philanthropy could play a crucial role in compensating for an increasingly insufficient state health care system. Various laws were enacted that facilitated the gradual revitalization of health philanthropy, with nongovernmental organizations developing alongside governmental ones, and international involvement increasing throughout the period. The overview is completed by a summary of developments since 2004, the year in which the Fourth Plenary Session of the 16th CCP Central Committee explicitly recognized the importance of the development of philanthropy to the state social security system. The chapter then concludes by identifying certain significant challenges for the current development of health philanthropy in China and offering some predictions for the future.

State Health Care Provision and the Elimination of Health Philanthropy in the People's Republic of China, 1949–1977

Soon after coming to power in 1949, the Chinese Communist Party (CCP) began implementing a new state welfare system. The institutional guideline, as articulated by leading CCP member Dong Biwu in 1950, was that "social relief and welfare should be in the hands of the government, while individuals and groups can participate in governmental relief activities and organizations" (Dong 1950). This indicated that future grassroots involvement would be coordinated by the state, and the role of nongovernmental philanthropic organizations was to be curtailed—a point emphasized in Dong's accompanying statement that charity should be considered as "an icing that deceives and anesthetizes the people," and a "conspiracy to sabotage the PRC by imperialists" (Dong 1950).

Private health charities had been one of the main driving forces behind the development of medical care in China in the turbulent transition period of the early twentieth century, but rather than continuing to operate as independent entities they became subsumed under government control. This process can be demonstrated by the fate of the nine largest *shantang* in Guangzhou. Shantang were benevolent societies, first arising in the late Ming dynasty, typically founded by Chinese gentry and merchants. The Guangzhou shantang (Aiyu, Guangji, Fangbian, Guangren, Huixing, Chongzheng, Runshen Society, Shushan, and Mingshan) provided various forms of medical treatment and medicine for free. Within the first few years of the PRC they were all either integrated and reformed into government-controlled structures or closed down. Some were transformed into hospitals or clinics and others into schools. For example, Huixing and Aiyu were placed under unified leadership and integrated into the Guangzhou Public Welfare Associations Union in 1954, as the First Clinic and Second Clinic of the Municipal Public Welfare Associations Union, respectively. In 1952 Fangbian Hospital was expanded, becoming Guangzhou First People's Hospital. Guangji Hospital was closed down in 1954 due to dilapidation. Its building was converted into Guangji Non-Staple Food General Market. Runshen Society came under the leadership of the Municipal Public Welfare Associations Union in 1954 and ceased offering medical services, becoming instead the Ronghua Street Primary School (Tan 2008). This was a pattern repeated across the country and by November 1953 over 1,600 old charitable organizations in 21 cities had been reorganized under state control.[1]

The role of international philanthropy in China during this period was also greatly diminished—especially following the outbreak of the Korean War in 1950 and the ensuing decline in Sino-U.S. relations, as almost half of the relief agencies and religious organizations that received foreign grants were subsidized by the United States. Following new government rulings in 1950 that effectively cut ties with the United States and other foreign philanthropic entities, the government began to integrate, adjust, and reform the existing international health philanthropies operating in China (Zhongyang Renmin Zhengfu fazhi weiyuanhui 1982, 724–727). For example, the China Medical Board, an American organization created by the Rockefeller Foundation, had to cut its ties with the institution it had built when the Peking Union Medical College (PUMC) was nationalized in 1951. The new government took charge of other institutions that had been established by international charities; hence when the American Friends Service Committee ceased operating in 1951, its properties were transferred to the Department of Civil Affairs. These various adjustments effectively resulted in the extinction of foreign charities operating in China.

In addition, the government determined that it would turn down future offers of international assistance. On August 21, 1954, in "Answering Foreign Journalists' Questions," the General Administrative Office of the Ministry of Internal Affairs elaborated on the guidelines of the Chinese government for the acceptance of foreign aid and donations for disaster relief, stating that "in principle, China welcomes the friendly assistance from international friends, however, Chinese people can pull through disasters, helping ourselves by engaging in production" (Fang 1995, 383).

Alongside the integration of both domestic and foreign-funded organizations into state-controlled structures, several new government-run welfare and relief agencies were established to perform the function of social assistance (Zhou and Zeng 2006, 363). These included the China Association for the Blind (1953) and the China Association for the Deaf (1956), which later merged in 1960. Meanwhile, collective welfare facilities such as sanatoriums, nursing homes, orphanages, and rest homes for the disabled were built into the Trade Union system. According to statistics, between 1949 and 1954, 666 welfare agencies for the disabled, the elderly, and children were built or reformed (Su 2011, 107). These welfare relief agencies were included in the financial budget at all levels under government administration. Overall government administration of charities was coordinated by the Chinese People's Relief Association from 1950 to 1956, at which time its undertakings were transferred to the Ministry of Internal Affairs.

Such organizations functioned as a supplement to the national health care security system that was being implemented by the government, and which was divided along urban and rural lines. The majority of urban residents were covered by two insurance schemes. From 1951, a state-funded Government Insurance Scheme provided free medical and health care services for serving and retired state officials, staff at government agencies, public institutions and universities, and handicapped military officers (Wong and Chiu 1997, 77). This was later extended to the dependents of the aforementioned groups and also to university students. A Labor Insurance Scheme covered employees of state-owned factories and enterprises (and subsequently their dependents), with the costs borne mainly by the enterprises, and requiring only a small contribution from workers (Ma, Lu, and Quan 2008, 939). The majority of China's vast rural population was insured under the Cooperative Medical System (CMS). This was a prepaid, collectivized health security program funded by contributions from individual peasant households and brigade (village) and commune (county) welfare funds, with an additional government subsidy. Much rural health care was provided by barefoot doctors—physicians with only a few months' training who offered a range of basic medical services to the rural populace, utilizing both Western and Chinese medicine (Wong and Chiu 1997, 77–78). By 1956 there were over 2,100 hospitals at the county level, 20,000 rural medical centers, and 41,000 clinics. By 1976, 90 percent of administrative villages (production brigades) had adopted the CMS, accounting for over 80 percent of the rural population (Xu 2009, 11). The achievements of this new health care system should not be underestimated: from 1952 to 1982 average life expectancy in China rose from 35 to 68 years, while infant mortality fell from 200 to 34 deaths per one thousand live births. The success of public health projects is reflected in the fact that, by the 1980s, chronic illnesses rather than infectious diseases were the main cause of death (Blumenthal and Hsiao 2005, 1166).

In theory, a fully realized social security system negated the need for health philanthropy, which was, after all, ideologically anathema to a communist project that believed the state itself could provide equal cradle-to-grave care for all. However, the health care security system was not without its flaws. There was great urban-rural disparity between the standards of care offered, and medical services were frequently limited, falling short of satisfying all the people's needs. In particular, with the rural CMS—where the main source of funding was from money paid into the system by farmers—as grassroots collective economic productivity decreased, there was an increased fiscal burden placed on farmers and the raising of sufficient funds to finance the system became more difficult. In addition to such systemic failings within the health care security system, China also suffered a series of large-scale natural disasters during this period, including the Three Years of Great Chinese Famine (which was much exacerbated by policy failings) from 1958 to 1961 and later the Tangshan earthquake of 1976. The ten years of the Cultural Revolution (1966–1976), meanwhile, only served to worsen an already severe lack of medicine, medical equipment, and doctors. During those years class struggle was rife and there was no exemption for the medical world: various medical facilities were destroyed and many doctors fell victims to political purges.

The great irony is that both the regular shortfall experienced in health care services, particularly in the countryside, and the more extreme instances of natural disasters were very much the contexts within which philanthropic health organizations might have played a significant ameliorating role. Yet throughout this period an ideologically hidebound government attempted to shoulder all the responsibilities regarding public health, despite this exceeding its financial and organizational capacity. Indeed, rather than coming to the fore in these times of crisis, the notion of philanthropy and private charity was further stigmatized as sugarcoated bullets from the bourgeoisie. A small but striking example is the case of a Shanghainese worker in the 1970s who mailed two hundred renminbi as a disaster relief donation to the local governments of the disaster-stricken Anhui and Guizhou Provinces, only to be rebuked as "harboring evil intentions and ulterior motives" (Zhu 1997). On a larger scale, in 1976, after the Tangshan earthquake, various countries offered emergency aid and medical supplies to China, but these offers were all refused by the Chinese government (Zhou and Zeng 2006, 365).

Furthermore, during the Cultural Revolution the many charities and official welfare and relief agencies that had been established or reorganized during the early years of the PRC were all dissolved. The Red Cross Society of China had developed rapidly in its organization and service capacity since being reformed and made subject to the Ministry of Health in 1950, and by 1966 it had more than five thousand grassroots organizations throughout the country and over five hundred thousand members. But after the Cultural Revolution began, the society was excoriated as a "feudal, capitalistic, and revisionist" force. Its branch offices at all levels were abolished and its main staff were dismissed or transferred to Cadre Schools (Red Cross Society of China 2008). The China Association for the Blind and Deaf stagnated, and in 1969 the Ministry of Internal Affairs, which administered governmental charitable agencies, was dissolved (Zhou and Zeng 2006, 379).

Philanthropy was beholden to the political ideology of the time. It was curtailed not only by direct policies, which abrogated the existence of philanthropic organizations, but also indirectly by wider economic and social policy: as economic development foundered in the wake of a series of misguided political campaigns there was a scarcity of social wealth. Even if there had been political space allowed for the operation of (domestic) health philanthropies, their efficacy would have been severely limited by a lack of resources. Philanthropy had become a river without a source and it would require significant political and economic transformation for this situation to change.

The Rehabilitation of Health Philanthropy, 1978–2003

Such transformation did begin to take shape from 1978 onward, as Deng Xiaoping pressed forward with a series of institutional reforms following the Third Plenary Session of the 11th CCP Central Committee. The reshaping of the state-society relationship precipitated by the Reform and Open Up policy was to have far-reaching ramifications for health philanthropy in China. The development of the market economy brought an end to the putative equal distribution of wealth in the country and weakened ideological resistance to the notion of philanthropy. The potential for more grassroots control of wealth laid the financial basis for the development of new philanthropy. Meanwhile increasing international interaction with China offered the possibility of renewed cooperation with foreign medical and philanthropic groups.

Crucially, at the same time as the potential for philanthropic development emerged, the need for its existence became more pressing, particularly in the case of philanthropy for health. After 1978, central government funding of both health care and public health initiatives fell greatly, with the financial burden transferred to provincial and local authorities. From 1978 to 1999 the central government's share of national health care spending fell from 32 percent to 15 percent. Inevitably this led to growing disparity between richer and poorer provinces, alongside increasing privatization of the health care system (Blumenthal and Hsiao 2005, 1166). In urban areas the transition to a market economy saw many state-owned enterprises either shut down or become private or joint-venture enterprises. A new urban employee health insurance program was introduced to replace the former Government Insurance and Labor Insurance Schemes. This covered employees of both state-owned and private enterprises, but required greater employee contributions, and did not cover employee's dependents (Ma, Lu, and Quan 2008, 940). The most dramatic change, though, occurred in rural areas where the CMS collapsed due to the dismantling of the agricultural communes, which had provided the financial basis for the rural medical system. No longer able to pool finances to insure against risk, individual households were forced to cover expenses themselves and "900 million rural, mostly poor citizens became, in effect, uninsured overnight" (Blumenthal and Hsiao 2005, 1166). Between 1979 and 1989 the percentage of villages with cooperative medical insurance schemes fell from 90 percent to less than 5 percent (Wong and Chiu 1997, 78).[2]

In 1985, the government promulgated several health reform policy issues, which approved for the first time the operation of private medical services. Furthermore, with political dogma no longer strictly opposed to the concept of private charity, and against the backdrop of an ever-increasing wealth gap and the collapse of the former health security system, new philanthropic organizations began to emerge. In 1981, the China Children and Teenagers' Fund (CCTF), which describes itself as "the first independent nonprofit charity organization in China" (China Children and Teenagers' Fund 2013), was founded, and the following year the Soong Ching Ling Foundation was established, with Deng Xiaoping as honorary president. To what extent foundations such as these can truly be described as "independent" is debatable. They may more accurately be termed government-organized nongovernmental organizations (known as GONGOs), operating with a degree of autonomy but still under the supervision of the government. The CCTF, for instance, was primarily endowed and is still supervised by the All-China Women's Federation (originally a mass organization supported by the CCP) and regulated by the Ministry of Civil Affairs. The place of GONGOs in the Chinese philanthropic landscape is discussed at greater length in Deng Guosheng and Zhao Xiaoping's chapter in this volume. However, irrespective of the level of independence these new organizations had from state intervention, they clearly marked a significant development from the Maoist era. Charitable organizations were no longer regarded as "an icing that deceives and anesthetizes the people," but were being recognized as a helpful and necessary addition to a struggling state health care service.

In November 1984, a nationwide municipal welfare institution adjustment exchange conference was held in Fujian. The conference proposed that social welfare should be transferred from the hands of the Ministry of Civil Affairs alone to the efforts of multiple channels, various levels, and different forms via a combination of state, collective group, and private individual input. A development direction for welfare was settled, "transforming from being arranged by the state to being held by society," (Zhou and Zeng 2006, 384), which marked the official recovery of nongovernmental philanthropy in China after more than 30 years. In practice, though, philanthropic ventures, at least initially, were almost entirely government-run.

A range of government directives and legislation followed, which would begin to form a regulatory environment for the evolution of health philanthropy in China. In 1988, the State Council issued its Measures for the Management of Foundations, which defined for the first time the nature and legal status of foundations in China (Song 2008). In 1994, with approval from the government, the China Charity Federation was legally registered as an independent entity. In 1998, the State Council issued its Regulations on the Registration and Management of Social Organizations and Interim Regulations on the Registration and Management of Civil Non-Enterprise Institutions, which clearly stipulated the definition of people-run non-enterprise units (*minban fei qiye danwei*) and social organizations (*shehui tuanti*). These two regulations framed the rights and duties, as well as the registration, administration, and supervision processes, for these entities.[3]

The potential for grassroots contributions to welfare and relief projects was demonstrated that same year: after serious flooding of the Yangtze, Songhua, and Nen Rivers, all walks of society were mobilized to offer financial aid and supplies, with donations surpassing seven billion renminbi—the largest donation since the foundation of the PRC. The fundraising effort, including appeals screened on CCTV, the state broadcaster, was a remarkable demonstration of how far official attitudes toward charitable giving had shifted since the 1970s. Following this, in 1999, the Public Welfare Donations Law was adopted at the 10th Meeting of the Standing Committee of the Ninth National People's Congress. This law clarified the rights and obligations of donors and recipients, the usage and management of donated properties, and favorable measures such as tax exemption for donors, and also regulated various activities deriving from donations. Article 8 of the law stipulated that "the State encourages natural persons, legal persons or organizations to donate to public welfare," ushering in a new era of public welfare giving in China. Also in 1999, the government issued new stipulations defining the payable income tax and the qualification and scope for tax exemption for institutional units, social organizations, and private non-enterprise entities. In 2001, the Ministry of Finance and State Administration of Taxation (SAT) jointly issued new tax policies for pilot regions, which marked the beginning of public welfare tax exemption legislation in China.

These new tax measures and the aforementioned legal documents began the normalization and safeguarding of philanthropy as a whole and both responded to and fostered the development of numerous health and medical organizations, including semi-official charities, nongovernmental charities, and international charities. By 2003, according to the statistics of China Social Organizations, 26,795 medical social organizations were registered in the country (China NPO 2005).

With the implementation of the Reform and Opening Up policy and the increasing demands for philanthropic intervention in the health sector, the state also began to open its gates to international development organizations. The United Nations, as the largest international organization in the world, began to exert tremendous influence on the health sector, with its subsidiaries carrying out specific activities in China. From 1978 to 1981, the World Health Organization (WHO), United Nations Populations Fund (UNFPA), United Nations International Children's Emergency Fund (UNICEF), and United Nations Development Programme (UNDP) set up offices in China one by one, and cooperated with the Chinese government in the health sector.

Alongside these UN organizations, a great number of other international organizations and foundations entered China, including the Rockefeller Foundation (1978) and the return of the China Medical Board (1981), the Li Ka Shing Foundation and VSO (1981), Project HOPE (1983), the Amity Foundation (1985), Oxfam (1987), the Ford Foundation (1988), Médicins Sans Frontières (1988), Health Unlimited (1993), Smile Train (1999), and Marie Stopes International (2000). The work of these projects tended to operate on the basis of Chinese-Western cooperation, with domestic organizations relying on international institutions in terms of funding and technology, and international organizations in turn relying on domestic ones to implement their projects utilizing local knowledge and expertise.

As the scale of international philanthropic involvement increased, the state moved to legislate this area more clearly. In 1998 the Ministry of Health issued a notice concerning the activity of foreign philanthropies that set regulations concerning the application, approval procedure, and authentication of professional qualifications of overseas charities to carry out health philanthropic activities in China. This notice also stipulated that overseas charities should focus on poorer patients and ensure technological advancement that would supplement local medical services. The document provided the legal basis for the supervision of international organizations' activities in China, regulating their medical activities and guaranteeing the quality of their medical service. In 2001, provisional measures were issued, defining both the qualifications for tax exemption for overseas donors and recipients, and the regulations regarding the import of donated materials for poverty-relief and charity purposes.

The legislation and political directives discussed in this section responded to, and stimulated, the development of the philanthropic sector, yet they emerged in somewhat piecemeal fashion. The speed of social and economic change in China following the Reform and Open Up policy has frequently resulted in legal and regulatory provisions having to play catch-up, and this was certainly the case with philanthropy during the period 1978–2003. It was not until 2004 that the importance of the development of philanthropy to the social security system became explicitly written into key CCP documents following the Fourth Plenary Session of the 16th CCP Central Committee, where it was proposed to "perfect the social security system in which social insurance, social assistance and social welfare are linked up with philanthropy" (Li 2005). Although in many ways modern philanthropy in China is still in a relatively early phase, with legislation and government regulation constantly evolving, it is this official recognition that philanthropy could play a crucial role in "continuously improving the ability to construct the harmonious socialist society" that has led 2004 to be identified as a watershed year for the development of philanthropy in China (Li 2005).

The Institutional Improvement Period of Health Philanthropy, 2004–2012

The state's commitment to the development of the philanthropic sector was reemphasized in various ways following the Fourth Plenary Session of the 16th CCP Central Committee. The *2005 Report on the Work of the Government of the State Council* officially proclaimed that "the development of philanthropy is supported" (Wen 2006). The Sixth Plenary Session of the 16th CCP Central Committee in 2006 proposed a policy of special tax reduction and exemption for social donations, and at the 17th CCP National Congress in 2007, philanthropy was identified as an important element and strategic step in the construction of a social security system with Chinese characteristics (Jin 2008, 46). That same year, the Ministry of Civil Affairs set up a Philanthropy Coordination Office within the Department of Disaster and Social Relief, and in September 2008 it established the Department of Social Welfare and Charity Promotion, which specializes in administrating social charities. Legislation since 2004 has also assisted the development of philanthropy, with draft regulations still underway.[4]

Table 1.1. The Medical Security System in China (2011)

Security System	Target	Population Coverage (millions)	Characteristics
Basic Medical Insurance for Urban Employees	All urban employees of enterprises	252.26	Mandatory; both the employer and the employee pay medical insurance fees
Basic Medical Insurance for Non-Working Urban Residents	All urban residents not covered by Basic Medical Insurance for Urban Employees, including students at primary schools and middle schools, infants, and other unemployed urban residents	220.66	Voluntary; insurance fee borne mainly by individuals (households), with some governmental subsidy
New Rural Residents Cooperative Medical Service	Rural residents	831.63	Medical fee borne jointly by individuals, community, and government, with low guarantee level of 200 RMB of subsidy per capita
Urban-Rural Medical Assistance System	Low-income individuals in urban and rural areas	21.44	Mainly targeted at several major diseases, with different aid standards in different areas, and different aid levels according to individual income

Source: National Health and Family Planning Commission of the People's Republic of China. 2012. *2012 China Public Health Statistical Yearbook.* http://www.nhfpc.gov.cn/htmlfiles/zwgkzt/ptjnj /year2012/index2012.html.

Before considering the specific development of health philanthropy since 2004, it is worth looking briefly at the state of the national health security system in China during this period. After the collapse of a comprehensive security system during the 1980s, in recent years the situation has improved, with a new multilevel system now established. Table 1.1 summarizes the basic types of state coverage offered in 2010.

After 15 years of development, the number of private medical institutions had increased to 447,995 by 2010, amounting to 48 percent of all medical institutions in China. However, they occupied a far smaller portion of the medical service market than public-owned medical institutions. In 2010, private medical institutions accounted for 17 percent of all medical service staff, 9 percent of all hospital beds, and 7 percent of total medical institution assets (Ministry of Health 2012). Most private medical institutions are classified as "profitable," meaning they are subject to a more stringent registration process and enjoy far fewer tax breaks than nonprofit institutions.[5]

Although China has completed the preliminary establishment of a medical security system, it is still faced with the problems of uneven distribution of medical resources and relatively low levels of care provision. In rural areas particularly there remains a shortfall in medical services and supplies, and people with financial difficulties are confronted with problems of expensive medical bills and difficulty in accessing quality health care. The supply of medical insurance can only meet people's basic medical demands and so health philanthropy is a vital supplement. Recognizing this, the government has issued pronouncements relating specifically to health philanthropy. In 2009 the CCP Central Committee issued opinions on deepening the reform of the medical and health care system, stating that efforts should be made "to encourage trade unions and other social organizations to engage in various forms of medical assistance activities, to encourage and guide organizations and individuals to develop charitable social medical assistance . . . [and] to vigorously develop health philanthropy, to formulate preferential policies, encourage social forces to set up charitable medical institutions or donate to medical assistance and medical institutions" (CCP Central Committee 2009). That same year, the Ministry of Civil Affairs explicitly pointed out that civil administration departments should "research and formulate policies related to, organize the implementation of, and link up medical assistance with, social charity aid" in opinions issued on the further improvement of the urban and rural medical assistance system (Ministry of Civil Affairs 2009).

Against this backdrop, the number of health-focused organizations has risen greatly. According to statistics from China Public Organization, by 2009 there were 38,828 nonprofit health organizations registered in China, comprising 27,237 nongovernmental organizations, 11,521 social organizations, and 70 foundations (China NPO 2009). This number would be considerably higher if those nongovernmental and foreign health philanthropic organizations with business registrations or without any registration were added. These health organizations represented the fourth-largest share of registered nonprofits in China in 2009 (see figure 1.1). Health philanthropies also receive a significant share of

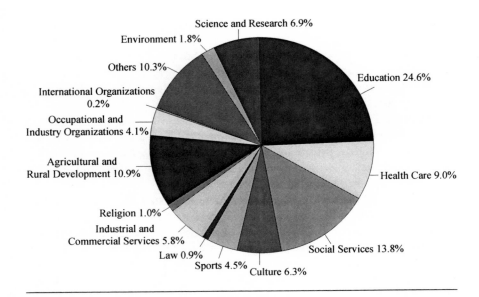

Figure 1.1. Distribution of Target Areas for Registered NPOs in China (2009).
Source: China NPO (2011).

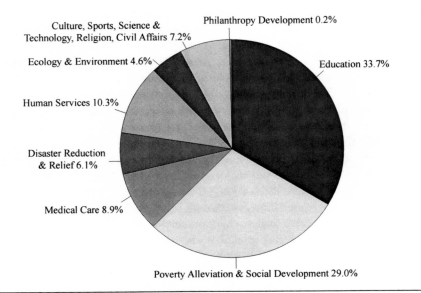

Figure 1.2. Distribution of Donations from Domestic Sources (2011). *Source: Yang (2012, 37).*

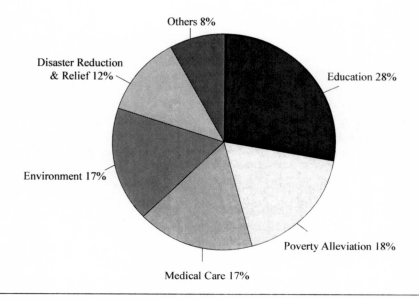

Figure 1.3. Distribution of Donations from Foreign NGOs (2010). *Source: Meng, Peng, and Liu (2011, 63–64).*

overall national charitable donations, although those do not approach the levels given to education and poverty alleviation, which are market leaders. According to the sample analysis of the overall donations in 2011, out of a total amount of 27.8 billion RMB, 2.5 billion RMB (9 percent) was invested in medical care (see figure 1.2). Public awareness of grave public health incidents and natural disasters during recent years, such as the SARS outbreak in 2003, the southern China snow damage and Wenchuan earthquake of 2008, and the Yushu earthquake and Gansu mudslide in 2010, is likely to have stimulated a rise in general donations.

Foreign NGOs in China have particularly focused on the medical and health sector in recent years, with many large-scale international foundations entering the country. In 2010, out of 1.67 billion RMB in donations from foreign NGOs, 17 percent was put into the health sector (Meng, Peng, and Liu 2011, 63–64), ranking third in terms of investment amount, after education and poverty alleviation (see figure 1.3). Perhaps most notably, although health philanthropy does not currently command the main share in terms of overseas financial donations, the largest proportion of foreign NGOs' activities in China are concentrated in the medical and health sector (23 percent), suggesting significant potential for further financial growth. According to recent research conducted by the China Development Brief (2013), of the 203 international NGOs operating in China in

2012, 69 launched medical and health programs. In 2012, 6 of the 14 international NGOs officially registered at the Ministry of Civil Affairs were involved in the medical and health sector (China NPO 2013).

High-profile international organizations have concentrated their efforts in a number of ways: (1) the development of new technologies and treatments; for example, Foundation Merieux focused on tuberculosis diagnosis and treatment technology, while the Bill & Melinda Gates Foundation and MSD HIV/AIDS Public-Private Partnership concentrated on the research and development of vaccines; (2) capacity building, such as talent development and training, lab construction, and capability improvement; (3) general management of patients; for example, MSD HIV/AIDS Public-Private Partnership creates profiles for those infected, does follow-up examinations and treatments, and provides new rural cooperative medical care subsidies, and the Bill & Melinda Gates Foundation provides consultation services, examinations, care and support, and projects aimed at reducing social discrimination; (4) the promotion of international research and cooperation; and (5) the development of national-level prevention and control schemes and the exertion of influence on the government's policy and development plan in certain areas through cooperation and negotiation with the Ministry of Health. As these projects suggest, large international philanthropic organizations are increasingly valuing the replacement of pure financial support with cooperative development, combining treatment with prevention initiatives, publicity and education, capacity building, and research innovation.

In China, international charities largely cooperate with the Ministry of Health and its affiliates such as the Chinese Center for Disease Control and Prevention and the State Council AIDS Working Committee Office in their major health programs. The relationship between these international organizations and the state has exhibited a game- or dance-like dynamic. For the Chinese government, cooperation with well-resourced international charities helps make up for the shortfall in public investment in the health sector, while allowing for close monitoring of these organizations and limiting the opportunities for them to work independently with local NGOs. For international organizations, since state approval is a precondition of entering China, direct collaboration on projects with the government is an effective approach to acquiring this permission. Collaboration with local NGOs is also often less enticing as, compared to the government, they lack the infrastructure to undertake large-scale nationwide projects. Besides, through cooperating with the government, international organizations can more directly influence the government's decision-making and policy orientation. Nonetheless it is often an important objective for the international stakeholders to promote the development of civil society in China when participating in China's health sector. Hence international organizations have sometimes made the commitment to developing local NGOs a prerequisite for providing financial support to the Chinese government. For instance, in 2011, the Global Fund froze its aid for HIV/AIDS, tuberculosis, and malaria programs in China (with the exception of medical supplies) due to dissatisfaction with funds management and the failure of the Country Coordination Mechanism of China to fulfill its pledge that at least 35 percent of project activity funds would be allocated to civil society organizations (20 percent in the first year, increasing progressively thereafter) (China Global Watch Initiative 2011, 3). Such negotiation and compromise is one of the features of modern health philanthropy in China, which is growing within a multilateral cooperation framework, "guided by government, sponsored by enterprises or international foundations, executed by health charities, and participated in by media and the public" (Yang and Ge 2009, 70).

Today the prospects for health philanthropy in China seem encouraging. It has undoubtedly become a valuable supplement to the welfare system, developing synchronously with the new medical security system. Nongovernmental health philanthropy and international organizations are being granted more opportunities and will continue to play an important role in China. In particular, international philanthropy work has been an important driving force in terms of research and breakthroughs in the treatment of diseases, the popularization of new technologies, the improvement of medical conditions in remote areas, capacity building, and epidemic prevention. Meanwhile, its promotion and interaction with the government can be of positive guiding significance for the design of national health policy. Nongovernmental grassroots philanthropy has been able to focus its attention on vulnerable groups, remote areas, and difficult fields, often emphasizing the role of health education. In addition, due to specific advantages such as the ability to respond rapidly to local situations, flexible mobility, and a willingness to endure hardships, grassroots NGOs have made significant contributions to medical assistance during natural disasters and epidemic outbreaks as well as in post-disaster reconstruction. The range of health activities pursued by health philanthropies has also diversified, particularly with projects now devoted to mental health issues, occupational illnesses (e.g., pneumoconiosis), and rare illnesses (e.g., hemophilia, osteogenesis imperfecta); and while health charities have continued caring for traditional groups such as the diseased and the disabled, teenagers, and social groups in danger and difficulty, they have also taken more minority groups as their service objects and partners, directing more attention to the participatory cooperation of these groups. Health charities have also become more innovative in providing services such as support groups and online assistance.

Alongside all these encouraging trends, though, various challenges remain. It is to these that the final section of this chapter now turns, as certain key challenges confronting contemporary health philanthropy in China are identified and several predictions offered for how this field may continue to develop, particularly if these hurdles can be overcome.

Challenges

Institutional Restrictions Hinder the Independence and Efficiency of Health Philanthropy Bodies

For nongovernmental organizations and international organizations the biggest institutional restriction is the difficulty of official registration, which represents a barrier for them in raising funds, seeking tax exemption, receiving legal protection, gaining public recognition, and carrying out activities smoothly.[6] State-run philanthropic organizations are subject to many layers of bureaucracy and interference, which can hamper efficient implementation of projects.

A Law-Governed Environment Has Not Been Fully Realized

Compared with those in developed countries, philanthropy laws and regulations in China still lag behind the development needs of the sector. The maintenance of order and the registration process for philanthropies is assigned higher priority than their ongoing management. Consequently, the government tends to interfere with charities instead of supporting them, and tends to restrict rather than facilitate (He and Ma 2004, 4).

The Sector Faces a Disparity in Resource Allocation

Looking at the entire philanthropic sector, nongovernmental health philanthropy receives relatively fewer domestic donations than other areas such as education, disaster relief, and support for vulnerable groups, and it is frequently hard for grassroots activities to be financed. The Ministry of Health and other government departments hold fast to their leading position in health philanthropy. In terms of resources, there is a stark imbalance between the near monopoly of state-run medical charities and poorly funded grassroots organizations.

The Sector Lacks an Effective Supervising Mechanism

At the state level, there is currently no unified supervision approach, nor overall platform to keep the public informed. The sector also has significant problems with a lack of transparency regarding the activities and finances of organizations. A 2011 survey suggested that 92 percent of the public was unsatisfied with the transparency of Chinese charities (Peng and Liu 2011, 9). The China Foundation Transparency Index's report on 2,213 foundations in China revealed that in 2012, 63 percent of the information provided was not fully substantiated (China Foundation Center 2012).

Capacity Building Is Insufficient inside Organizations

As treatment and research areas often require a high level of expertise, which nongovernmental organizations lack, nongovernmental bodies tend to crowd into the relatively easy areas of promotion and public awareness, resulting in repeated labor at a low level. Consequently they often cannot then meet the more high-level technical requirements of international organizations, and are therefore also unable to attract overseas funding.

Predictions

The Role of the Nongovernmental Sector Will Grow, and Cooperation between the Two Actors Will Increase

Given the demands of diversified development in the medical sector, the grassroots will play a larger role. The government will likely shoulder the main responsibility and seek to direct the development of the medical sector, but grassroots and international participants will become more involved, exerting increasing influence on the government in terms of policies and implementation. Already domestic Chinese donations have increased from 30.9 billion RMB in 2007 to over 60 billion RMB yearly following the 2008 Wenchuan earthquake (Meng, Peng, and Liu 2011, 14). Total nongovernmental organizations rose from 260,000 in 2003 to over 460,000 in 2011 (Ministry of Civil Affairs 2012, 155). Proposals related to philanthropy are receiving more time and attention from the National People's Congress (NPC) and Chinese People's Political Consultative Conference (CPPCC). In addition, the Chinese government is directing more financial support to social organizations. In 2012, the government provided 200 million RMB to purchase services from NGOs. Eighteen percent of the government's experimental social service programs and 12 percent of social service demonstration programs are health-related (Wang 2013, 32–33).

New Legislation Will Bring Increasing Legitimization of Nongovernmental Organizations

Political legitimacy is the precondition for nongovernmental and international organizations to successfully launch activities. It is likely that new legislation related to the health and philanthropy sectors will increasingly foster a more liberalized, less restricted space for philanthropic health organizations to develop. With the development of civil society in China and the government's recognition of grassroots forces, in time a more active and open management mode will replace the passive restriction of the past. One positive sign is that dual management, which has been the biggest obstacle for the legitimization of NGOs, will most likely be abolished. At the end of 2012, 19 provinces in China approved the trial registering of NGOs at their provincial-level civil affairs departments. In March 2013, the General Office of the State Council distributed a notice on its institutional restructuring, which promoted the direct registration of NGOs with local civil affairs departments. This means it will henceforth be much easier for NGOs to register as official entities.

Health Philanthropy Will Serve as an Incentive for the Development of the Health Sector as a Whole

In addition to potentially influencing policy decisions, health philanthropy constantly explores new service areas, especially in the research of cures for difficult and complicated diseases, the promotion of epidemic prevention, the improvement of medical conditions in remote regions, and capacity building. Moreover, health philanthropy introduces innovative management modes alongside advanced new technologies. In July 2012, Chinese Rural Kids Care (CRKC) was founded. This program provides up to twenty thousand renminbi to every needy child living in a rural area suffering from a major disease through a form of business insurance. So far it has been launched in several trial counties, covering more than 115,000 children (Chinese Rural Kids Care 2013). This program covers many kinds of major diseases, while the state medical security system covers only twenty diseases. CRKC covers the insurance fee for the children, and the insurance company pays for any medical expenses.

Philanthropic Donations from the Wealthy Will Continue to Increase

Individuals who have become wealthy earlier than others and private enterprises that have been successful are likely to place increasing emphasis on charitable giving. In 2011, the top one hundred donors gave about 12 billion RMB, and in 2012 this number rose to 15 billion RMB, a donation increase of 3 billion RMB in just one year (Beijing Normal University China Philanthropy Research Institute 2013).

Health Philanthropy Will Witness Growing International Communication and Cooperation against the Backdrop of Globalization

With the advancement of globalization and international cooperation in the health sector, international partners will provide health philanthropy in China with more resources, technical support, and innovative ideas, playing a greater role in this cause. At the same time, health philanthropy in China will continue to increasingly open up to international collaborations. China will engage in discussions on global health developments, and will likely provide increasing assistance to other countries and regions as suggested by the aid offered after events such as the Indian Ocean tsunami in 2004, the Haiti earthquake of 2009, and the Tohoku earthquake of 2011 (Yang and Ge 2009, 69).

In short, with its remarkable pace of development, not only may China soon be further improving its own health care sector with the assistance of international philanthropy and increasingly well-coordinated domestic philanthropic projects, but also, in the not too distant future, it will have become a significant player in the wider global context, bringing much experience and insight to bear on the development of global health, not least because of its own current steep learning curve.

Notes

1. "Chengdu Social Groups Investigation," 1951, 85-1-64, Chengdu Archives.
2. For a more detailed discussion of the impact of the post-1978 reforms of the health care sector, see Wong and Chiu (1997, 78–80), and Blumenthal and Hsiao (2005, 1166–1169).
3. For a more detailed discussion of legislative issues see Mark Sidel's chapter in this volume.
4. Mark Sidel's chapter in this volume provides an in-depth discussion of the legislation relating to philanthropy during this period, as well as further detail on some of the earlier legislation already mentioned.
5. In February 2000, the State Council put forward the Guiding Opinion on Health System Reform in Cities and Towns, prepared by the System Reform Office of the State Council and other departments. According to this document, medical institutions are classified as either profitable or nonprofit institutions.
6. At present 61 percent of the international organizations operating in China remain unregistered. Most of those with registration were registered at the industrial and commercial departments, and few at the civil departments (Wu Yuzhang 2010, 330).

References

Beijing Normal University China Philanthropy Research Institute. 2013. "2012 Top 100 Chinese Donors List." http://www.bnu1.org/research/donated/year/1055.html.

Blumenthal, David, and William Hsiao. 2005. "Privatization and Its Discontents: The Evolving Chinese Healthcare System." *New England Journal of Medicine* 353:1165–1170.

China Children and Teenagers' Fund. 2013. "About CCTF." http://www.cctf.org.cn/aboutus.html.

China Development Brief. 2013. "International NGO Directory." http://www.chinadevelopmentbrief.cn/?page_id=455.

China Foundation Center. 2012. "China Foundation Center Distributes Transparency Index of China Foundation Charts (2012)." http://news.foundationcenter.org.cn/html/2012-12/58668.html.

China Global Watch Initiative. 2011. *China Global Fund Watch.* No. 14. http://www.cgfwatch.org/files/pdf/China_Global_Fund_Watch_Newsletter__Issue_14_cn_Final.pdf.

China NPO (Nonprofit Organization Net). 2005. "The Development of NGOs within the Previous Year." http://www.chinanpo.gov.cn/2201/20152/yjzlkindex.html.

———. 2009. "Nonprofit Organization Statistics on a Regional Basis." http://www.chinanpo.gov.cn/2201/48277/yjzlkindex.htm.

———. 2011. "2009 Nonprofit Organization Statistics on a Regional Basis." http://www.chinanpo.gov.cn/2201/48277/yjzlkindex.html.

———. 2013. "Nationwide Inquiry into Civil Society Organizations." http://swshzz.chinanpo.gov.cn/search/searchOrgList.do?action=searchOrgList.

Chinese Rural Kids Care. 2013. "Program" section, http://www.dbyb.org.

Dong Biwu. 1950. "Relief Welfare of PRC." *People's Daily* (Beijing), May 5, sec. 1.

Fang Zhangshun. 1995. *Zhou Enlai and Earthquake and Disaster Prevention.* Beijing: Central Party Literature Press.

He Yunfeng, and Ma Kai. 2004. "Major Problems in the Development of NGOs in China." *Shanghai Normal University Journal* 2:1–6.

Jin Huanyu. 2008. "Several Theoretical Problems in the Development of Philanthropy." *Journal of Hunan Business College* 3:46–49.

Li Peilin. 2005. "The Status and Function of Philanthropy in the Social Development in China." *Chinese Academy of Social Sciences Review,* January 11, sec. 003.

Ma, Jin, Mingshan Lu, and Hude Quan. 2008. "From a National, Centrally Planned Health System to a System Based on the Market: Lessons from China." *Health Affairs* 27 (4): 937–948.

Meng Zhiqiang, Peng Jianmei, and Liu Youping, eds. 2011. *China Charity Donation Report.* Beijing: China Society Press.

Ministry of Civil Affairs. 2012. *China Civil Affairs Statistical Yearbook.* Beijing: China Statistics Press.

Ministry of Health. 2012. *2011 China Health Statistics Yearbook.* Beijing: Peking Union Medical College Press. http://wsb.moh.gov.cn/htmlfiles/zwgkzt/ptjnj/year2011/index2011.html.

Peng Jianmei, and Liu Youping, eds. 2011. "China Philanthropy Transparency Report (2011)." http://www.charity.gov.cn/fsm/sites/diaphanous/preview1.jsp?ColumnID=743&TID=20111130171920062640912.

Red Cross Society of China. 2008. "The Birth and Historical Development of Red Cross Society in China." http://www.redcross.org.cn/hhzh/zh/hsigk/lsyg/200806/t20080622_901.html.

Song Yang. 2008. "Philanthropy Law Boosts Philanthropy." *China Philanthropy Times.* http://www.gongyishibao.com/zhuan/30years/fagui.html.

Su Zhenfang. 2011. *Introduction to Social Security.* Beijing: China Audit Publishing House, China Society Press.

Tan Buxia. 2008. "Basic Facts and Changes of the Nine Shantang in Guangzhou." *Guangzhou Cultural and Historical Accounts.* http://www.gzzxws.gov.cn/gzws/cg/cgml/cg9/200808/t20080826_4053.htm.

Wang Zhenyao. 2013. *Philanthropy and Social Services: The 2012 Annual Report of China's Charity Sector.* Beijing: Social Sciences Academic Press (China).

Wen Jiabao. 2006. "The 2005 Report on the Work of the Government of the State Council." Central People's Government of the People's Republic of China. http://www.gov.cn/test/2006-02/16/content_201218.htm.

Wong, Victor C. W., and Sammy W. S. Chiu. 2007. "Health-Care Reforms in the People's Republic of China: Strategies and Social Implications." *International Journal of Public Sector Management* 10 (1/2): 76–92.

Wu Yuzhang. 2010. *Big Events of NGOs in China (2010).* Beijing: Social Sciences Academic Press (China).

Xu Qingzhao. 2009. "Devlopment, Achievements and Experience of the Development of Rural China Cooperative Health System Since the Founding of PRC." *China Collective Economy* 9:11–12.

Yang Tuan. 2012. *China Philanthropy Development Report 2012.* Beijing: Social Sciences Academic Press (China).

Yang Tuan, and Ge Daoshun. 2009. *Report on the Philanthropy Development in China (2009).* Beijing: Social Sciences Academic Press (China).

Zhongyang Renmin Zhengfu fazhi weiyuanhui [Legal Committee of the Central Government]. 1982. *Zhongyang Renmin Zhengfu fa-ling huibian* [Decree compilation of the Central Government]. Beijing: Lawpress China.

Zhou Qiuguang, and Zeng Guilin. 2006. *A Brief History of Philanthropy in China.* Beijing: People's Publishing House.

Zhu Lingen. 1997. "Donations 26 Years Ago." *Xinmin Evening News* (Shanghai), February 15. Quoted in Tao Haiyang. 2008. "Governmental Charity and Challenges in Modernization." *Studies on the Socialism with Chinese Characteristics,* no. 4: 104.

2 The Shifting Balance of Philanthropic Policies and Regulations in China

Mark Sidel

As other chapters in this volume show clearly, the philanthropic arena is developing with extraordinary speed in China. There are now several thousand Chinese foundations, both private foundations and the so-called public fundraising foundations (most more closely associated with the government than the newer private foundations), and a rapidly increasing community of wealthy and middle-class donors. Health care and medicine are one of the interests of these new donors and their institutions, and a strong interest of the growing community of foreign foundations and other donors in China. At the same time, philanthropy and giving have received a great deal of the media's attention as well, for both positive and negative reasons. Philanthropy and charitable giving played a major role in the public response to the Wenchuan earthquake in Sichuan in 2008, while recent scandals in the charitable sector have brought negative attention as well to problems of accountability, transparency, and disclosure. And as this volume is being completed in December 2013, charitable giving—now primarily to nonstate nonprofit organizations directly—has been playing a significant role in relief from yet other Chinese natural disasters as well.[1]

Chinese policy and regulation has sought to keep up with, mold, and control these developments and growth in domestic, diaspora, and foreign giving, including giving for health. This chapter surveys the landscape for philanthropy policy and law in China, on the basis of extensive interviews and discussions in China as well as a review of news reports, academic research, and data on philanthropy.[2] It is future-oriented, recognizing that policy and the legal environment for philanthropy will play a major role in the development of charitable giving as China transitions in its leadership and continues the growth of philanthropy, and as the health sectors come to incorporate philanthropy more and more into their work and resourcing. It is also geared toward a general understanding of changes in philanthropic policies and regulations in China and not intended for specialists.[3] In all of these decisions and transitions, China faces the continuing tension between a policy and legal framework that facilitates civic participation, and a policy and legal environment that controls, constrains, and squelches civil society and independent giving. The ways in which that key policy and legal tension are balanced and resolved will play a decisive role in the development of philanthropy and civil society in China over the next several decades.

This chapter thus covers, first, the current policy, legal, and regulatory environment affecting philanthropy in China, including the national policies, regulations, and laws that impact philanthropy and the emergence of key local philanthropy policies, regulations, laws, and pilot programs—a particularly important set of developments in recent years. It further discusses the next steps in the enabling environment for philanthropy in China, particularly the current laws and regulations that are under revision, the shape and pace of those shifts in the legal and policy environment, and the key provisions, process, timeline, and institutional actors in this broad shift in the legal and policy framework that will have an impact on philanthropy across the board, including in the health sector. Diaspora and foreign philanthropic organizations are discussed elsewhere in this volume.

The Overall Structure and Legal Framework for Philanthropy in China

For an understanding of how political and policy decisions on the legal framework for philanthropy and civil society organizations may impact the health sector in future years, a brief introduction to the structure of and framework for philanthropy in China may be useful. There are multiple forms of nongovernmental, not-for-profit organizations (NPOs), including philanthropic organizations, in China (ICNL 2013a, 2013b). They include social organizations (SOs) (*shehui tuanti*); foundations (*jijinhui*); civil non-enterprise units (*minban fei qiye danwei*); unregistered, local organizations (including small grassroots organizations), and others. Some NPOs have a special status and exist under individual statutes, regulations, or other forms of permission; the Red Cross Society of China is one example.

The legal, regulatory, and fiscal framework for the broader nonprofit sector—which is described in outline terms here—has become increasingly complex in China in recent years, fueled by the government's political aim of both encouraging and also molding, constraining, and controlling the directions that philanthropy and the nonprofit sector will take. We will continue to see intensive regulatory activity by the government and key ministries (such as the Ministry of Civil Affairs, the Ministry of Finance, and others) and by increasing provincial and local regulation of nonprofit activity at the subnational level.

The roots of all that policymaking and regulation lie in the Chinese Constitution of 1982, which provided for a freedom of association. Article 35 of the 1982 Constitution states, "Citizens of the People's Republic of China enjoy freedom of speech, of the press, of assembly, of association, of procession and of demonstration."[4] Of course the official Chinese notion of "freedom of association" is certainly not the same as in other countries, and it is not too bold a statement to indicate that the official Chinese definition of what a right to "freedom of association" means is considerably more limited than in some other countries. But the constitutional framework for freedom of association is how China frames its policy and legal efforts in these areas, even though the reality of policy and law does not generally live up to the freedom promised in the Constitution.

That basic constitutional reference has fueled a number of regulatory efforts over the years, including highly restrictive provisions on philanthropy and the nonprofit sector in the 1950s that made it very difficult for foundations and other charitable entities to register and operate, and gradually more facilitative documents in the 1980s and 1990s. The current policy and legal framework for the philanthropic and nonprofit sector in China is rooted in several regulatory documents issued in the 1990s, including the Regulations on the Registration and Management of Social Organizations issued by the State Council in 1998; the Interim Regulations on the Registration and Management of Civil Non-Enterprise Institutions, also issued by the State Council in 1998; the Public Welfare Donations Law, enacted by the Standing Committee of the National People's Congress in 1999; and the Regulations on the Management of Foundations issued by the State Council in 2004.

There are of course many other policy and legal documents governing the sector, but those are some of the key ones, along with a variety of tax laws and documents which begin the process of outlining tax exemption and deductibility issues. Those basic documents and the more specific implementing documents under them have provided an initial framework for the formation, registration, governance, oversight, tax status, and other key elements of nonprofits.[5] The fiscal framework for this activity has rapidly become considerably more complex as well, yet it still mirrors the political policy of encouraging nonprofit and philanthropic activity that the government favors (particularly in service provision), while serving to discourage, control, and constrain nonprofit activity that the government does not want to see occur. The International Center for Not-for-Profit Law (ICNL) describes the current fiscal framework succinctly:

> In practice, donations, state subsidies, and some other forms of income are tax exempt. Contributions to NPOs are deductible from income tax, with limits depending on the type of taxpayer, the type of beneficiary, and the use of the contribution. . . . Contributions to informal NPOs, however, are [generally] not tax deductible. . . . NPOs that engage in nursing, medical, educational, cultural, or religious activities or activities in which services are performed by the disabled are exempted from the Business Tax on the sale of services. However, informal NPOs that are registered as businesses are required to pay the Business Tax. (ICNL 2013a)[6]

In the philanthropic framework, the available legal documents are somewhat more sparse. There are, as mentioned above, the Regulations on the Management of Foundations (2004), as well as the Public Welfare Donations Law (1999), and some more specific implementing documents issued over the years that deal with specific foundation and other philanthropic issues. They govern the basics of the philanthropic sector, at least as envisioned in the early part of the last decade. These include the differentiation of two types of foundations: "public fundraising foundations" (*gongmu jijinhui*), generally closer to the government, which are allowed to raise funds from the public, and "non-public fundraising foundations" (*feigongmu jijinhui*), akin to private foundations in other countries, which receive funds largely from key donors and are generally not permitted to raise funds from the public.

As ICNL notes, Chinese "foundations, like social organizations, are regulated by both a registration and administration agency, usually the Ministry of Civil Affairs in Beijing or a provincial, municipal, or local Civil Affairs bureau or office, and by a professional agency such as the relevant government ministry or agency at the national, provincial, municipal, or local level" (ICNL 2013a). That philanthropic regulatory framework—which is beginning to shift toward single reporting mechanisms in some parts of the country—also includes (particularly in the 2004 Foundation Regulations) general principles expressed in regulatory form for governance of foundations, reporting, audits and the like, and government oversight and reporting requirements and responsibilities. In addition, more specific implementing documents issued over the years on philanthropic issues include, for example, regulations on foundation names (Provisions on the Administration of Names of Foundations, 2004), on information disclosure by foundations (Measures for the Information Disclosure of Foundations, 2006), on annual inspection of foundations (Measures for the Annual Inspection of Foundations, 2006), and on audit guidelines for foundations, in part a response to scandals involving foundations (Notice on Strengthening and Perfecting the Audit System of Foundations, 2011; Hu 2011). And we have even more specific regulatory documents on particular issues in the philanthropic arena, such as documents on foreign philanthropy (Notice of the General Office of the Ministry of Health, 2008), or on donations of foreign exchange to domestic organizations (Notice of the State Administration of Foreign Exchange on Issues Concerning the Administration of Foreign Exchange Donated to or by Domestic Institutions, 2009). Most of these regulations and documents in turn have been substantially supplemented or amended over the years.

Yet despite all this regulation-making, virtually all seem to agree that the framework for legal regulation of both the broader nonprofit sector and the specific philanthropic part of it began incompletely, could not be completed through the promulgation of implementing rules and notices, are now increasingly rickety and out of date, and have been difficult to implement and enforce, particularly in light of inappropriate practices and the occasional charity or philanthropic scandal.

That framework has been made either overly general or directly obsolete by the march of time and developments around China and, perhaps ironically, by the increasing tendency to explore different approaches and reforms in this sector in recent years. This inevitable obsolescence comes from some positive developments, including the growth of the sector and its increasing roles in Chinese society. At the same time, the regulatory structure and the broader legal framework outside of nonprofits have been unable to fully respond to emerging problems, such as more instances of fraud or inappropriate practices in the sector. And many would agree on another conclusion as well: the legal framework for the nonprofit sector has done a considerably better job at facilitating state control of the growth and programmatic directions of the sector than at safeguarding the rights of those who try to form and register organizations or work in them.

The Current Policy, Legal, and Regulatory Environment Affecting Philanthropy in China

In both health philanthropy and the broader giving environment, Chinese government policy, and thus the legal environment, has sought to encourage the growth of service-oriented philanthropy while discouraging, constraining, and controlling the development of independent civil society, advocacy, and overly independent philanthropic practices. That broad policy framework—a political decision by the Chinese leadership-has remained relatively stable for a number of years, though emphases may have changed at particular moments, some regions of the country may display either more policy flexibility or greater policy hardness, and implementation has remained somewhat flexible, particularly outside Beijing and some other major cities. Indeed, implementation of a political policy that seeks both to encourage the growth of philanthropy and to constrain the emergence of independent civil society ranges across a spectrum that at times confounds foreign and even some Chinese observers: even within specific fields (such as AIDS services and policy), government policy implementation at national and local levels ranges from broad latitude and encouragement for the work of a wide range of philanthropic and nongovernmental groups within the strict bureaucratic requirements of the state, to the smashing and jailing (and worse) of NGO organizations and personnel that are perceived to threaten the state or key policies. What emerges is what some Chinese scholars call "differentiated management," in which the policy and legal framework enables a wide range of responses by the state to the activities of nongovernmental and philanthropic groups depending on whether they are pursuing activities, services, policy advocacy, and other work that the state approves of or seeks to discourage.

Within that broad policy framework of encouragement with controls and "differentiated management," the current legal environment is important—and its impact is not underestimated by the domestic Chinese philanthropic community. The key legal framework for the management and administration of philanthropy, including health philanthropy, in China focuses on the three basic forms of organizations in the Chinese nonprofit sector: foundations (*jijinhui*), social organizations (*shehui tuanti*), and civil non-enterprise units (*minban fei qiye danwei*). The basic framework includes the following:

National-Level Policy and Regulation

For health, medical, and other foundations in China, the Regulations on the Management of Foundations, issued in 2004 with many supplementary documents since then, remain the guiding legal and policy document. The regulations specify two basic types of foundations: public fundraising and non-public fundraising foundations (the latter of which would often be called private foundations elsewhere). There are specific minimum capital, governance, and other requirements, including strict provisions on registering foundations—a key method for control and government decision-making regarding which philanthropic entities should be permitted. This key but relatively basic document is now awaiting the issuance of revised regulations that were completed by the Ministry of Civil Affairs and the State Council Legal Affairs Office in 2011 and further revised in 2012 and 2013. The regulations are discussed further below because they and their future are of particular importance to philanthropy, both health-related and otherwise, in China.

The Regulations on the Registration and Management of Social Organizations and the Interim Regulations on the Registration and Management of Civil Non-Enterprise Institutions (both issued by the State Council in 1998, and both supplemented with additional regulatory documents over the years) are less directly related to philanthropy but bear significantly on some of the nonstate (or "lesser-state") organizations that domestic, diaspora, and foreign philanthropy support in China. Those include a myriad of health and medical social organizations and civil enterprises. These framework rules also make registration complicated, until recently required the "dual management" of both a professional supervisory body (such as the Ministry of Health or a provincial health bureau) and an administrative supervisory body (such as the Ministry of Civil Affairs or a provincial civil affairs bureau) for a significant range of organizations, and have enabled the government to encourage and mold the development of various forms of nongovernmental organizations in the health field, and other fields, that support the government's provision of health and social services while not undertaking—at least for the most part—more independent advocacy activity. These policy documents are also now well out of date; each has also been revised by the Ministry of Civil Affairs and the State Council Legal Affairs Office and are awaiting promulgation, which has been delayed.

On the increasingly important issue of charitable donations and fundraising, the Public Welfare Donations Law, enacted by the Standing Committee of the National People's Congress in 1999, is the key national policy and legal document, supplemented by specific rules for various types of organizations and by increasingly (though not sufficiently) favorable tax incentives for giving. Like the other policy and legal documents, the Public Welfare Donations Law is significantly out of date, left behind by major developments in the Chinese giving environment, particularly after the 2008 Wenchuan earthquake. It is not clear whether the law will be revised, or donation provisions inserted into the national framework Charity Law that is now in draft, or a separate statute on fundraising enacted. But the currently restrictive rules on fundraising, which formally bar most Chinese foundations, social organizations, and other groups from public fundraising, are proving to be complex and difficult policy issues in an economic, social, and political environment in which more and more Chinese both want to give to independent groups and have the resources to do so.

A national framework Charity Law has been in draft since 2004, and is now with the State Council Legal Affairs Office for detailed review before going to the National People's Congress (through its Legislative Affairs Commission) for legislative review in 2013 or 2014. Discussion and adoption of the Charity Law has been delayed on a number of occasions, for reasons and over issues discussed in more detail below.

National-level tax legislation dealing with entity income tax, tax deductions for charitable donations, and the possibility of an estate tax has been gradually developing in China. China has a developing infrastructure that permits tax deductions for charitable donations (up to prescribed levels), and tax exemptions for various kinds of charitable organizations. That tax infrastructure will continue to be modified in the years ahead, with extensive conflict possible over calls from society to increase the incentives for giving and over misgivings on the part of tax and other officials. This is a complex area, and one that will see continuing change (ICNL 2013a and 2013b).

Other regulatory documents affect the domestic, diaspora, or international philanthropic and nonprofit sectors. Examples of these abound; one recent and important example is Notice 63, issued by the State Administration of Exchange Control in December 2009 (effective March 1, 2010), which makes it more difficult for some, especially unregistered, social organizations to receive foreign funding. And, of course, specific thematic sectors sometimes have specific rules on philanthropy in their area. The Ministry of Health, for example, is empowered to issue certain rules on domestic, diaspora, and international philanthropy for health, and has been active in this area, particularly with respect to foundations, social organizations, and civil non-enterprise organizations in the health and medical arenas. As national framework policies, laws, and regulations are updated, we can also expect to see more devolution of policymaking and rulemaking in specific areas—like health—to the key national ministries that work in those particular areas.

Key Local Philanthropy Policy, Regulation, Law, and Pilot Programs

In recent years, and consistent with national political policy that seeks to encourage, constrain, and mold the development of civil society and philanthropy, local policy and regulatory activity on philanthropy has emerged as a key area of development and experimentation. Legal and policy documents on philanthropy, charitable giving, donations, and foundations have now been issued in many provinces and centrally administered municipalities, and in some cases they are used to explore new and more flexible approaches to state regulation of the philanthropic sector. Some provinces and municipalities (such as Guangdong, Shenzhen, Shanghai, Jiangsu, Beijing, and others) have become well known for their progress in this area, including local experimentation with new forms of administration for the central authorities in Beijing to watch and learn from.

A full cataloguing of local regulatory and experimental efforts is beyond the scope of this chapter, in part because not all—or even necessarily most—of the local efforts are targeted at philanthropy in the health arena. But some of the more important such local legal and policy documents include the following. Most of these are regarded as sector-neutral or somewhat more favorable toward the sector (i.e., by reducing registration requirements or the mandates of state administration). Some are regarded as more restrictive, like the Yunnan regulations on international NGOs. This new wave of local regulation and policymaking, approved by Beijing, is now expanding constantly. Some of the early examples included:

- New policies and regulations on registration and management of social organizations, social contracting for the provision of social services by NPOs, and other regulations in Shenzhen and Guangdong Provinces
- Expanded experiments and procedures for "social contracting" (delegating the provision of social services to nonprofit organizations by government through contract) in Shanghai, and new draft charitable donation and charitable transparency rules in Shanghai
- New regulations on supervision and management of local foundations, and on the promotion of charity in Jiangsu Province (Jiangsu Province Regulations on Charity Promotion, 2010)
- New regulations on fundraising in Hunan Province (Hunan Province Regulations on Fundraising, 2011)
- Regulations or amended earlier regulations on the registration of social organizations in Beijing and many other provinces and cities around China;

experiments with registration in Guangdong led to national changes that simplified registration procedures for a significant range of NPOs

- 2010 regulations on the management of international NGOs in Yunnan Province (which many interpret to be relatively restrictive in nature) (Yunnan Province Interim Provisions on the Activities of Foreign Nongovernmental Organizations, 2010)
- A number of other provincial and local regulations on philanthropy and nonprofit organizations around the country

The willingness of Beijing central government authorities to allow provincial and subnational implementation and, in some cases, experimentation with new procedures on the registration, management, and oversight of foundations, social organizations, and other entities is an important area for observation by domestic, diaspora, and international donors. But it does not yet rise to the level of provincial or other subnational "competition" for philanthropic resources that such subnational regulation has, in the past, represented for foreign investors interested in arbitraging the differences between local incentives for foreign investment. In short, local developments in philanthropy and other nongovernmental policymaking and regulation represent some local specificity and, at times, local experimentation with approaches, which may or may not be scaled up for other provinces or cities or even national promulgation as Beijing carefully watches progress in local areas. As ICNL has stated, "Over the last few years, there have been important local policy experiments in the Chinese nonprofit and philanthropic sector, mostly at the provincial level. These policy experiments are important because they provide the central authorities with policy ideas and experiences that play a role in shaping national-level legislation. They therefore [may] serve as harbingers of changes in national-level legislation" (ICNL 2013b).

The role of local regulation of philanthropy and social organizations in policy experimentation and information provision to national policymakers in Beijing, though it began earlier, is now generally traced most publicly to mid-2009, when the Ministry of Civil Affairs announced a Cooperative Agreement on Advancing Integrated Reforms in Civil Affairs with the municipal government of Shenzhen, a major economic area in the southern province of Guangdong and China's original special economic zone (SEZ). In early 2012, Guangdong also announced—in part as a result of the local regulatory experiment—that the requirement of finding a professional supervisory unit that would sponsor a nonprofit organization's registration would be eliminated in 2012. Guangdong is also moving toward eliminating or reducing restrictions on social organizations engaging in public fundraising, and perhaps to allow new nonprofit tax incentives as well (ICNL 2013b). In 2012 and 2013, still other reforms were announced, including a shift away from the much-disliked "dual management" system in which many Chinese nonprofits needed to register both through a "professional" agency (such as a provincial health bureau) and through an administrative agency (i.e., the provincial civil affairs bureau), and be directed by both.

Looking toward the Future

This is a time of significant change for philanthropy and its legal and policy framework, including for health and medical organizations. The current legal framework is under revision, with the shape and pace of those shifts in the legal and policy environment still not entirely clear, in part because the political policy toward the nonprofit sector and philanthropy determines the shape of specific legal and policy initiatives. The key provisions, process, timeline, and institutional actors in this broad shift in the legal and policy framework will certainly have an impact on philanthropy across the board, including in the health sector.

A multistage set of policy and regulatory responses to the combined problems of obsolescence, generality, and difficulty in implementation in the current legal framework for philanthropy and the nonprofit sector is now underway in China. Each of these shifts will have implications for philanthropy, and for philanthropy in the health arena.

Policy and Regulatory Responses in Philanthropy

The first policy and regulatory response is to revise the key original enactments, the regulations first issued in 1998 and 2004, to maintain some relevance and detail under present, greatly changed circumstances. For example, the national enactment on social organizations, the 1998 Regulations on the Registration and Management of Social Organizations, has been under review for amendment for a number of years. The same is the case for the Interim Regulations on the Registration and Management of Civil Non-Enterprise Institutions, also issued by the State Council in 1998. Differences in approach and view, and the onward march of events and developments that cause new problems for drafting as soon as earlier issues are resolved, have delayed the reemergence of these much-needed sectoral framework revisions.

This policy and regulatory response has been used with respect to the Regulations on the Management of Foundations (2004) as well. A revision of these regulations has been underway for a number of years. As the philanthropic situation has developed and become more complicated, new issues have arisen in this revision, contributing to a delay in the release of a new version or new regulations. Some of those issues have been identified in discussions with foreign specialists, or in the Chinese press, and each has the potential for significant impact on growth and programmatic priorities in the health philanthropic sector. They include:

- Whether to maintain the current, but quickly weakening, "dual management" reporting system for some foundations (the decision currently reported on that question is to eliminate the dual management system for foundations and have foundations be specifically overseen only by the civil affairs network)
- Investment of assets by foundations and whether a minimum portion of assets should be required to be held in safe instruments such as state bonds or bank accounts (i.e., 90 percent), and whether to require a minimum return on saved assets, both early regulatory means to control asset investment
- Whether major donors to private foundations should be required to donate a minimum portion of the annual donations to such foundations, as early regulation required
- Whether to give donors a right to check on the use of their funds, and how to do that
- How to strengthen foundation information disclosure mechanisms, through a combination of government regulation and industry self-regulation, a significant priority in light of recent charity scandals in China
- The relative power of the board over investments
- Whether to require minimum outlays (donations) by foundations for public benefit purposes
- The current dual definition of foundations (public fundraising foundations and non-public fundraising foundations), which has caused confusion and imposed limits on fundraising by some groups
- Whether to allow non-public fundraising foundations (now usually termed "private foundations" in China) to raise funds from the public
- The scope of internal foundation governance and external state oversight to be provided in the regulations
- Whether enhanced provisions on foundation tax exemption and tax deductibility should be included in the foundations regulations or deferred for tax legislation (or included in the Charity Law)
- Whether private foundations should be permitted to register at lower levels of government (below the provincial civil affairs bureau level), and some other issues as well[7]

The second policy and regulatory response to the obsolescence, generality, and difficulty of enforcement in that first generation of legal framework regulation has been to try to achieve an overall Charity Law governing the sector. Such a law would of course encompass health philanthropy within its scope. And so for many years, going back to the 1990s, a Charity Law (*Cishan zujinfa*)[8] has been in draft in Beijing, as an overall framework law for the sector. The Charity Law has yet to be enacted, but numerous drafts have been produced and reviewed or discarded as debates proceed in China on key issues in the law and rapidly changing circumstances overtake the terms of the various drafts, while demands for its promulgation come back each year.[9]

There are a number of issues, difficulties, and disputes in the finalization of the Charity Law, and a number of provisions that have not been decided upon. They include:

- Whether to maintain any residual form of the dual management reporting system for any charitable organizations
- Whether to allow social organizations and other forms of charitable organizations to raise funds from the public (a right generally now only available to public fundraising foundations, though a number of social organizations have found ways to do this in connection with foundations)
- How to regulate the business activities and investment activities of charitable organizations in general, and whether to differentiate among them in these areas
- Whether to give donors a right to check on the use of their funds, and how to do that
- How to strengthen charitable information disclosure and transparency mechanisms, through a combination of government regulation and industry self-regulation
- Whether enhanced provisions on charitable tax exemption and tax deductibility should be included in the Charity Law or deferred for tax legislation and regulation
- Whether and how to facilitate the formation of charitable trusts, a topic of inquiry among some wealthy Chinese donors, and some other issues as well

The third policy and regulatory response to the obsolescence, generality, and difficulty of enforcement in that first generation of legal framework regulation has been to try to supplement government regulation with various forms of industry-generated (philanthropy-generated) self-regulation and information disclosure. The move to supplement government regulation with robust self-regulation and information disclosure would of course also have significant implications for domestic health philanthropy, and perhaps for some aspects of diaspora giving as well.

The Chinese discussion of nonprofit self-regulation has its roots in business self-regulation, with initial principles for nonprofit self-regulation issued by Shang Yusheng and the China NPO Alliance in 2001. On the philanthropic front, the Private Foundation Forum issued self-regulatory principles for private foundations in 2009, asking the new private foundation community to abide by those (China Private Foundation Forum, 2009). In 2012 and 2013, a host of new transparency, disclosure, and accountability measures and frameworks have been initiated by the Chinese nonprofit and foundation sector as well as by government-linked associational groups, intended both to forestall further government regulation and to strengthen governance, transparency, and accountability in the nonprofit and foundation sector. In Chinese NPO and philanthropic circles—including in the health and medical arena—there remains strong interest in self-regulation, and discussion of its feasibility and potential forms can be expected to grow further in the years ahead.

Organizational disclosure and transparency is also closely related to self-regulation and to organizational autonomy, and thus in recent years we have seen the emergence of several forms of organizational disclosure. For foundations, information disclosure is required, and has been strengthened, under the Regulations on the Management of Foundations (2004), and through multiple implementing documents issued since. Information disclosure is now also accomplished through the China Charity Donation and Information Center (CCDIC), a mandated mechanism, and through a self-regulatory mechanism, the China Foundation Center. The multiple jurisdictions seeking information disclosure seem problematic to an outsider, but may not seem so from a Chinese view closer to the action.

The Roles of Key Party, Government, and Legislative Institutions

All of these regulatory shifts are led by several key government agencies and their leading officials, and—with inevitable institutional and organizational shifts— they will continue to be guided by such key agencies and officials in the future. There are a number of Chinese government agencies and individuals involved with formulating philanthropic sector policy and regulation. In the national government, the key ministry is the Ministry of Civil Affairs, which has primary responsibility for philanthropic and nonprofit policy and legal issues through at least four departments. The Ministry of Civil Affairs is generally responsible for the initial drafting of much of the non-tax regulation and legislation in the field. But other ministries are also crucially important in this process. They include, for tax issues, the Ministry of Finance and associated tax administration units and, on security issues, the Ministry of Public Security and Ministry of State Security. Other relevant ministries, such as the Ministry of Health, Ministry of Education, Ministry of Environmental Protection, Ministry of Commerce, Ministry of Foreign Affairs, State Administration of Foreign Exchange Control, National Audit Office, and others, weigh in on topics, regulations, and rules specific to their jurisdictions. It is in this context that the Ministry of Health is empowered to play a role in regulating significant areas of health philanthropy (including some activities of foreign foundations involved in health-related grant-making in China).

Above the Ministry of Civil Affairs and other ministries, the State Council reviews draft regulation and legislation on the philanthropic and nonprofit sector and has become increasingly assertive in formulating philanthropic policy above the to-and-fro of the ministries and agencies. Within the State Council, the State Council Legal Affairs Office is the crucial agency for review and promulgation of draft regulation, and review and forwarding of draft legislation to the National People's Congress. In addition to the legal research and drafting work of the Legal Affairs Office, other organizations within the State Council also contribute to philanthropy and nonprofit sector policy, including the Development Research Center of the State Council.

For national law on the philanthropic and nonprofit sector (including the draft Charity Law), the National People's Congress is the key site for debate and enactment. Within the National People's Congress, the Legislative Affairs Commission is primarily responsible for this research and drafting work. Review of draft legislation is conducted through the Law Committee of the National People's Congress and other substantive committees.

The Communist Party remains a crucially important site for policy on the social sector and philanthropy. A number of Communist Party organizations are involved in this policymaking process. They include the Central Propaganda Department, the Central Policy Research Office, the Central Compilation and Translation Bureau, and other Communist Party offices.

Reform Scenarios in Chinese Philanthropic Policy and Regulation

The best possible outcome for the intensive discussions of policy and regulatory reform in Chinese philanthropy would probably see the promulgation of revised and liberalized regulations on foundations, social organizations, and civil non-enterprise units that undertake a series of reforms, some of which have been pioneered at the local level, as well as a Charity Law that loosens restrictions on the sector. Under a best-case scenario, reforms that would benefit the entire philanthropic sector, including the domestic health philanthropy field, include:

- One-agency management of social organizations and foundations (which is occurring over time, as the dual management system erodes as a result of local experimentation and national reforms)
- Loosened restrictions on registering (legalizing) organizations
- Loosened restrictions on fundraising that allow social organizations (NGOs and nonprofits of various kinds) to raise funds from the public
- More relaxed restrictions on investments by foundations
- Substantially increased tax incentives for donors and nonprofits, and investment options for nonprofits
- Other reforms

But these scenarios are not all certain to occur. If none of the current proposals pass, China is left with a situation in which the current regulatory and policy framework is increasingly out of date and ineffective, unable to respond to rapid changes in the sector. That offers flexibility to the philanthropic sector, including health philanthropy, in the regulatory gaps. But it also offers risks, as the government and the Communist Party may be even more willing to step into those regulatory gaps with arbitrary decisions in the absence of an up-to-date legal framework. These matters should become clearer, with respect to the Foundation Regulations, the Charity Law, and other legal documents after the Party Congress scheduled for fall 2013. Eventually we can expect to see the revisions of the three key regulations (on foundations, social organizations, and civil non-enterprise institutions) adopted, along with the national framework Charity Law, and amendments that gradually provide greater tax benefits in terms of deductions for donors and exemptions for charitable organizations.

Beyond reforms in the current framework, policymakers and legal drafters are faced—one might say beset—with new forms of giving that have significantly strained regulatory capacity. These are directly relevant to health philanthropy, whether undertaken within China by domestic donors and organizations or from outside, via the diaspora or others. For example, online giving is growing rapidly in China, but with little policy or legal framework to control it. Yet new areas like online giving add regulatory actors to this list—in this case the government and policy regulators of online activity, social media, banking, and other relevant areas—making the policy and legal process even more complicated. Similarly, various forms of social enterprise are growing rapidly in China, another area directly relevant to health philanthropy. Here a somewhat different situation guides us, for Chinese social entrepreneurs have generally chosen one of a number of legal forms and channels for registration and operations, including commercial forms. Social enterprise-specific regulation is only now emerging at the national and subnational levels, but will likely accelerate in the years ahead.

Conclusion

China continues to pursue a nuanced if constrained policy toward the development of civil society and philanthropy. The policy and legal framework encourages the growth and, in some cases, registration of social service organizations and other groups undertaking activities favored by the state, while discouraging through a range of means the formation and activities of advocacy and other groups that the state disfavors. That policy of guided development is likely to continue. In the health arena, the focus of this volume, philanthropic and civil society groups working on medicine and health are likely to find complex but feasible channels to registration and activities, with the Chinese state continuing to monitor and channel activities toward state-approved goals. For foreign foundations and other organizations working in the health arena, a direct link to the Ministry of Health, provincial health bureaus, or Ministry of Health–related organizations is likely to be either necessary or highly facilitative for new or continuing activities. Health and medicine are areas in which the Chinese government is likely to continue to encourage engagement by domestic and foreign groups, and so while policy and legal processes are complex in China, the future should continue to allow such activities. As the past indicates, however, these policies and legal processes are complex and are subject to change and rebalancing, and domestic and foreign organizations working in the health arena in China must always continue to be aware of the policy and legal frameworks within which they work.

Notes

1. The development of domestic philanthropy is accompanied by continuing progress in foreign and diaspora giving to China as well. Though the Chinese diaspora and foreign foundations have been active in China since the end of the 1970s, accelerating in the 1980s and 1990s, significant new sources of both diaspora and foreign foundation giving have joined these streams in the past decade. They are dealt with in other chapters.

2. I am grateful to the China Medical Board, Beijing Normal University Capitol Philanthropy Research Institute, Golden Bridges, and the International Center for Not-for-Profit Law (ICNL) for support in enabling me to write this chapter and to attend the CMB/BNU workshops on health philanthropy in February and December 2012, and to Peter Geithner at CMB for commissioning it. This work has been supported by the University of Wisconsin-Madison, ICNL, and the MacArthur Foundation, none of which are responsible for views expressed here.

3. Specialists in Chinese philanthropic policy and regulation may find the treatment here overly abbreviated in some respects or more general than would be desired. For a more detailed treatment of these issues, see, e.g., Simon (2013). China Development Brief, based in Beijing, publishes very useful work on nonprofit and philanthropic policy and regulation in China as well.

4. Earlier Chinese Constitutions of 1954 (Article 87), 1975 (Article 28), and 1978 each included formal rights to freedom of association as well, in generally similar terms.

5. There is of course a wide array of regulatory documents on specific issues and subsectors, including in health—too many to list here, though the ICNL USIG Note and others provide a longer list. To offer just one example of the tendency to regulate on specific topics or subsectors as needed, we have—and many others could be mentioned—the Select Opinions of the General Office of the State Council on Accelerating and Promoting the Reform and Development of Trade Associations and Chambers of Commerce (2007).

6. There has also been some interest over the years, both in China and abroad, in the prospects for an estate tax in China and whether, if an estate tax were to be enacted, it would include a provision for charitable gifts and deductions. Inquiries in 2012 and 2013 produced a consistent response on this question: there have been discussions of an estate tax in China, and of charitable deductions as part of that, but no forward movement has been made on enacting an estate tax and no movement is expected for years to come, if at all. One senior official answered this question by saying, "People with significant interests and wealth are opposed to this and nothing is going to happen with it for the foreseeable future." Others interviewed concurred, indicating very clearly that they expected no movement on an estate tax for years to come and that there is no unanimity or confluence of views on it that would lead toward legislative action.

7. This list of issues to be resolved is derived from multiple conversations over a number of years in China, and extensive review of press sources, which now identify these issues on a frequent and frank basis.

8. The *Cishan cujinfa* is usually translated as "Charity Law" rather than using the complete terminology, which would come out as "Charity Promotion Law." A more complete translation of the title of the draft law might bring with it better foreign understanding of the purposes of the law, and thus some further thought on the criticisms that have been aimed at various drafts of it.

9. For an English translation of the September 15, 2006, draft of the Charity Law obtained by the U.S. Embassy from the American Chamber of Commerce in China, see http://dazzlepod.com/cable/07BEIJING3884/?rss=1. A draft marked September 15, 2006, was also provided to the International Center for Civil Society Law (ICCSL), which provided detailed "Comments on the Draft Charity Law of the People's Republic of China," *International Journal of Civil Society Law* 5, no. 1 (2007): 12–27. In 2008, the International Center for Not-for-Profit Law also obtained and provided detailed comments on a later draft of the law. I note, for those who may be interested, that somewhat similar drafting and a similar set of debates have been underway in Vietnam for many years on what is there called the Law on Associations (*Luat ve Hoi*). For more information on that, see, among other sources, Sidel (2010).

References

China Private Foundation Forum. 2010. "Self-Regulatory Principles for Private Foundations." http://gongyi.qq.com/a/20101027/000026.htm.

Hu, Xing. 2011. "Foundations Are Required to Publish Audit Reports." http://hausercenter.org/chinanpo/2011/12/foundations-are-required-to-publish-audit-reports.

ICNL (International Center for Not-for-Profit Law). 2013a. "United States International Grantmaking, China." http://www.usig.org/countryinfo/china.asp.

———. 2013b. "NGO Law Monitor: China." http://www.icnl.org/research/monitor/china.html.

Sidel, Mark. 2010. "Maintaining Firm Control: Recent Developments in Nonprofit Law and Regulation in Vietnam." *International Journal of Not-for-Profit Law* 12 (3) http://www.icnl.org/research/journal/vol12iss3/art_1.htm.

Simon, Karla. 2013. *Civil Society in China: The Legal Framework from Ancient Times to the "New Reform Era."* New York: Oxford University Press.

3 Changing Health Problems and Health Systems

Challenges for Philanthropy in China

Vivian Lin and Bronwyn Carter

Introduction

The World Health Organization (WHO) defines health as not merely the absence of disease, but also physical and mental well-being (WHO 1948). It also recognizes the importance of social and economic factors in shaping population health status (WHO 2008). Definitions of public health further recognize that the protection and improvement of health requires an organized effort by society (Lin et al. 2007). Thus, the health of a country or a community reveals not only the array of factors that determine the pattern of health and illness, but also the nature of the collective societal effort at improving the health of the population.

Between the 1940s and the late 1990s, life expectancy in China more than doubled, from 35 to 73 (Lin et al. 2010). The major burden of disease has also shifted from infectious to noncommunicable diseases (NCDs). The positive results reflect in part a more equitable path of social and economic development, and in part a shift from a highly chaotic health system to one with a strong degree of organization. In the past three decades, however, market-based economic reforms have led to the collapse of universal health care coverage, rising health inequities, and, ultimately, new comprehensive health system reforms announced in 2009. During this period of tremendous social and economic change, challenges and opportunities have emerged for the development of China's health system. The sector's actors, including health professionals, government policymakers, and development partners, are vital to the successful development of the system. Those concerned with health in civil society—both from within and outside China—also have critical roles to play in service provision and shaping the direction of change.

This chapter discusses China's health challenges, including the epidemiological and demographic transitions that have brought about new trends in disease, injuries, and risk factors. It then discusses the concerns and problems for China's health system in regard to current health care reforms and the changing burden of disease. The chapter then turns to philanthropy's contributions throughout the twentieth century and the increasing role of Chinese civil society in addressing these new health and health system challenges. It closes with a brief discussion of the obstacles and opportunities that government, civil society, and philanthropy meet in facing China's complex health landscape in the twenty-first century.

Health Challenges

China's Epidemiological Transition

Globally, the highest disease burden in developing countries results from traditional problems of communicable, maternal, perinatal, and nutritional disorders, whereas the highest disease burden in developed countries results from NCDs, including mental health and injury (WHO 2012). Few similar studies have been carried out in China (Zhou et al. 2011), but the burden of disease in China is now consistent with that of developed countries (Vos et al. 2012). With the improvement in health status in China resulting from a decline of infectious diseases and improved maternal and infant mortality, noncommunicable diseases began to emerge as the major cause of death (World Bank 1990). Chronic diseases now account for 80 percent of deaths and 70 percent of disability-adjusted life years (DALYs[1]) lost in China. Cardiovascular disease, cancer, and chronic respiratory disease are the top causes of burden of disease (See figure 3.1). These chronic NCDs are the major cause of mortality in both urban and rural China, and for both men and women. Moreover, rates of death from chronic disease in middle-aged people are higher in China than in some high-income countries. Identified risk factors for chronic disease in China are the same as those in developed countries, including low activity levels, overnutrition, and tobacco (Wang et al. 2005). Tobacco use is particularly high among males; in 2009, 51 percent of adult males in China smoked tobacco, compared to just 2 percent of adult females (World Bank 2012).

In addition to tobacco use, air pollution is also recognized as contributing to high rates of respiratory disease (Kan, Chen, and Hong 2009). Nonsmoking women living in the largest cities in China have been shown to have the highest rates of lung cancer ever recorded anywhere in the world among women who do not smoke (World Resources Institute 1998–1999). Air pollution in China is at much higher levels than in developed countries; therefore the importance of the increased health risk is even greater (Kan, Chen, and Hong 2009). After cardiovascular disease, cancer, and chronic respiratory disease, injury is the fourth-highest cause of death in China, but it causes greater loss of DALYs than those

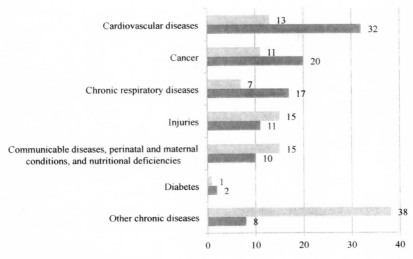

Cardiovascular diseases — 13 / 32

Cancer — 11 / 20

Chronic respiratory diseases — 7 / 17

Injuries — 15 / 11

Communicable diseases, perinatal and maternal conditions, and nutritional deficiencies — 15 / 10

Diabetes — 1 / 2

Other chronic diseases — 38 / 8

% DALYs lost (total 195.7 million)

% Deaths (total 10.3 million)

Figure 3.1. Estimated Proportions of Total Deaths and DALYs Lost for All Ages in China, 2005. *Source: Wang et al. (2005).*

diseases (See figure 3.1). The leading causes of high mortality and morbidity rates due to injury are suicide, road traffic injury, and drowning. The suicide rate in China is one of the highest in the world (Phillips, Liu, and Zhang 1999). Approximately 286,000 fatalities due to suicide occur each year, with the rate in rural areas three times the rate in urban areas (Phillips, Liu, and Zhang 1999) and with the majority of deaths resulting from the intentional ingestion of agricultural pesticide. China is one of only a few countries in the world where the female suicide rate is higher than that of men—it is estimated to be higher by as much as 25 percent (WHO 2009). As Ray Yip discusses in chapter 7, HIV/AIDS has been a public health concern for China since 1989—one in one thousand people between the ages of 15 and 49 are infected with HIV (World Bank 2012) and its prevalence is increasing (WHO 2006). In 2010, 20 to 39 percent of eligible people with HIV in China were receiving antiretroviral therapy (UNAIDS 2011).

China's Demographic Transition

Determinants of health in China, as in other countries, include social, political, environmental, and economic factors. Income, access to education and health care, environmental hazards, and social support are all underlying determinants of health status. Differences in disease prevalence between rural and urban populations in China, including HIV, injuries, and chronic diseases such as diabetes and cardiovascular and respiratory disease, reveal the extent to which these factors affect health outcomes.

The fundamental drivers of current health challenges for China include major demographic transitions such as an aging population, unprecedented urbanization caused by human migration out of rural areas into the cities, and growing income inequality. The Organisation for Economic Cooperation and Development (OECD) data for China for the years 2003–2010 show an increase in the percentage of the population over 65 years old, from 7.4 percent to 8.2 percent, and a decrease in the percentage of the population aged zero to 14, from 23.3 percent to 19.5 percent (OECD 2012). In addition to this rising longevity combined with low fertility, the urban population is quickly increasing as millions of migrant workers, China's "floating population," flock to the cities seeking employment. The 2010 census showed that China's urban and rural populations were approximately 666 million and 674 million, respectively, which is approximately 50 percent each. This reflects a 14-percentage-point increase in the urban population over a period of 10 years (Ma 2011). If this trend continues as currently projected, China's urban population will easily reach over 60 percent by 2020, according to China's 12th Five-Year Plan.

In addition to an increasing income gap between urban and rural areas, there have also been increasing intraregional gaps within rural areas and within urban areas, with the income gap within urban areas increasing more than the gap within rural areas (Wu and Perloff 2005, Chen and Ravallion 2007). The Gini index measures the gap between actual variations in income for each household and a hypothetical line of absolute income equality. During the period 1980–2000, when the national income distribution gap increased by 12 points, the increase in the gap was larger in urban areas (14 points) and lower in rural areas (11 points) (figure 3.2).

The demographics of income inequality show that access to health care, housing, and education is an issue of special importance for millions of children in rural China as well as migrant children living in urban areas. Out of around 367 million children, approximately 50 million live in poverty, 570,000 are orphans, more than 20 million are migrant children without access to basic survival needs and health care, and 58 million rural children are left behind with relatives while their parents migrate to the city to work (Save the Children 2011).

China's Changing Health Care System

Twentieth-Century Successes

The social and political chaos of the first half of the twentieth century took its toll on the health of the population as well as the structure for health administration in the young Republic of China. By 1949, the Chinese health system was characterized by inadequacy and misdistribution of health resources and underdevelop-

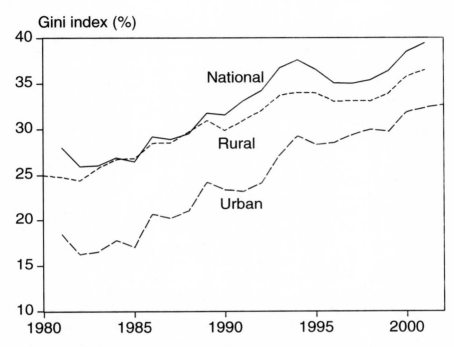

Figure 3.2. Income Inequality in Rural and Urban Areas and Nationally. *Source: Chen and Ravallion (2007).*

ment of public health infrastructure (Lin et al. 2010). After 1949, under top-down government leadership and control, marked improvements in population health as well as in health policy development occurred as the government organized the health care system through central planning mechanisms. Between the 1930s and the 1970s, life expectancy in China improved from 35 years to 65 years (63 for males and 66 for females) (Lin et al. 2010). This extraordinary achievement relates to both political and social stability, as well as the health policy framework established by the Chinese government under the Communist Party. Near-universal health insurance coverage achieved during this time is credited with contributing to improved health outcomes. During the 1970s, urban workers could count on health care as part of their so-called "iron rice bowl" of social services provided by the state while the rural cooperative medical service (CMS), with basic health services provided by the "barefoot doctors" at the village level, covered an estimated 90 percent of the rural population (World Bank 2005).

Implementation of health policy and health outcomes achieved during this period relied largely on the vertical hierarchical system (Zhao 2005) and the prevailing administrative culture of political solidarity and practices of the planned economy. Under the ideological framework of equity, health care was to be widely available, accessible, and affordable for all. Ethical indoctrination ensured conformity to what was thought to be good practice and good behavior. For example, the Patriotic Health Campaign that began in the 1950s facilitated multisectoral social mobilization, which was the key to tackling environmental health and infectious disease problems. The main efforts were directed to improving water and sanitation, vector control for infectious diseases, and personal hygiene (Lin et al. 2010).

Regionalized health care delivery systems established in urban and rural areas built upon the collective enterprises in each setting, such as state-owned enterprises in the cities and people's communes in the countryside, and linked the different levels through clinical referrals and supervision. Low-cost basic primary care was made accessible, financially and geographically, through the wide dispersion of health care workers with basic training. A major campaign to spread health care to rural settings sent doctors to the countryside in the late 1960s through the early 1980s. These barefoot doctors were the predecessors to today's village doctors, who still provide basic medical services, but of whom there is a dearth due to lack of both adequate infrastructure and financial incentives to practice medicine in rural areas. All things considered, China's basic socialist health care system was dismantled without a commensurate replacement. Within a 30-year period, due to failed attempts to share health care responsibility through a mix of planning and market approaches, health care—from the village to the city level—has been severely hindered by both high-cost, limited access, and the corollary problem of quality of care.

Challenges of Reform

During the transition out of a planned economy in the 1980s through China's market-based economic reforms, new problems associated with high health care costs and distorted financing arrangements at the system level emerged out of China's previously successful health care system. An upheaval of the primary health care system caused the breakdown of equal access to health care for urban and rural areas. The dismantling of the commune system led to the collapse of primary health care in rural areas, as there was no longer a system for mobilizing finances and organizing health care delivery. Some barefoot doctors who had previously provided low-cost medical care in rural areas drifted into cities or away from medical work, while others became private village doctors reliant on user fees and drug profits. Public hospitals became the mainstay of China's medical institutions, whereby changes in financing turned health care providers into profit-seekers, resulting in so-called "public identity, private behavior." Perverse incentives at the system level that encouraged inappropriate sales of medication and overservicing by doctors reflected the tension between the imperative to earn revenue and public subsidization (Zhao 2005).

Inadequate government financing of health care due to fiscal decentralization and corporatization of state-owned enterprises during the economic restructuring process also ushered in the first stage of reforms to the health care system. The Chinese Ministry of Health was tasked with increasing hospital efficiency while being confronted with decreasing government financing. In attempting to manage these challenges, such policies as the reintroduction of private practice, increased pricing of services, implementation of service contracts, and allowing sideline commercial activities were aimed at getting hospitals to focus on recovering costs and increasing income by expanding revenue (Gu et al. 1993). Consequently, charges increased for patients, with doctors favoring multiple prescriptions (drugs allow profit margins of up to 15 percent), increased use of diagnostic tests, new medical technologies, and extended hospital stays (Lin and Zhao 2008). Health workers were given performance incentives by their institutions to make up for low salaries (Bloom 2001), such as bonuses related to raising revenue. One significant unintended consequence has been the growing distrust and tensions between doctors and patients, with increasing episodes of violence against doctors in hospitals—over 17,000 cases in 2010 alone. High-cost yet poor-quality care is a crisis for both the medical profession and sick patients seeking care (Hesketh et al. 2012).

In addition to these deficiencies in medical service provisions, medical insurance was also affected. By 1993, less than 10 percent of the rural population had health insurance (World Bank 2005), and by 2003, more than 70 percent of the total population was without any health insurance coverage. Between 1986 and 2002, the share of government spending on health declined from 39 percent to 16 percent while personal spending on health increased accordingly. Rural-urban disparities worsened. Migrants from rural areas flocking into the cities for work had no entitlement to services but often found themselves in risky work environments, including construction, factories, and prostitution. By 2004, almost 80 percent of government spending on health was allocated to urban institutions, even though city dwellers represented only 42 percent of the country's population (Huang 2011). It was not just the number of people covered by health insurance which fell—by 1998 nearly half the urban population lacked health insurance—but the depth of coverage also declined. By 1997, more than one-third of inpatient costs for insured patients were out-of-pocket expenses, resulting in decreased access for those with lower incomes (World Bank 2005) and catastrophic health costs for an increasing number of people. Between 20 and 50 percent of those who fell into poverty in rural areas did so because of health care costs.

During this period of failed health system changes, inter- and intraregional health inequalities began to reflect the inequitable distribution of health resources, particularly in terms of the availability and accessibility of primary health care services (Fang et al. 2010). Old problems reemerged—tuberculosis (TB), schistosomiasis, vaccine-preventable illnesses, and sexually transmitted infections (STIs)—while the gains in maternal and infant mortality were beginning to be reversed (Lee et al. 2003).

By the late 1990s, the government began to grapple with the problems in the health system in a second stage of health reforms. Recognizing that health care was a matter of public welfare, along with the need to balance social and economic benefits, a series of reforms were introduced through pilot programs. The reform pilots included licensing doctors, regulating drug prices, urban health insurance, a health safety net to protect the very poor from catastrophic health costs, creating regional health planning and health surveillance, supporting rural facilities and cooperatives, strengthening community health services, providing general practitioner (GP) training, and increasing contributions to the new rural health insurance scheme from provincial and local governments.

While some of the pilots during this ten-year period were successful, and programs were disseminated to multiple locations, there was little impact on the health system as a whole. The reforms were implemented in a piecemeal manner and failed to curb the rising popular discontent with the increasing cost and poor quality of health care (Fang, Chen, and Rizzo 2009; Song 2008). Improvements in reestablishing rural cooperative medical services were difficult to sustain while rural-urban disparities grew even further. None of the reforms could begin to tackle the new health challenges of noncommunicable diseases.

In 2002, with concern for social harmony and an overall policy framework based on "people-centered development" and the "Five Balances" (urban/rural, coastal/hinterland, social/economic development, built/natural environment, and external/internal markets), the government announced new policies in relation to rural cooperatives, and health insurance for the very poor and urban residents. At the same time, government funding was provided to strengthen public health surveillance and a range of public health treatment programs. The advent of China's SARS epidemic, along with a change of government administration in 2003, provided the impetus for more serious deliberations of system-wide reforms. Poor infection control helped spread the infection in a primary-care system dominated by hospitals. Structural weaknesses in the system were identified, such as lack of coordination due to fragmentation and territoriality, lack of resources, and poor communication of risk. The fragility of the health system was the result of earlier economic reforms of hospitals and public health institutions. This weakened capacity had been recognized in the 1990s, but the government did not address it with system-wide reforms of the health sector. SARS also demonstrated how the tradition of community-based political mobilization in earlier public health efforts had not been lost (Liu 2003), such as the multisectoral structure of the Patriotic Health Campaign. Such community-based interventions are not without historical precedent in China, where government's relationship with international and domestic philanthropy and civil society—from cooperation to suppression and now control—has varied. Nevertheless, the interests and actions of these groups have laid the foundation for China's health system today.

Philanthropy's Contributions to Health Systems Challenges

Early Foundations

Chinese medical texts reveal patterns of health and illness in China in the late Qing dynasty and early Republican periods were not dissimilar to European countries of the same time, with major problems related to infectious diseases, infant and maternal mortality, and malnutrition, along with natural disasters, famine, war, and civil conflict (Lin et al. 2010). Droughts as well as floods in China in the late nineteenth and early twentieth centuries resulted in major famines, poverty, and loss of life. From 1876 to 1879, during the worst famine in imperial Chinese history, tens of millions of people died due to the absence of an organized response—by government or the commercial sector—to natural disasters and lack of food reserves. In the 1900s, government action helped to reduce the impact of famine through the extension of railway networks. When droughts and floods caused poverty and triggered mass migration, successful emigrants sent help back home via train.

During the nineteenth and twentieth centuries, within the context of political disruptions and the absence of an organized governmental response to public health challenges such as infant mortality, famine, malnutrition, and the impact of natural disasters, Western philanthropic organizations helped to develop systematic approaches to and established infrastructure for medicine and public health in China to address these issues. The efforts of Western philanthropic organizations such as the Rockefeller Foundation and the United Church of Canada introduced new ways of providing health care, namely, establishing Western medicine and its associated organizational forms, and as such helped to lay the foundation for China's health system of today. Western-style institutions offered new service models for the provision of primary care and public health services and developed a generation of health practitioners and health leaders in China. Significant early developments with wider implications for the development of the health care system include the introduction of Western medicine, development of hospitals, training of the medical and nursing workforce, knowledge and technology transfer in areas such as surgery and public health, and the development of service models used in hospitals, primary care clinics, and public health service.

Western philanthropy inspired participation from the local Chinese philanthropic community as well. As treaty settlements led to the growth of missionaries and the establishment of missionary hospitals and the popularity of Western hospitals grew, Protestant medics won over the support of indigenous authorities and merchants, whose charitable giving also contributed to the establishment of missionary medicine in the nineteenth century (Kalusa 2008). Missionary hospitals practicing Western medicine led to the establishment of connected educational institutions. Doctors who trained and practiced medicine in connection with missionary hospitals came to earn the trust of the local population through their skills in surgery and public health and mediated the interests between the Chinese and foreign communities (Chapman and Plumb 2001). Because of Western philanthropic investments and focus on training, Chinese medical leaders of the time were products of Western medical education. The knowledge transfer between American institutions and Chinese scientists and educators was important in establishing foundational perspectives in life sciences (Dikötter 2004).

The Rockefeller Foundation was particularly important among Western philanthropic and educational institutions in the development of medical and nursing education in the first part of the twentieth century. The Peking Union Medical College (PUMC), founded by Protestant missionaries in 1906, provided the training basis for Western medicine and the model for medical education (Brown 1979; Legge, Lin, and Guo 2010). The United Church of Canada was actively involved in China from the early 1890s and established many hospitals and universities continuing in China today, and through its mission-inspired philanthropy has provided training in medicine as well as nursing, dentistry, and pharmacy, as well as medical treatment to thousands of people. Moreover, it has undertaken public health initiatives serving a wide array of interests in Chinese society.

Civil society action on health and social development was not limited to missionary, charitable, and educational organizations. During the 1800s, the nature of opium addiction as a public health concern was debated between colonial governments, overseas reformists, and Chinese citizens (Baumler 2007). In 1899, anti-opium crusaders mobilized over one hundred physicians, denouncing the opium trade on public health grounds. In 1938, a government-instigated treatment and rehabilitation effort was unsuccessful in eradicating the widespread use of opium. A civil society organization, the Society for the Elimination of Opium Trade, mobilized Chinese citizens arguing for prohibition simply on moral grounds. Through the organized action of various Chinese anti-opium groups working together, state-run opium farms were abolished (Baumler 2007). The successful role of the society in the abolition of opium farms is an example of strong Chinese civil society participation in combating a public health problem in Republican China. During this period, various organized civil society groups were active, addressing issues for rural workers and for women, such as the anti-foot binding league. Professional groups were also active, such as the Guangzhou Municipal Doctors Union, which promoted public sanitation (Fitzgerald 1996).

Another example of successful public action during this period is the collective action of both native physicians and modern doctors' associations in the battle for the legitimization of native medicine. This debate was held in the public sphere, through newspapers, professional journals and meetings, open letters, and public rallies. Both groups built voluntary associations, lobbied government officials, and shaped public opinion (Xu 1997).

Beginning in 1949, for 40 years there was little role for nongovernment input, nor was there a role for philanthropy in the health system over this period, other than the following: welfare assistance for the very poor in the tradition of mutual help; the beginnings of corporate philanthropy whereby Chinese entrepreneurs donated to government welfare projects and gained political access and social status in exchange (Ma and Parish 2006); and overseas Chinese projects for improvements in ancestral localities.

System Preparedness for New Health Challenges

Although the burden of NCDs has been around for several decades, there has been limited government action as NCDs have been viewed as an inevitable part of old age. Similarly, there has been a lack of initiative regarding sexually transmitted infections (STIs), HIV/AIDS, drug abuse, and road and industrial accidents, because, even though they are on the rise, they have been seen as the problems of recalcitrant individuals. Yet international evidence points to these issues not as individual problems but rather as problems with social roots, with patterns of distribution reflecting daily social and economic conditions of different groups in society (Brunner and Marmot 2006; WHO 2008).

Recent health reforms announced in 2009 begin to address widespread popular concerns about the cost and quality of health care, particularly equitable access to primary health care and preventive services. The reforms restate previous concerns, but have concentrated previous efforts in a more systematic manner in relation to health insurance for urban residents; medical cooperatives for rural dwellers; assistance for those living in poverty in both urban and rural areas; public health services including maternal and child health care, immunization, and mental health; aged care and chronic disease management; community health services integrated with Chinese medicine; an essential drug list; and hospital reforms (Xinhua 2009). There was also further recognition of the need for action on regional planning, budgeting, pricing, provider regulation, information systems, health laws, research, and workforce.

The policy reform process behind the reforms was innovative, with an open process that included both public consultation and debate, as well as input from domestic and international experts. The government released a white paper in 2008 for public discussion, which stimulated extensive debate in a variety of media and forums (Lin 2011). However, the question remains as to the capability of a top-down health care system in meeting the needs of special and vulnerable population groups and the complex social and health issues that are emerging in a changing Chinese society. Continuing health challenges for China indicate an ongoing role for philanthropic and civil society organizations in addressing current public health issues.

Opportunities for International Philanthropy and the Rising Role of Chinese Civil Society

After a lacuna for philanthropy in China during the heyday of collectivism in socialist China (discussed in chapter 1 by Wang Zhenyao and Zhao Yanhui) international philanthropy and development organizations began to again exert influence in China in the 1980s (Legge, Lin, and Guo 2010). In the last two decades of the twentieth century, the World Bank has become the most significant external influence on China's health system, through its substantial loans for multisite projects, as well as its highly influential analytical reports, which identified options for policy and service delivery reform and tested models that were adopted as policy. UN agencies have also played important roles in addressing health challenges, for example UNICEF's aid to improve maternal and child health; WHO's technical support in infectious disease surveillance, prevention, and control; and from the 1990s, UNAIDS's work in HIV/AIDS prevention and control (WHO 2011). World Bank projects introduced into China's health care system regional health planning and health promotion (World Bank 2005), both of which required a systems perspective and working across sectors. Moreover, these international aid agencies partnered with Chinese domestic resources. World Bank and UK Department for International Development (DFID) projects related to HIV (Lin and Yates 2009), and later the Global Fund for AIDS, Tuberculosis and Malaria, enlisted participation by Chinese domestic grassroots organizations. World Bank health sector projects also incorporated participation by non–health sector actors (such as women's federations) through "democratic" structures and peer education. Social assessment and participatory arrangements were introduced as mandatory project features, to address gender and equity issues.

In reproductive health, Ford Foundation seeded notable projects outside of government, which led to further involvement in family planning, promotion of human rights for people living with or at risk of HIV/AIDS, sex education, and gender issues in a range of settings. In the late 1990s, Ford partnered with the World Bank and DFID to scale up its successful models in reproductive health for poverty-stricken counties in central and western China (Ford Foundation 2013).

Since the 1990s, foreign philanthropies and international nongovernmental organizations (NGOs) have increased their presence, largely working on specific health issues rather than health sector development while the civil society sector in China has been undergoing substantial and complex changes. Although increased regulation by government of the charity sector is seen as beneficial in increasing transparency, concerns have been expressed that recent changes to the law may be counterproductive, such as a requirement to publish reports about income every three months during a fundraising drive, a ban on profit-making, and a ban on endorsing any business or commercial product (Chen 2012; Yu 2012). But the emergence of private foundations and social enterprises has created new opportunities for funding nonprofit endeavors, government has begun purchasing public services from NGOs (Wang 2011), and opportunities for cooperation with the international community are developing. These trends point to ongoing growth in the civil sector (Shieh 2011). Most philanthropic organizations work in a limited number of localities or with vulnerable populations in more disadvantaged areas. Some organizations, such as Save the Children, are working at national and provincial levels in partnership with government bodies such as the Ministry of Foreign Affairs, Ministry of Civil Affairs, and education and health bureaus, as well as with civil society organizations, to address the health needs of rural and migrant children. Similarly, the Environmental Defense Fund, headquartered in the United States, is now working with government officials in China on economic incentives and proposed changes to air pollution laws (EDF 2012). By 2005, international philanthropic funding had reached $229 million (China Daily 2005), which included $134 million for HIV/AIDS from the Global Fund to Fight AIDS, Tuberculosis and Malaria, which provided $14 million to strengthen civil society organizations' ability to reach high-risk populations (Bates and Okie 2007). There is also an unmet need for more widely available modern treatments for opiate dependence in China, which presents another opportunity for philanthropic assistance (Tang et al. 2006).

With China's opening up after over three decades of market-oriented reforms, philanthropy and civil society groups are playing an increasing role in public health. Philanthropic organizations have made significant contributions to medical education reform, the development of service models in response to local health needs, capacity building such as leadership training, the development of policy models such as regional planning and health insurance, and multisectoral and consultative policy research. Valuable experiences in these fields have been gained, indicating that successful particular service models can be used as models for new projects, programs can be targeted to address equity and the needs of vulnerable groups, successful pilot programs can be scaled up, and NGOs can foster community participation. Capacity building, both of institutions and health workers, remains the most lasting contribution. New ways of working and particular projects undertaken by official donors and philanthropic organizations are summarized in table 3.1.

Many of the service models adopted in the new health reforms developed in response to China's changing epidemiological profile have been supported by projects and training programs that began in the 1990s with donor support,

Table 3.1. Notable Late Twentieth-Century Contributions of Philanthropy/Donors

Projects/Issues—International NGOs	Ways of Working
• Reproductive health—Ford Foundation • Health promotion—World Bank, AusAID • HIV/AIDS—UNAIDS, World Bank, UK DFID, Ford Foundation • Rural health (including health safety net)—World Bank • Urban community health (including basic health insurance)—UK DFID • Health system reform—UK DFID • Academic/research partnerships—World Bank Institute, Harvard, IDS, La Trobe, Yale	• Multisite/ large scale • Multistakeholder (central/local, multiple sectors, academics) • Capacity building—new concepts and skills for people working within existing institutions • Capacity building—new concepts and skills for people working within existing institutions • Evaluation of pilots and policy engagement/advocacy • Donor collaboration

such as health promotion and programs for HIV/AIDS. Stand-alone programs addressing specific health issues such as maternal and child health, reproductive health, TB, and schistosomiasis have offered new approaches for old problems. Programs addressing equity and the needs of vulnerable groups have been scaled up from pilots seeded by donors, including providing a health security safety net for the very poor. NGOs have been quite active in health promotion, notably in response to specific health issues and events and in mobilizing community participation in response to gaps occurring in the health system.

Donors have also been important in supporting policy change, particularly the new health reforms announced in 2009. As debate raged between ministries about appropriate measures for health sector reform, DFID funded a unique project called Health Policy Support Project (HPSP) (UK Department for International Development 2012), which provided critical and strategic support for the health sector reform process, including a platform for dialogue between China and international organizations about health reforms and between researchers and policymakers on evidence for health policy, along with the development of positive informal relationships between ministries (Lin and Yates 2009). In particular, the project ensured there was a forum for pro-poor policy stakeholders to dialogue, and therefore a pro-poor focus was maintained throughout the policy process. This made it a rather unique process for social policymaking in China.

Philanthropy has been growing, particularly in support of civil society organizations. Notable NGOs involved in China in recent years include the China Foundation, supporting the development of rural health centers and addressing problems such as hepatitis B; the Soros Foundation, supporting civil society involvement in AIDS/HIV; and the Bloomberg Foundation and the China Medical

Board, funding projects in tobacco control (Legge, Lin, and Guo 2010). The Bill & Melinda Gates Foundation has committed $57 million for HIV prevention efforts, $33 million toward TB testing and treatment in 2009, and $24 million for tobacco control (Bill & Melinda Gates Foundation 2009). The Narada Foundation, a domestic Chinese philanthropy, has been providing grants for social innovation projects funded by wealthy Chinese donors, with a particular focus on education for migrant children (Nicholas 2012).

The Sichuan earthquake of 2008, the worst in China in 30 years, further unleashed corporate philanthropy, as well as charity action from the citizenry. In response, 703 companies, 47 percent of those listed in the Chinese stock market, donated more than $645 million in cash and goods (Zhang et al. 2010).

Charitable giving is increasing in China: the average donation from the most generous one hundred donors was $16 million in 2012, having increased fivefold since 2004 (Hurun Report 2012). The first charity hospital opened in Hangzhou in 2007, followed in 2012 by a second. The Beijing Smile Angel Hospital is supported by a foundation established by the parents of a child born with a cleft palate, following their experiences trying to get treatment (this is discussed further in chapter 12). This general children's hospital is financed mainly through donations and is staffed by 180 doctors and nurses, 10 percent of whom are volunteers. The 13 board members are each required to donate 1.5 million RMB ($235,000) per year for the first five years (Yang 2012). These efforts, along with the revival of Buddhist philanthropy, may reflect a delayed response to the state's disengagement from the social sector (Laliberté 2009) as well as the development of a more open and pluralist society. More than two hundred NGOs are now listed as working in China in public health–related fields (China Development Brief n.d.). Grassroots NGOs now operate in almost every sector in China.

Local programs supported by overseas charities help to address social determinants of health for particular population groups. For example, since 2007, laid-off impoverished workers in Qingyuan's rural areas, most of whom are females, have been assisted by Give2Asia through the provision of loans and technical training (Give2Asia 2013). In this way, the provision of social services enables this group to be gainfully employed, prevents detrimental health effects associated with unemployment and poverty, and improves health outcomes for this population group.

Another example of philanthropic activity in China that addresses social determinants of health and where there is potential for ongoing further development is the cooperative movement. Since the 1930s in China, cooperatives have served workers and local communities, mostly in industrial and agricultural production, enabling safe and productive employment and promoting health. Recent changes to the law in China are facilitating the work of cooperatives. With legal recognition and political support, they can operate in an established network, although the current law is limited to agricultural cooperatives (Ware 2011). The

International Committee for the Promotion of Chinese Industrial Cooperatives, originally named Gung Ho (ICCIC 2013) and supported now by international donors, aims to promote further laws that would apply to other parts of the economy and is now working in rural primary health care, offering education and training in health promotion to rural women. The New Zealand China Friendship Society, together with the New Zealand government, contributed funds to rural health cooperative projects. In 2001, the Women's Cooperative Health Center was established in Songjia Village at the Kathleen Hall ICCIC Clinic. Hundreds of women have participated in preventive health training.

Government-sponsored philanthropy—so-called government-organized nongovernmental organizations, or GONGOs, discussed by Deng Guosheng and Zhao Xiaoping in part III of this volume—has been increasingly operating in partnership with private domestic donors in the field of health philanthropy. For example, the quasi-governmental philanthropy China Soong Ching Ling Foundation (CSCLF) has begun to work in the health sector in poverty areas as well. Seven of the top eight listed donors of CSCLF support health- and poverty-related needs. These include: pediatric medical research sponsored by an overseas car manufacturer; tertiary education for women from various ethnic groups sponsored by a Chinese technology company; health and welfare services for children and families funded by an international fast food charity; education for schoolchildren sponsored by a Chinese bottled water company and overseas movie star; programs for the integration of intellectually and physically disabled children sponsored by Taiwan's second-largest financial holding company; education, public health, and medical services in rural and urban areas funded by a Chinese transport-related company; and earthquake recovery for children funded by a Chinese car company (China Soong Ching Ling Foundation n.d.).

Implications for the Future

The solutions to China's current and future health challenges are likely to rest with a partnership across government sectors as well as between government, civil society, and philanthropy. Lessons from the past may well inform the role of philanthropy in the future.

The current demographic and epidemiological transitions (aging, urbanization, and migration) pose many challenges for the Chinese health system. Healthy aging requires not only access to health care throughout the course of one's life (Gu, Zhang, and Zeng 2009), but also other positive social and economic conditions—including education, employment, secure housing and retirement income, social support, and opportunities for social participation. Migrant workers need access to health care as well as social welfare, housing, and psychological support (Wei et al. 2009). Occupational rehabilitation service system development for the injured and disabled needs to be based on bio-psychosocial and work disability prevention models (Tang et al. 2011). Injury prevention requires engineering controls, state regulation, and strategic communication to influence changes in behavior, as well as responsive emergency services. The prevention and control of noncommunicable diseases need a well-coordinated continuum of care across the health system—with primary prevention involving schools, community organizations and workplaces, early detection and management in the primary care setting, and self-management and self-help groups in the community setting, along with cost-effective treatment in acute care as needed (World Bank 2011). Community-based outreach and peer support services have been shown to be effective for people with HIV/AIDS and drug problems. People with mental health problems need not only legal protection and sensitive services from the health system, but also the removal of stigma in order to receive the community support they require.

The essential public health service package announced as part of the 2009 national health system reforms starts to address some of these concerns, such as aging and mental health. The current reforms may improve health service delivery by lowering the financial barriers to health care access, but given the top-down nature of the system, it is questionable how well the system is prepared to offer new service models that are person-centered and community-based. The extent to which responsive, people-centered health services based on multidisciplinary teams can be offered depends not only on the financing and regulatory incentives in the system, but also on the way in which the health workforce is educated and socialized (WHO 2007) and how the health providers relate to the broader community system, including NGOs and social care organizations. Whether health and social services can be seamlessly coordinated for the most needy population groups is a further challenge for a system that has traditionally been run on the basis of vertical programs and strong territorial battles across ministries.

These health challenges are fundamentally social challenges. Actions on social determinants of health require a collective effort, rather than government acting alone. An increasing number of grassroots organizations have been complementing the work of Chinese GONGOs, whether related to cancer, diabetes, or AIDS self-help (Mok 2001; Wilson and Gyi 2010). Local individual and corporate philanthropy have also been on the rise, variously acting out of social responsibility, communal relationship building, enlightened self-interest, or reputation management (Ho and Hallahan 2004).

In this space of emerging health challenges and the changing nature of government–civil society relations, the philanthropic sector will thrive and fill crucial roles. Philanthropy in the past has shown that it can fill the gaps to develop and pilot new service models, update and refresh health personnel education, support partnership approaches between sectors and civil society organizations,

Table 3.2. Contribution of Philanthropy

Pre-Liberation (before 1949)	Post–Economic Reforms (after 1980)
• Introduction of Western medicine • Infrastructure—hospitals • Medical and nursing workforce • Knowledge and technology transfer—surgery, public health • Service models—hospitals, public health, primary care	• System reconstruction—medical education • Service models—emergency services, community health/GPs, rehabilitation, health promotion (IEC and settings) • Capacity building, leadership development, and institutional strengthening—training, study tours • Policy models—regional planning, health safety net, health insurance • Safe policy space—multisectoral, consultative, policy research

and demonstrate innovative strategies that can make a difference to health and social equity and prepare for and tackle new health and social challenges.

Both earlier and contemporary history of philanthropic involvement suggest that the contributions of philanthropy include introducing new concepts about health care and new service models, maintaining a focus on equity issues, and fostering the development of civil society organizations. Key contributions of philanthropic organizations and donors in the first part and following the economic reforms of the 1980s are suggested in table 3.2.

Conclusion

The twentieth century has seen extraordinary transformations in the health status of China's population, as well as the evolution of China's health care system. International philanthropies, including missionaries and educational institutions, laid the foundation for the development of China's health system and health workforce of today. While the Chinese government has taken the lead since 1949 in the transformation of health and health care institutions, international donors, including philanthropies, have continued to transfer knowledge (Legge, Lin, and Guo 2010), just as domestic and international philanthropies played a role in the earlier part of the twentieth century. From the late 1800s to the late 1900s, Western philanthropies debated the emphasis of their work—relief or long-term development; elitist education or grassroots support; capital and technology gifts or institution-building (Minden 1989). The legacy that remains is one of capacity building and institutional development. Particularly since the last part of the twentieth century, through pilot projects and time-limited programs, donor and philanthropic organizations have introduced further new concepts, models, and techniques in health care delivery. They have also fostered the development of NGOs working on health issues, and advocated for attention to health equity.

The role of civil society can be expected to become even more important as the new health challenges experienced by China are also shared in many other countries. The health reforms of 2009 are paving the way for a health care system that is better prepared to address the challenges of prevention, primary care, equitable access, and chronic disease. Removing financial barriers to access and providing public funding of essential public health services are key measures to address equity and population health improvement, and these are appropriately accompanied by other health system strengthening measures, such as regional health planning, legislation and regulation, and workforce education. Yet the health challenges of the twenty-first century are likely to exceed the capacity of any government, as they are also rooted in the broader social and economic changes that are part and parcel of China's transition to a more globalized economy and society. Facilitating learning between sectors and countries will be a new contribution by philanthropy to China in the twenty-first century.

With the aim of reducing the death rates from chronic disease, China can benefit from successes in developed countries in addressing lifestyle risk factors and broader social determinants of health. Similarly, approaches used overseas to achieve gains in STI, HIV/AIDS, drug abuse, and road and industrial accidents can be shared. Working in partnership with local universities, philanthropies could provide consultation on the development of innovative program models, support research such as evaluation of pilot programs, and provide teaching to update health personnel education.

Philanthropies can continue to work in partnership with government and civil society, within China and also in the global health policy arena, participating in intersectoral dialogue and engaging in policy debates at the global level. Philanthropies can contribute to capacity building for local charity groups. Projects operating across sectors can be developed and supported, with the aim of addressing social determinants of health such as the increasing income gaps within and between rural and urban areas.

In addressing the health challenges of the future for China, local social organizations and international philanthropies in China have a particular contribution to make. Working in partnership and complementing the role of government and business in the current health reforms, the philanthropic sector in China can pilot new service models and help strengthen the connection between health and social care, thereby enabling the provision of person-centered programs responsive to local community needs. Strategic investments from the philanthropy sector can help break down the funding and organizational silos that exist within and between the health and social welfare systems, and open up space for social and health innovation from civil society organizations. Outcomes from such projects will contribute knowledge to other countries facing similar public health challenges and more broadly to global health policy development. The challenge in a more open and pluralist China, however, is whether new models can be as easily scaled up, be as influential, and have as much transformational influence as those in the last century.

Note

1. DALYs are calculated by the sum of years of life lost due to premature mortality (YLLs) and years lived with disability (YLDs); they reflect the number of individuals who die or have nonfatal illness or impairment (Murray et al. 2012).

References

Bates, Gill, and Susan Okie. 2007. "China and HIV—A Window of Opportunity." *New England Journal of Medicine* 356:1801–1805.

Baumler, Alan. 2007. *The Chinese and Opium under the Republic: Worse than Floods and Wild Beasts.* Albany: State Universtiy of New York Press.

Bill & Melinda Gates Foundation. 2009. "China Office Fact Sheet." http://docs.gates foundation.org/global-health/documents/china-office-fact-sheet.pdf.

Bloom, Gerald. 2001. "Equity in Health in Unequal Societies: Meeting Health Needs in Contexts of Social Change." *Health Policy* 57 (3): 205–224.

Brown, E. Richard. 1979. *Rockefeller Medicine Men: Medicine and Capitalism in America.* Berkeley: University of California Press.

Brunner, Eric, and Michael Marmot. 2006. "Social Organization, Stress, and Health." In *Social Determinants of Health,* edited by Michael Marmot and Richard G. Wilkinson, 6–30. Oxford: Oxford University Press.

Chapman, Nancy E., and Jessica C. Plumb. 2001. *The Yale-China Association: A Centennial History.* Hong Kong: China University Press.

Chen Shaohua, and Martin Ravallion. 2007. "China's (Uneven) Progress against Poverty." *Journal of Development Economics* 82:1–42.

Chen Weijun. 2012. "Government Wants More Transparency, i.e. More Control over NGOs." http://www.asianews.it/news-en/Government-wants-more-transparency,-i.e.-more -control-over-NGOs-25456.html.

China Daily. 2005. "New Rules to Combat AIDS Spread." http://www.china.org.cn/english /government/146791.htm.

China Development Brief. n.d. "Directory of International NGOs (DINGO): China Development Brief's Database of over 200 International NGOs Operating in China." Accessed August 2013. http://nickyoung.chinadevelopmentbrief.com/dingo/.

China Medical Board. n.d. "China Programs." Accessed August 2013. http://www.china medicalboard.org/index.php?option=com_content&view=article&id=54&Itemid=152.

China Soong Ching Ling Foundation. n.d. "Charity and Welfare." Accessed August 2013. http://sclf.cri.cn/commonweal.htm.

Dikötter, Frank. 2004. "Biology and Revolution in Twentieth-Century China by Laurence Schneider." *China Quarterly* 180:1114–1115.

Environmental Defense Fund. 2012. "EDF's Beijing Office Helps China Merge Its Goals: China's Challenge; Growth with Less Pollution." http://archive-org.com/page/418842/2012-10-12/http://www.edf.org/climate/edfs-beijing-office-helps-china-merge-its-goals.

Fang Hai, Chen Jie, and John A. Rizzo. 2009. "Explaining Urban-Rural Health Disparities in China." *Medical Care* 47 (12): 1209–1216.

Fang Pengqian, Siping Dong, Jingjing Xiao, Chaojie Liu, Xianwei Feng, and Yiping Wang. 2010. "Regional Inequality in Health and Its Determinants: Evidence from China." *Health Policy* 94 (1): 14–25.

Fitzgerald, John. 1996. *Awakening China: Politics, Culture and Class in the Nationalist Revolution.* Stanford, CA: Stanford University Press.

Ford Foundation. 2013. "China." http://www.fordfoundation.org/regions/china/.

Give2Asia. 2013. "Give2Asia in China." http://give2asia.org/documents/Give2Asia-China-Overview.pdf.

Gu, Danan, Zhenmei Zhang, and Yi Zeng. 2009. "Access to Healthcare Services Makes a Difference in Healthy Longevity among Older Chinese Adults." *Social Science & Medicine* 68 (2): 210–219.

Gu Xingyuan, Gerald Bloom, Tang Shenglan, Zhu Yingya, Zhou Shouqi, and Chen Xingbao. 1993. "Financing Health Care in Rural China: Preliminary Report of a Nationwide Study." *Social Science and Medicine* 36 (4): 385–391.

Hesketh, Therese, Dan Wu, Linan Mao, and Nan Ma. 2012. "Violence against Doctors in China." *British Medical Journal* 345:e5730.

Ho, Fei-Wen, and Kirk Hallahan. 2004. "Post-Earthquake Crisis Communications in Taiwan: An Examination of Corporate Advertising and Strategy Motives." *Journal of Communication Management* 8 (3): 291–306.

Huang Yanzhong. 2011. "The Sick Man of Asia: China's Health Crisis." *Foreign Affairs* 90:119–136.

Hurun Report. 2012. "Hurun Philanthropy List 2012." http://www.hurun.net/usen/NewsShow.aspx?nid=215.

ICCIC (International Committee for the Promotion of Chinese Industrial Cooperatives). 2013. "The International Committee for the Promotion of Chinese Industrial Cooperatives (Gung Ho-ICCIC)." http://www.gungho.org.cn/en-danye.php?id=11.

Kalusa, Walima T. 2008. "Healing Bodies, Saving Souls: Medical Missions in Asia and Africa." *Bulletin of the History of Medicine* 82 (3): 749–751.

Kan Haidong, Chen Bingheng, and Hong Chuanjie. 2009. "Health Impact of Outdoor Air Pollution in China: Current Knowledge and Future Research Needs." *Environmental Health Perspectives* 117 (5): A187.

Laliberté, André. 2009. "The Institutionalization of Buddhist Philanthropy in China." In *State and Society Responses to Social Welfare Needs in China: Serving the People*, edited by Jonathan Schwartz and Shawn Shieh, 113–134. London: Routledge.

Lee, Liming, Vivian Lin, Wang Ruotao, and Zhao Hongwen. 2003. "Public Health in China: History and Contemporary Challenges." In *Global Public Health: A New Era*, edited by Robert Beaglehole, 156–171. Oxford: Oxford University Press.

Legge, David, Vivian Lin, and Guo Yan. 2010. "Global Influences on Health and Health Services in China." In *Health Policy in and for China*, edited by Vivian Lin, Guo Yan, David Legge, and Wu Quhong, 368–381. Beijing: Peking University Medical Press.

Lin, Vivian. 2011. "Transformations in the Healthcare System in China." *Current Sociology* 60 (4): 427–440.

Lin, Vivian, James Smith, Sally Fawkes, Priscilla Robinson, and Susan Chaplin. 2007. *Public Health Practice in Australia: The Organised Effort.* Sydney: Allen & Unwin.

Lin, Vivian, and Hongwen Zhao. 2008. "Public Identify and Private Behavior: Causes, Consequences and Remedies for Health Sector Reform in China." In *International Health Law: Solidarity and Justice in Health Care Access*, edited by A. P. den Exeter, 201–216. Antwerp: Maklu.

Lin, Vivian, Hongwen Zhao, Hui Yang, and Rachel Canaway. 2010. "History of Health Policy in China." In *Health Policy in and for China*, edited by Vivian Lin, Guo Yan, David Legge, and Wu Quhong, 294–311. Beijing: Peking University Medical Press.

Lin, Vivian, and Rob Yates. 2009. "Health Policy Support Project: Project Completion Review." UK Department for International Development. http://projects.dfid.gov.uk/project.aspx?Project=107802.

Liu Chaojie. 2003. "The Battle against SARS: A Chinese Story." *Australian Health Review* 26 (3): 3–13.

Ma, Dali, and William L. Parish. 2006. "Tocquevillian Moments: Charitable Contributions by Chinese Private Entrepreneurs." *Social Forces* 85 (2): 943–964.

Ma Jiantang. 2011. "Press Release on Major Figures of the 2010 National Population Census." National Bureau of Statistics of China. http://www.stats.gov.cn/english/newsandcomingevents/t20110428_402722237.htm.

Minden, Karen. 1989. *Canadian Development Assistance: The Medical Missionary Model in West China, 1910–1952.* Toronto: University of Toronto-York University Joint Centre for Asia Pacific Studies.

Mok Bong-Ho. 2001. "Cancer Self-Help Groups in China: A Study of Individual Change, Perceived Benefit, and Community Impact." *Small Group Research* 32 (2):115–132.

Murray, Christopher J. L., and Alan D. Lopez. 1997. "Global Mortality, Disability, and the Contribution of Risk Factors: Global Burden of Disease Study." *Lancet* 17:1436–1442.

Murray, Christopher J. L., Theo Vos, Rafael Lozano, Mohsen Naghavi, Abraham D. Flaxman, Catherine Michaud, Majid Ezzati et al. 2012. "Disability-Adjusted Life Years (DALYs) for 291 Diseases and Injuries in 21 Regions, 1990–2010: A Systematic Analysis for the Global Burden of Disease Study 2010." *Lancet* 380 (9859): 2197–2223.

Nicholas, Jenna. 2012. "The Development of Civil Society in China." Stanford Social Innovation Review. http://www.ssireview.org/blog/entry/the_development_of_civil_society_in_china.

Organisation for Economic Cooperation and Development. 2012. "Country Statistical Profile: China 2011–2012." http://www.oecd-ilibrary.org/economics/country-statistical-profile-china-2011_csp-chn-table-2011-1-en.

Phillips, Michael R., Liu Huaqing, and Zhang Yanping. 1999. "Suicide and Social Change in China." *Culture, Medicine and Psychiatry* 23 (1): 25–50.

Save the Children. 2011. "Save the Children: China Programme Brief '11." http://www.amcham-shanghai.org/amchamportal/infovault_library/2011/Save_the_Children_China_Programme_Brief_11.pdf.

Shieh, Shawn. 2011. "Good News for 2011: Starting Up China Development Brief." NGOs in China: A Blog about Developments in the Nongovernmental, Nonprofit, Charitable Sector in China. http://ngochina.blogspot.com/2011/01/good-news-for-2011-starting-up-china.html.

Song Shutao. 2008. "Government Promises Equitable Healthcare for All." *China Daily.* http://english.gov.cn/2008-01/08/content_852428.htm.

Tang Dan, Gang Chen, Xu Yan-Wen, Karen Y. L. Hui-Lo, Luo Xiao-Yuan, and Chetwyn C. H. Chan. 2011. "An Emerging Occupational Rehabilitation System in the People's Republic of China." *Journal of Occupational Rehabilitation* 21 (suppl. 1): S35–S43.

Tang Yi-Lang, Zhao Dong, Zhao Chengzheng, and Joseph F. Cubells. 2006. "Opiate Addiction in China: Current Situation and Treatments." *Addiction* 101 (5): 657–665.

UK Department for International Development. 2012. "Health Policy and Support Project: Increased Capacity in GoC for Evidence-Based, Integrated, Pro-Poor Health Policy-Making." http://projects.dfid.gov.uk/project.aspx?Project=107715.

UNAIDS. 2011. *World Aids Day Report.* http://www.unaids.org/en/media/unaids/contentassets/documents/unaidspublication/2011/jc2216_worldaidsday_report_2011_en.pdf.

Vos, Theo, Abraham D. Flaxman, Mohsen Naghavi, Rafael Lozano, Catherine Michaud, and Majid Ezzati. 2012. "Years Lived with Disability (YLDs) for 1160 Sequelae of 289 Diseases and Injuries: A Systematic Analysis for the Global Burden of Disease Study 2010." *Lancet* 380 (9859): 2163–2196.

Wang, Cindy. 2011. "The Growing Third Sector in China." Hauser Center for Nonprofit Organizations at Harvard University. http://hausercenter.org/chinanpo/2011/05/the-growing-third-sector-in-china/.

Wang Longde, Kong Lingzhi, Wu Fan, Bai Yamin, and Robert Burton. 2005. "Preventing Chronic Diseases in China." *Lancet* 366 (9499): 1821–1824.

Ware, Robert. 2011. "Gung Ho and Cooperatives in China." *Grassroots Economic Organizing (GEO) Newsletter* 2 (7). http://geo.coop/node/603.

Wei Xiaolin, Chen Jing, Chen Ping, James N. Newell, Li Hongdi, Sun Chenguang, Mei Jian, and John D. Walley. 2009. "Barriers to TB Care for Rural-to-Urban Migrant TB Patients in Shanghai: A Qualitative Study." *Tropical Medicine & International Health* 14 (7): 754–760.

WHO (World Health Organization). 1948. "Constitution of the World Health Organization." http://apps.who.int/gb/bd/PDF/bd47/EN/constitution-en.pdf.

———. 2006. "New HIV Data Show Growing AIDS Epidemic in China." http://www.who.int/mediacentre/news/releases/2006/china_hiv_aids/en/index.html.

———. 2007. "People-Centred Health Care: A Policy Framework." http://www.wpro.who.int/health_services/people_at_the_centre_of_care/documents/ENG-PCIPolicyFramework.pdf.

———. 2008. "Commission on Social Determinants of Health—Final Report: Closing the Gap in a Generation; Health Equity through Action on the Social Determinants of Health." http://www.who.int/social_determinants/thecommission/finalreport/en/index.html.

———. 2009. "Women and Suicide in Rural China." *Bulletin of the World Health Organization* 87 (12): 885–964. http://www.who.int/bulletin/volumes/87/12/09-011209.pdf.

———. 2011. "Progress Report 2011: Global HIV/AIDS Response; Epidemic Update and Health Sector Progress towards Universal Access." http://www.who.int/hiv/pub/progress_report2011/en/.

———. 2012. "Projections of Mortality and Burden of Disease, 2004–2030." http://www.who.int/healthinfo/global_burden_disease/projections/en/.

Wilson, Anne, and Aye Aye Gyi. 2010. "The Status and Perspective of Diabetes Health Education in China: Inspiration from Australia." *International Journal of Nursing Practice* 16 (2): 92–98.

World Bank. 1990. "China Long-Term Issues and Options in the Health Transition." http://documents.worldbank.org/curated/en/1998/04/693588/china-basic-health-services-project.

———. 2005. "Rural Health Insurance—Rising to the Challenge." http://documents
.worldbank.org/curated/en/2005/05/6217256/rural-health-insurance-rising-challenge.

———. 2011. "China-Basic Health Services Project." http://www.worldbank.org/projects
/documents/1998/04/693588/china-basic-health-services-project.

———. 2012. "Health Nutrition and Population Statistics: China." http://datatopics
.worldbank.org/hnp/country/china.

World Resources Institute. 1998–1999. "The Environment and China Water and Air Pollution: Water and Health." http://www.wri.org/publication/content/7833.

Wu Ximing, and Jeffrey M. Perloff. 2005. "China's Income Distribution, 1985–2001." *Review
of Economics and Statistics* 87 (4): 763–775.

Xinhua. 2009. "China to Set Up Essential Medicine System to Curb Rising Drug Prices."
http://english.gov.cn/2009-04/07/content_1279671.htm.

Xu Xiaoqun. 1997. "'National Essence' vs 'Science': Chinese Native Physicians' Fight for
Legitimacy, 1912–37." *Modern Asian Studies* 31 (4): 847–877.

Yang Wangli. 2012. "China's Two Charity Hospitals Focus on Children's Well-Being." *China
Daily* (Beijing). http://www.chinadaily.com.cn/cndy/2012-08/22/content_15694937.htm.

Yu Qian. 2012. "Charities Get New Rules to Improve Their Transparency." *Global Times*
(Beijing). http://www.globaltimes.cn/content/724057.shtml.

Zhang Ran, Zhu Jigao, Yue Heng, and Zhu Chunyan. 2010. "Corporate Philanthropic Giving,
Advertising Intensity, and Industry Competition Level." *Journal of Business Ethics* 94
(1): 39–52.

Zhao Hongwen. 2005. "Governing the Healthcare Market: Regulatory Challenges and Options in the Transitional China." DrPH diss., La Trobe University.

Zhou Shang-Cheng, Cai Le, Wang Jing, Cui Shao-Guo, Chai Yun, Liu Bing, and Wan Chong-
Hua. 2011. "Measuring the Burden of Disease Using Disability-Adjusted Life Years
in Shilin County of Yunnan Province, China." *Environmental Health and Preventive
Medicine* 16 (3): 148–154.

PART II
CHINESE ROOTS AND
FOREIGN ENGAGEMENT

4 Medicine with a Mission

Chinese Roots and Foreign Engagement in Health Philanthropy

Zhang Xiulan and Zhang Lu

THE EARLIEST SUSTAINED foreign philanthropic involvement in China came from a wide array of church-sponsored philanthropies. Although such philanthropies are no longer prominent in China, their legacy has been considerable. Drawing on a range of archival sources, this chapter first briefly sketches the Chinese charitable landscape in which Western church-sponsored initiatives arrived. It then provides examples of the wide variety of projects that developed, considering both how these ventures were funded and their relationship with the state. Finally, it considers their legacy: paving the way for other foreign philanthropic engagement, establishing medical institutions that continue to thrive today (although they are no longer linked to their original church heritage), and, most significantly, acting as an initial point of contact for Western and Chinese health care practices, influencing medical education and management models that have carried through to the present day.

Context: Indigenous Chinese Charitable Organizations in the Nineteenth Century

The concept of charity was not something imported into China from the West. Offering charity to the poor is called *shan* in Chinese, and this principle has existed in Chinese culture for thousands of years. Social organizations that provided assistance to the needy existed before the Qin dynasty (211 BCE). During the time of the Song dynasty (960–1127), a range of avenues for charitable deeds emerged, particularly in response to the need for famine relief, including gruel kitchens funded by local elites, medical facilities and food stations provided by Buddhist temples, and welfare activities sponsored by local granaries. Alongside these, the government introduced a system of medical financial aid and sponsored a number of poorhouses and medical bureaus (Handlin Smith 1987, 310). State medical aid continued in the Ming dynasty (1368–1644) with the establishment of the Hui Min Medical Bureau. Over time, though, such government aid decreased, particularly in the wake of war, and by the beginning of the Qing dynasty (1644–1912), it was abolished altogether as the government ceased providing health services to the poor (Renmin zhengxie wang 2009).

As state-sponsored medical provisions declined, a new influential form of charitable organization emerged during the Ming dynasty, the *shantang* and *shanhui*, both of which may be translated into English as "benevolent society." These societies first appeared in the more developed Yangtze River Delta region and were replicated in other parts of the nation through the course of the Qing dynasty. Liang Qizi estimates that there were 222 such organizations by the end of the Daoguang regime (1821–1850) of the Qing dynasty (Liang 2001), with many more established during the Tongzhi regime (1861–1875), as local resources increased and greater financial support became available (Yu 2003, 267). These societies were supported, monitored, and regulated by local elites. It is important to note that this encompassed not only the more traditional elite strata of society—scholars and the gentry—but also newly wealthy merchants and farmers. The centrality of wealth rather than land or time-honored social standing in the establishment of these societies relates to the changing socioeconomic landscape of late Ming and Qing dynasty China. Joanna Handlin Smith (1987) has argued that

> the growing importance of merchant wealth, the acquiescence on the part of scholars to the rhetoric of commerce, and the tightening of bonds between merchants and gentry were the fundamental reasons for the new charitable institutions. . . . Highly visible, tolerated by the state, and sponsored by the local community, the benevolent societies expressed widespread public beliefs that wealth could serve noble causes and a spirit of civic pride. (330–331)

Although a distinction between "charity" (immediate succor given to the needy) and "philanthropy" (giving aimed at a more sustained, systematic improvement of public life) is not drawn in Chinese in the same way it often is in English, a case can be made for regarding these benevolent societies as the earliest widespread examples of modern philanthropic institutions within China. Privately founded and funded rather than government-run, they provided welfare assistance, which, in time, extended beyond emergency provisions for the most vulnerable to encompass a range of social services that benefited the community. While many of the benevolent societies were what might be termed "comprehensive" in nature (offering various services, including education and food assistance), health care services were one of the key elements provided. The following examples may provide an indication of the type of philanthropic institutions that had developed by the mid-nineteenth century, when Western medical missionaries began to have an impact in China.

One of China's first modern medical philanthropies was Puji Hall in Hangzhou. It began as a comprehensive charitable organization offering medical assistance and later evolved into a full medical center. Fuyuan Hall in Shanghai was established in 1844. It provided medication and coffins on credit during seasonal epidemics, and doctors there provided free services to the public every day from 7:00 AM to noon. (Fuma 2005, 468, 470, 566).

Guangren Hall in Tianjin was established in the 1870s during a large famine in northern China. Its purpose was to look after widows and orphans. In 1881, the patron of Guangren Hall set up a medical center to address the seasonal epidemics that occurred every summer and fall. For two months during the summer, the medical center hired doctors to provide free medical services. Every day from 7:00 AM to 10:00 AM and 3:00 PM to 6:00 PM, Tianjin's poor could visit the medical center for free treatment. According to its records, Guangren Hall provided medical assistance to 26,000 poor people between 1881 and 1882. In the spring of 1883, hot weather hit the region, followed by heavy rains in the summer. When many people contracted cholera and malaria, the medical center responded effectively by treating 11,300 people in one hundred days.[1] In 1884, Guangren Hall established a year-round inpatient center that treated around 10,000 patients annually.[2]

Some benevolent societies also sponsored branch hospitals and clinics. Xianghouren Hall in the Yinxiang area of Shanghai sponsored Yinxiang Hospital, while Xinpuyu Hall in Shanghai established an inpatient hospital and also launched four clinics in the Wusong, Jiangwan, Zhabei, and Yangshupu areas. By 1921, Xinyupu Hall was sponsoring eight clinics and had established a hospital in the Nanshi area during the summer to treat seasonal epidemics. Lianyishan Organization and Pushan Mountain Villa in Shanghai also launched hospitals to provide free health care services and medicine during seasonal epidemics (Tao 2004).

Alongside the health care aspects of the comprehensive services funded by various benevolent societies, charitable ventures with a specific medical focus also emerged in the late nineteenth century and early twentieth century. By the end of the Guangxu regime (1875–1908), Yang Jun, a wealthy philanthropist, had established a hospital for seasonal epidemics in the city of Suzhou in Jiangsu Province (Zhang 1991), and in 1893, the Dantu Clinic in Jiangsu was established by two local businessmen, Yang Hanwen and Zhang Yangchan, providing year-round medication and free health care to the poor. In 1903, the clinic was expanded into a hospital with several departments (Zhang, Weng, and Gao [1991 (1925), 332]). In 1921, Zhu Baosan and Wang Yiting established Guangyi Chinese Medicine Hospital in Shanghai, which included inpatient and outpatient departments.

Later, it became the Common People's Hospital of Chinese Medicine. In the same year, the Siming Hospital, established by the Ningbo business community, offered traditional Chinese medicine to Ningbo's poor. Severely ill patients were also provided with free accommodations. For those who died at the hospital, free coffins and burial plots were made available. Patients who came from outside the Ningbo area could also receive free medication and treatment depending on their means and their illnesses.

The funding for these initiatives came from individual and corporate donors, with supplementary money obtained through special fundraising activities such as performances, bazaars, lotteries, and door-to-door collecting (Zhou and Zeng 2007). Yet even though public funding had declined, there was still, at times, an intersection with the state. For example, when it was established in 1882, the Medical Bureau of Nanxun in Zhejiang initially depended heavily on donations from wealthy local donors, but later, it also received money from silk taxes and rent from government properties that were collected locally (Zhou 1991, 397). Money was sometimes raised by linking funding for medical care with business development and the growth of the financial sector, which the state had fostered. This was called "Business Development Interest." In 1884, the Qing dynasty provided ten thousand silver coins (about four million renminbi in today's currency) to Shanghai's Huasheng Machinery Textile Factory with the understanding that 0.6 percent of the annual interest would be paid to finance health care for the poor.[3]

Such examples reinforce Vivienne Shue's observation that charitable activities in late imperial China "tended to blur the distinction between public (or state) welfare and private philanthropy." Shue draws attention to

> [a] moral and social vision shared by members of both the political-official and the non-official social elites which posited the comprehensive and harmonious integration of the upright conduct of social life and of state programs and actions. . . . Where individual philanthropy activists were concerned, the line dividing official from personal roles was likewise blurred, as was the line between a demonstration of moral duty or social responsibility on their part, and a demonstration of personal kindness or magnanimity. (1998, 334)

Echoes of this private-public overlap are apparent in the contemporary landscape of Chinese health philanthropy. For the present chapter, though, the overlap that is more relevant is with the Western church-sponsored medical philanthropies that arrived in China during the nineteenth century. There were similarities with indigenous Chinese philanthropies in that the health care services were being offered within the framework of a wider moral purpose. It was not an exact parallel, of course, as the medical missionaries were ultimately hoping to save souls through conversion (viewed as a philanthropic venture in itself), not just extend temporal life through medical treatment. While Buddhist-inspired charity often extended to the afterlife as well (including burials, coffins, and funerals), the moral imperative to improve life was compatible with both Confucian and Buddhist principles underpinning much local charitable work, in which benefactors both provided a demonstration of their own piety and sought to strengthen the wider fabric of society. The educative purpose of the church-sponsored philanthropies—which, as will be discussed later, became primarily medical rather than religious—also shared some common ground with the instructive nature of local philanthropies. Many early Chinese philanthropists were intellectuals, and, in addition to establishing charitable halls, hospitals, and clinics, they printed popular books intended to educate the public about health and medicine (Jizhaijushi 2002 [ca. 1715], 115). Such similarities facilitated the successful spread of Western church-sponsored philanthropies. Some of the differences and innovations they brought with them, meanwhile, would go on to have a lasting influence on Chinese health care.

Development: The Spread of Western Church-Sponsored Health Philanthropies in China

Western missionaries working in China recognized medical philanthropy as a potent tool for gaining acceptance and establishing a foothold in local communities. As the missionary doctor William Lockhart wrote in 1861,

> In opening a new station where foreigners have not previously resided . . . it is very important to adopt a course which will speedily win the confidence of the people. No course has been found more likely to effect this than the opening [of] a dispensary and a hospital, where the relief afforded shows at once our object to be the welfare of those about us. The influence of a mission thus begun is immediate, and remains permanently in the memory of the people. (116–117)

From the early nineteenth century, churches established by Western missionaries were operating small clinics and dispensaries. In 1835 in Canton (now Guangzhou), the Yale University–educated missionary physician Peter Parker founded the first Western-style hospital in China. Parker's Canton Hospital specialized in ophthalmology and operated out of premises owned by a philanthropically minded local merchant who waived the rent on the property. A total of 1,061 patients were treated during the first three months, of whom 1,020 (96 percent) had ocular illnesses. The hospital was temporarily closed in 1840 due to the hostilities of the First Opium War, but it reopened in 1842 and was soon thriving again. In his records, Parker noted that between July 1845 and December 1848, 7,571 patients were examined. The range of ailments treated had diversified, but ocular complaints (75 percent) were still predominant. The hospital was later renamed the Boji Hospital, and in 1866, it established its own medical school—a trend that also took place in many of the other church-supported hospitals. In

1886, Sun Yat-sen, the future first president of the Republic of China, received medical training at the school (Chan, Liu, and Tsai 2011, 791–793).

A great number of church-sponsored hospitals were founded over the next hundred years, initially in coastal areas and then spreading inland. In Shanghai alone, there were 14 hospitals with a total of 2,000 beds established between 1844 and 1911. Church-led philanthropy flourished further still following the collapse of the Qing dynasty, and between 1911 and 1925, more than 50 hospitals with 4,000 beds were opened in Shanghai (Ni Hong 2008). A similar trend occurred in Beijing where many different Christian denominations launched medical activities at the start of the twentieth century. The first church hospital was established by the Catholic Church in 1900 and could treat 850 inpatients and 90,000 outpatients annually. French churches opened a French Hospital in 1902 with outpatient services, a radiology department, 34 inpatient beds, an electrotherapy room, and a pharmacy. By 1920, it had grown to 50 hospital beds and was able to provide treatment to 550 inpatients and 25,000 outpatients. In 1902, the American Presbyterian Church founded Duow Hospital, and in 1903, the American Methodist Episcopal Church established Johns Hopkins Memorial Hospital. Finally, in 1906, the American Protestant Episcopal Church opened St. Luke's Hospital (Deng and Cheng 2000, 324–325).

By 1921, with the exception of Tibet and Qinghai, all provinces in China had church-sponsored hospitals (Deng and Cheng 2000, 340). According to the 1938 edition of *World Mission,* by the end of 1937, European and American church philanthropies had established three hundred hospitals with twenty-one thousand beds and opened six hundred clinics. Approximately half of these were managed by American Christian organizations, with the rest managed by British or European Christian organizations. A handful of hospitals were jointly established by British and American churches, including Qilu Hospital in Shandong and Huaxi Union University Hospital in Chengdu (Gu 1991, 279).

The funding for these church-sponsored hospitals came from a range of sources. Church organizations themselves, and their associated fundraising activities, provided the primary source of financing. Additional international funding came from secular donations, though the benefactors were frequently religiously motivated. This was particularly the case with the Rockefeller Foundation, which also endowed the China Medical Board. Together these two bodies provided the most significant secular international donations, offering financial support to church-sponsored hospitals in Beijing, Tianjin, Shanghai, Shenyang, Baoding, Dezhou, Yantai, Taiyuan, Suzhou, Nanjing, Nantong, Yangzhou, Ningbo, Wuhu, Anqing, Jiujiang, Changde, Yichang, Xiamen, and Guangzhou, with most of the money used to purchase X-ray, laboratory, and surgical equipment (Zhang 2009, 150). The Pasteur Institute also gave to church-sponsored hospitals, donating eight new American X-ray machines to China during the 1920s.[4] Beijing's Duow Hospital relied on church funding and international donations for 50 percent of its income and almost 100 percent of its medications. The salaries of its international staff were paid directly by the American Presbyterian Church in U.S. currency (Chen et al. 1998). The medical schools that frequently developed alongside the church-sponsored hospitals were particularly reliant on church financing and other international philanthropic donations: in the early twentieth century, 80 percent of medical school funding came from these sources. Rich Chinese donors also contributed to medical schools, but they typically sponsored individual prestige projects such as new buildings (Xu and Han 2003, 62).

Domestic Chinese donations became increasingly prominent in the twentieth century, as many missionary societies began raising funds in China to build new hospitals. For example, the Seventh-Day Adventist Church of America came to China in 1902 and built 12 hospitals in less than 30 years. Their hospitals were mainly funded by domestic Chinese donations with little help from the church or other international donors (Gu 1991, 279). Over time, fundraising from Chinese alumni of church-supported medical schools also became common practice. In 1933, direct church funding for St. John's Medical School declined by 75 percent due to the Great Depression in the United States. Then, the bankruptcy of Shanghai's American Oriental Bank led to the further loss of 70 percent of the school's savings. In 1933–1934, St. John's sent 257 fundraising letters to its graduates, and 155 graduates responded with donations. By 1941, donations from graduates had reached sixty thousand dollars. In 1946, the medical school raised an additional thirty-five thousand dollars from its graduates to maintain operations (Xu and Han 2003, 63).

Most church-supported hospitals originally provided free medical treatment. However, starting in the 1920s, with more patients seeking medical care and funding becoming more uncertain, many adopted the policy of charging service fees. Despite this, most hospitals continued to offer financial support by providing fee waivers or subsidies to the poor, while charging higher fees to the rich to make up the difference, raising charitable donations to establish relief funds for the poor, and regularly hosting clinics where free medical services were offered (Li 2008, 318–319). It became a common practice for church hospitals to divide inpatient beds into different classes, charging patients in first and second classes more to cover subsidies for poorer patients. Guangji Hospital, for example, had hospital beds classified into first class and general class according to gender.[5] Qilu Hospital classified its inpatient beds into first class, second class, and general wards. The cost of staying in the general ward was a third of the fee for the first-class ward and half the price of the second-class ward. Hospital records from 1935 reveal that 2–3 percent of patients were treated free of charge, with the payments covered by the wealthier patients (Shandong daxue Qilu yiyuan zhi bianji weiyuan hui 2000, 77).

Tuition fees became an important source of funding for the medical schools. For example, before the 1920s, students at Qilu University Medical School were charged for tuition and meals. In practice, these fees were paid by missionary societies. In the 1920s, when more students, especially non-Christian students, began entering the program, the university council asked the students to pay more tuition in order to cover costs. Despite the objections of local missionary societies, who believed that higher tuition would exclude students from Christian families, fees were significantly increased. Thereafter, local Christian medical philanthropies could only support a few poorer students, leaving the rest to pay their own way (Liu 1998, 92). Medical schools also received income generated by their affiliated hospitals. In the 1930s, after the Xiangya Medical School stopped receiving direct church funding, half of its income came from its affiliated hospitals (Liu and Li 1994).

During the early period of Christian medical philanthropy and up until the 1930s, international missionary societies remained the largest single source of funding for church hospitals and medical schools, but with the economic impact of the Great Depression, Western churches were forced to reduce or cease funding for overseas mission activities. The numbers of missionaries was also reduced: in 1920, there were 8,000 missionaries in China, but by 1936, this number had fallen to 4,250. By that time, overall financial support to missionary societies had been reduced by one-third and some societies received only half of the funding they had obtained in the 1920s (Deng and Cheng 2000, 326). Although the domestic fundraising channels outlined above sought to mitigate this loss of international funding, the flourishing of church hospitals was severely impacted by the Japanese invasion of China. The war restricted access to domestic funding and stifled the ability of the hospitals to recruit new doctors, while many church hospitals even had their buildings destroyed during the conflict (Zhou and Zeng, 2007).

During and after the war, certain medical facilities initiated by church philanthropies survived due to support from the Chinese Nationalist Government. This was indicative of the sympathetic stance of the state toward these institutions during the Republican era. Indeed, in addition to the various funding sources already mentioned, church-supported medical facilities also sometimes received government subsidies. For example, in 1914, Xiangya Medical School was jointly established by Hunan's Provincial Government and the Yale-China Association. According to their agreement, the Yale-China Association paid twenty thousand silver coins (eight million renminbi in today's currency), Hunan Provincial Government paid fifty thousand silver coins (twenty million renminbi), and the landowner donated ten thousand silver coins (four million renminbi) for the purchase of the land (Liu and Li, 1994). During and immediately after the war with Japan, the main source of financial support for this medical school was the Chinese Nationalist Government. Meanwhile, in 1931, the Ministry of Education provided financial assistance to Shandong's Qilu University Hospital, and in

1946, the Nationalist Government earmarked funding for reopening the hospital (Shandong University 2000, 77).

The state's stance toward church-sponsored health philanthropy changed greatly during the Qing dynasty and the Republican era. Prior to the First Opium War (1840–1842), the Qing government banned foreign religions from proselytizing in China, and so, missionaries relied on health philanthropy to gain acceptance. Generally, the Qing government didn't intervene in missionary organizations and allowed church-sponsored medical philanthropies to manage their own activities. But if the government discovered that a church or foreign hospital was engaged in proselytizing, "the hospital would be pulled down, and the missionaries forced to leave China" (Li 2008, 117). After the First Opium War, the Qing government was forced to relax its total prohibition against foreign religions, but its attitude toward Christian churches and foreign medical philanthropies remained ambivalent. On the one hand, Western medicine was highly regarded by the Chinese; on the other hand, the government was wary of the churches' intention to attract converts to Christianity.

Li Hongzhang, the Beiyang trade minister, was very supportive of Western medicine. He provided financial support for church hospitals and, in 1893, even established a large Western hospital, the Tianjin Zhuyaoshiyi Hospital, which had a Western school of medicine, an inpatient department, and a Western-style pharmacy (Zhou and Wang 2007, 150). The hospital served Li Hongzhang's navy, and graduates of the Western medical department were assigned to the navy as medical officers (Nihon Rikugun, Shinkoku Chūtongun, and Shireibu 1986 [1909], 318). Meanwhile, local governmental policies toward church hospitals varied greatly during the late Qing dynasty. The Boxer Rebellion destroyed many local church hospitals, especially in northern China, yet there were also cases of officials in southern China protecting church hospitals and doctors under threat (Li 2008, 123).

At the beginning of the twentieth century, in response to the demands of the Western powers, the Qing government began to safeguard missionary activities. Many local officials not only protected church hospitals and medical schools but also made donations and participated in ceremonies to show their support. When facing epidemics, officials often solicited help from local church hospitals. Guangzhou city officials even began paying the local church hospital a per-patient stipend for taking care of the city's mentally ill, and during the 1911 pandemic, the Qing government solicited help from medical missionaries (Li 2008, 124). In general, though, Qing government policies toward church-sponsored hospitals were piecemeal and inconsistent, which was symptomatic of its lack of a clear policy framework for nongovernment philanthropic work more generally.

When the Chinese Nationalists came to power, they issued a number of policies and regulations to promote and manage health philanthropy. The Nationalist government created the Ministry of Internal Affairs and the Bureau of

Civil Affairs in 1927 and charged them with organizing relief for the poor and managing the activities of philanthropies. At the same time, they issued specific guidelines for nongovernmental philanthropic organizations and brought all charitable and philanthropic initiatives under the central government's control (Yu 2003, 249–255).

The Nationalist Government established the Ministry of Health and began building the central and local Public Health System. The Ministry of Health issued a series of policies concerning Western medicine during the time when church health and medical institutions were under its jurisdiction, including the Regulations on Western Medicine and Licensing Procedures for Foreign Doctors in 1931, which required that foreign doctors who wished to practice Western medicine in China have a Medical Certificate from his or her country of origin and that the Medical Certificate be verified by the Ministry of Foreign Affairs before the foreign doctor was allowed to practice in China (Compilation Office of the Legislative Yuan 1935, 871–872).

Although the Chinese Nationalists abrogated many of the treaties with Western powers that they considered unjust, they did not ban church-sponsored health philanthropy. In the 1920s, however, the government did adopt a policy of promoting educational sovereignty. Churches complied with this policy by requiring their hospitals and medical schools to separate missionary functions from medical services (Deng and Cheng 2000, 326–327). The Ministry of Education, meanwhile, established a Medical Education Committee and a Midwife Education Committee and issued the Guidelines for the Establishment of Educational Institutions by Religious Groups in 1929, requiring any educational institution sponsored by a religious group to report to the Ministry of Education before enrolling students (Li 2008, 149). In addition to the evolution of Chinese and church policies, beginning in the 1930s, doctors also gradually became less willing to allow hospitals to conduct missionary activities. Increasingly, the quality and effectiveness of medical services became doctors' first priority, and separation of medical care from missionary activities became the new norm (Deng and Cheng 2000, 326–327). The diversification of funding sources and the growing financial independence of hospitals and medical schools from churches further increased the distance between missionary activities and secular health philanthropies (Tian 1995, 181–182), as did the growing scientific research advocacy by philanthropic bodies such as the Rockefeller Foundation (Bullock 1992).

The amenable attitude of the government toward church-sponsored health philanthropy may have partly been due to the fact that many Nationalist officials had close ties with the Christian religion. Both President Chiang Kai-shek and his wife Madame Soong May-ling were Christians and both contributed to church-sponsored health philanthropies. In 1932, the three Soong sisters donated three thousand silver dollars (1.2 million RMB in today's currency) to the Gospel Hospital of Wujing County in Zhejiang Province (Yang 1932, quoted in Li 2003,

157). But the most compelling reason was likely the sheer importance of medical missions to the nation's health program by the late 1920s and 1930s. It may
not be possible to verify the complete accuracy of statistics from the period, but
figures published in 1941 nonetheless provide an indication of the scale of church-
sponsored health care. The Chinese physician H. B. Chu reported that there were
38,159 hospital beds in China, 10,903 of which were government-operated and the
rest run by nongovernmental agencies including Protestant and Catholic missions and the Red Cross. The 231 Protestant missionary hospitals accounted for
19,572 beds—51.3 percent of all hospital beds in China and 8,669 beds more (79.5
percent more) than government-provided beds (Choa 1990, 115–116).

Writing in 1861 about his 20 years as a medical missionary, William Lockhart stressed the importance of deploying skilled doctors to medical missions:

> The decided opinion to which a somewhat extensive experience has led me, is
> that medical missionaries should be *laymen*,—surgeons, not ordained minis-
> ters. I believe it is a great mistake to suppose that an efficient medical mission-
> ary can be made out of a minister, by giving him a few months' attendance on
> lectures and hospital practice. (117)

He also quoted approvingly from an address given on behalf of the Medical Missionary Society in China in 1838, concerning the education of Chinese youths in
Western medicine by missionary doctors:

> "Young men thus instructed will gradually be dispersed over the empire. . . .
> The success of their measures will render them respectable, and of course will
> redound to the credit of those also from whom they learned their art. Their pa-
> tients will not only hear, but feel, that the people from the West are good men.
> The effect of such influence will be silent but powerful; for there is something
> irresistibly impressive in benevolent action, especially when it appears exempt
> from the imputation of interested motives." (139)

The enlightened attitude of missionary doctors such as Lockhart, who prioritized medical expertise over evangelical zeal, undoubtedly contributed to the
successful spread of church-supported health philanthropy. It also facilitated the
gradual unlinking of church-funded medical infrastructure from the proselytizing nature of their original conception. In fact, the medical missions had very
limited success in converting the local populace to Christianity. But, as the next
section discusses, the lasting impact they had on Chinese health care was vast.

Legacy: The Lasting Influence of Church-Supported
Philanthropy on Chinese Health Care

Church-supported health philanthropy very much paved the way for the work
of major foreign philanthropic foundations. Most significantly, the Rockefeller
Foundation, which endowed the China Medical Board, was motivated by religious inclinations and, as previously mentioned, church-supported hospitals fre-

quently became conduits for Rockefeller money. In terms of lasting influence, the Rockefeller Foundation made a significant contribution to China's modern medical system by giving grants to medical schools and providing scholarships to pay for the overseas training of Chinese medical students and teachers (Liu 1998, 88–89; Zhang 2009; Bullock 2011). The China Medical Board, at that time an arm of the Rockefeller Foundation, in 1915 secured the purchase of the Peking Union Medical College, which had been founded in 1906. It was initially maintained by six missionary societies: the London Missionary Society (which owned the property); the Society for the Propagation of the Gospel in Foreign Parts; the London Medical Missionary Association; the American Board of Commissioners for Foreign Missions; the Board of Foreign Missions of the (American) Methodist Episcopal Church; and the Board of Foreign Missions of the Presbyterian Church in the United States of America. After PUMC was reestablished by the China Medical Board, it greatly expanded its medical and teaching facilities and is still one of the most selective and highly regarded medical colleges in China. The transfer of property was detailed in the China Medical Board's *First Annual Report,* published by the Rockefeller Foundation in January 1916. The report opened with a letter from the president of the Rockefeller Foundation to the Missionary Societies in the United States and Great Britain, highlighting the pioneering work done in China by the medical missions:

> Happily the Foundation is not first in the field. Many and various missionary societies of America, Great Britain and the Continent have preceded it. Hundreds of physicians are now practicing in China under the auspices of these societies. Their patients number tens of thousands annually. . . . With these societies and with the work undertaken by them, the Foundation from the first has contemplated the most cordial and sympathetic cooperation. (5–6)

Alongside PUMC, various medical institutions specifically founded by medical missionaries have survived and flourished, though they no longer have a religious underpinning. For example, in 1844, William Lockhart founded the Chinese Hospital in Shanghai, which is now known as the Renji Hospital and is one of the most highly regarded medical facilities in China. Peter Parker's original Ophthalmic Hospital in Canton went through various incarnations following its establishment in 1835 and is known today as the Zhongshan Ophthalmic Center. It is an internationally renowned hospital and one of the leading ophthalmic centers in the world. In 2010, the hospital treated 80,499 outpatients and performed 34,428 operations, and its staff published 76 articles in Science Citation Index journals (Chan, Liu, and Tsai 2011, 796).

These modern-day facilities are tangible examples of the profound effect the medical missions had on helping to transform domestic health care practices. Starting in the mid-1800s, medical missionaries introduced to China the Western practice of treating diseases in a hospital setting (Tian 1995, 181–182).

Early on, medical missionaries noticed different illness patterns in China than in the West. Some illnesses that were common in Europe, such as appendicitis and pneumonia, were less common in China, while certain venereal diseases, digestive problems, and rectal and eye diseases were more prevalent in China. The research initiated and conducted by church hospitals into Chinese patterns of disease helped to establish a new emphasis on medical research in China (Balme 2009 [1921]).

The integration of medical schools with clinical practice in a hospital setting was another feature of the Western medical system that was introduced by the churches into China. Medical schools supplied the doctors and students for the hospitals, while the advanced equipment found in hospitals provided the training tools needed for medical schools. The church-supported hospitals also introduced China to the Western system of hospital management, including the keeping of systematic medical records (Balme 2009 [1921]). The advent of a more modern Western-style system of hospital management encouraged professionalization in doctors, and starting in the 1860s, specialization among medical doctors became increasingly common (He 2006, 126). Church-supported hospitals also led to changes in the doctor-patient relationship. In Chinese medicine, the family was traditionally the center of treatment and care. Patients would stay with their families and doctors would come visit them in their homes. The Western hospital-centered treatment model challenged this traditional approach and placed a new focus on patient management by a team of doctors and nurses in a hospital setting (Lei 2003).

Alongside the introduction of Western scientific medicine, a major achievement of the medical missions was the teaching of public health and hygiene awareness. Early church-supported medicine in China focused on four major areas—promoting smallpox vaccinations; prevention and treatment of eye diseases; surgery; and the control of epidemics such as plague, leprosy, and cholera—three of which were firmly tied to public health issues. Long before Western medicine was widely accepted in China, smallpox vaccination was the main medical service provided by missionary doctors and a major catalyst for the eventual embrace of Western medicine was the success of church smallpox programs (He 2006, 164). Before the 1920s, most vaccines were administered through church hospitals. After the 1920s, when more Western-trained Chinese doctors were practicing in China, church hospitals cooperated with Chinese doctors to advocate for public health and control of epidemic diseases (Deng and Cheng 2000, 313).

The merits of Western medical expertise were also demonstrated during a major outbreak of plague in northeast China in 1910–1911. Here, also, church-supported health philanthropy was influential. The Qing government sent two Western-trained Chinese doctors to study the situation. One of the doctors was Wu Liande. Wu earned his PhD and MD at Cambridge University and had also been exposed to Western medical practices in France and Germany. With Wu's guidance, doctors from church hospitals and students from PUMC Hospital successfully prevented the plague from spreading. Although the plague claimed sixty thousand victims, this was considered a great success given the huge population at risk. In April 1911, the International Conference for Plague Control was held in China with Wu as its chair. Public health experts from 11 countries attended. A major outcome of this conference was the creation of a Northeast China Division of Plague Control and the establishment of hospitals for plague prevention in Harbin City and other places (He 2006, 170).

By the summer of 1921, under the supervision of the Beijing Church Medical Association, the Chinese Nationalist Government began offering public health education in colleges and universities. Students from PUMC gave lectures on public health at summer schools hosted by Beijing universities (Deng and Cheng 2000, 325). Church hospitals and medical schools worked closely with various levels of the government to address public health issues. In 1935, the Health Bureau of the Chinese Nationalist Government convened a meeting of church hospitals and medical schools on enhancing the public health function of these institutions (Bureau of Public Health 1935).

The influence of Western medical practices introduced by the medical missionaries on local Chinese health philanthropies was particularly striking. The first section of this chapter discussed the work of Chinese benevolent societies, which frequently ran comprehensive health and aid centers. From the beginning of the twentieth century, Chinese philanthropies, influenced by the church medical missions, began experimenting with new syncretic models of medical management. One major change in traditional medical philanthropy was the transformation of temporary, seasonal institutions into permanent year-round medical facilities. Many benevolent society halls were effectively transformed into hospitals. Although they still provided traditional Chinese medicine, some also introduced Western medical services and established inpatient and outpatient departments. In 1906, Mai Xinjian, a wealthy Guangdong resident, proposed to Governor Yuan Shikai the establishment of a new medical school to train women gynecologists at Guangren Hall. This was China's first gynecological institution.[6] In 1916, businessmen Fan Shixun and Sheng Zhushu, who were both from the Zhenhai area of Zhejiang Province, renamed Gongshan Hall into the more modern Gongshan Hospital. Begun as a small epidemic hospital, in May 1921 Gongshan Hospital added a Department of Western Medicine and began providing free medical services to the poor. Pushan Mountain Villa in Shanghai, established in 1914, hosted both traditional Chinese medicine and Western medicine (Le 2007, 392). In 1929, Fuyuan Hall in Shanghai hired three traditional Chinese doctors and one Western doctor to provide free health services and medicine to a total of 13,576 patients (*Shanghai tebie shi shehui ju* 1929).

Alongside the reformation of health services provided by traditional Chinese benevolent societies, Chinese philanthropists, inspired by the successful work of church-supported hospitals, began to establish entirely new Western-style medical facilities. Indeed, in economically developed areas, it became fashionable and yielded kudos for successful businessmen to establish Western-style hospitals. There are several examples of this occurring with Ningbo businessmen: in 1909, Shanghai Hospital in the Nanshi area was founded with Ningbo businessman Yu Qiaqing as its director; in 1918, Ningbo philanthropists Zhu Baosan, Liu Hongsheng, and Shen Dun financed Shanghai's Seasonal Epidemic Hospital; in 1919, Zhu Baosan founded Shenzhou Hospital in southern Shanghai; and in 1920, Zhu Baosan and Yu Qiaqing jointly established Pudong Hospital. Another Ningbo businessman, Huang Chujiu, donated his house in Shanghai as an eye clinic for the poor. In 1926, when Shanghai's seasonal hospital was unable to cope with the huge number of patients during a serious epidemic, Huang Chujiu set up a temporary emergency hospital to provide free medical care. In 1928, with Huang Chujiu's financial help, the temporary hospital became a permanent hospital with over one hundred beds on four floors. Later, Huang established Huang Chujiu Hospital, which specialized in ophthalmology but also provided treatment for other illnesses. Huang Chujiu Hospital supported lower-income people with free or subsidized medical care and medications (Le 2007, 390).

Following the founding of the People's Republic in China in 1949, nongovernmental philanthropy was eliminated and foreign intervention refused. The country entered into a period of philanthropic eclipse, from which it only began to emerge after 1978 with the impact of the Open Door reform policies. Although Western medical missionary activity came to a halt, the impact of church-supported philanthropy on Chinese health care had been so great that its legacy remains today. By the time the medical missionary societies were forced to leave the country, they had been involved in China for over a century and their work—facilitated by the cross-pollination of the Western medical expertise they introduced and already-existing Chinese philanthropic practices—had helped permanently transform the landscape of Chinese health care.

Notes

1. "Guangxu liu nian 1881 choushe shiyaoju juan (shanshu shi yao cai fu)" [Sixth Year of Emperor Guanxu's Reign, 1881, the Volume of Preparation of Benevolent Pharmacy (Books of Benevolent Medicine Attached)], 1881, Benevolence Hall File 130-28, Tianjin Archives.

2. "Guangxu shi nian (1884) yi zong chuangshe yangbing suo bao ying ju ji guibing guangren tang fu juankuan" [Ten Years of Guangxu Emperor's Reign, 1884, a File on Establishing a Convalescent Home and a Children Protection Agency, Which Has Been Incorporated into Benevolence Hall, Donations Attached in the File], 1884, Benevolence Hall File 130-1-30, Tianjin Archives.

3. Ibid.

4. "Sili zhendan daxue yi lan di san bian yixueyuan gaikuang" [Overview of the Private Zhendan University, Vol. 3., Brief of the Medical College], n.d., Y8-1-189, Shanghai Archive.

5. Ibid.

6. "Guangxu sanshier nian (1906) er yue duxian yuan zha xingban nvyi xuetang juan" [Thirty-Two Years of Guangxu Emperor's Reign, 1906, a File on Establishing a Female Medical School by Yuan Shikai], n.d., Guangren Hall file J0130-1-93, Tianjin Archives.

References

Balme, Harold. 2009 [1921]. *China and Modern Medicine: A Study in Medical Missionary Development.* London: United Council for Missionary Education.

Bullock, Mary Brown. 1992. "Luokefeile jijinhui he zhongguo" [Rockefeller Foundation and China]. In *Ershi shiji meiguo yu ya-tai diqu guoji xueshu taolunhui lunwenj* [Twentieth-Century America and Pacific-Asia Region International Academic Symposium Papers], edited by Zhonghua meiguo xuehui [China and American Scociety] and Zhongguo shehui kexue xueyuan—meiguo yanjiusuo [Institute of American Studies, Chinese Academy of Social Sciences], 419–428. Beijing: *Xiandai chubanshe* [Modern Press Co., Ltd.].

———. 2011. *The Oil Prince's Legacy: Rockefeller Philanthropy in China.* Washington, DC: Woodrow Wilson Center and Stanford University Press.

Bureau of Public Health. 1935. "Weishu ducu jiaohui yiyuan zhuyi gonggong weisheng gongzuo" [Bureau of Public Health Urges Church Hospital to Pay Attention to Public Health]. *Zhonghua yiyuan zazhi* [Chinese Medical Journal] 21 (4): 437.

Chan Chi-Chao," Melissa M. Liu, and James C. Tsai. 2011. "The First Western-Style Hospital in China." *Archives of Ophthalmology* 129 (6): 791–797.

Chen Fenglin, Liu Shiying, Liang Jun, Yang Jinlin, and Jiang Yongxiang. 1998. "Beijing daoji yiyuan kaolüe" [An Investigation on Dow Hospital in Beijing (Peking)]. *Zhonghua yishi zazhi* [Chinese Journal of Medical History] 28 (3): 141–144.

Choa, Gerald H. 1990. *"Heal the Sick" Was Their Motto: The Protestant Medical Missionaries in China.* Hong Kong: Chinese University of Hong Kong Press.

Compilation Office of the Legislative Yuan. 1935. *Zhonghua minguo fagui huibian (ershisan nianji) disi bian—neizheng* [Republic of China Laws and Regulations, chapter 4, Domestic Affairs]. Shanghai: Zhonghua shuju [Zhonghua Book Company].

Deng Tietao, and Cheng Zhifan. 2000. *Zhongguo yixue tongshi: Jindaijuan* [History of Chinese Medicine: Modern Volume]. Beijing: Renmin weisheng chubanshe [People's Medical Publishing House].

Fuma Susumu. 2005 [1997]. *Zhongguo shanhui shantang shi yanjiu* [Research of Chinese Charitable Houses History]. Translated by Wu Yue, Yang Wenxin, and Zhang Xuefeng. Beijing: Shangwu yinshuguan [Commercial Press].

Gu Changsheng. 1991. *Chuanjiaoshi yu jindai zhongguo* [Missionaries and Modern China]. Shanghai: Shanghai renmin chubanshe [Shanghai People's Publishing House].

Handlin Smith, Joanna F. 1987. "Benevolent Societies: The Reshaping of Charity during the Late Ming and Early Ch'ing." *Journal of Asian Studies* 46 (2): 309–337.

He Xiaolian. 2006. *Xiyi dongjian yu wenhua tiaoshi* [Western Medicine to the East and Cultural Adaptation]. Shanghai: Shanghai guji chubanshe [Shanghai Classics Publishing House].

Jizhaijushi. 2002 [ca. 1715]. "Ba [Postscript]." Dasheng bian [edited by Dasheng]. In *Xuxiu siku quanshu* [Continuation of Completed Four House Books], Vol. 1008. Shanghai: Shanghai guji chubanshe [Shanghai Classics Publishing House].

Le Chengyao. 2007. *Jindai Ningbo shangren yu shehui jingji* [Modern Businessmen and Socio-economics of Ningbo]. Beijing: Renmin chubanshe [People's Publishing House].

Lei Xianglin. 2003. "Fuzeren de yisheng yu you xinyangde bingren—zhong-xi yi lunzheng yu yibing guanxi zai minguo shiqi de zhuanbian" [Responsible Doctors and Patients with Faith: The Debate between Traditional Chinese Medicine and Western Medicine and the Doctor-Patient Relationship during the Transitional Period of the Republic of China]. *Xin shi xue* [New History] 14:45–96.

Li Chuanbin. 2008. "Jiaohui yiliao shiye yu jindai Zhongguo de yiliao weisheng he cishan jiuji shiye" [Missionary Medical Undertaking and Health and Medical Charities in Modern China]. In *Jindai hunan yu jindai zhongguo* [Modern Hunan and Modern China], edited by Li Yumin, 286–315. 2nd ed. Changsha: Hunan shifan daxue chubanshe [Hunan Normal University Press].

Liang Qizi. 2001. *Shishan yu jiaohua—Ming-Qing de cishan zuzhi* [Charity and Enlightenment: Charity Organizations in Ming and Qing Dynasties]. Shijiazhuang: Hebei jiaoyu chubanshe [Hebei Education Publishing House].

Liu Jiafeng. 1998. "Qilu daxue jingfei laiyuan yu xuexiao fazhan: 1904–1952" [Qilu University Funding Sources and School Development: 1904–1952]. In *Shehui zhuanxing yu jiaohui daxue* [Social Transformation and Church Universities], edited by Zhang Kaiyuan and Ma Min, 88–89. Wuhan: Hubei jiaoyu chubanshe [Hubei Education Publishing House].

Liu Xiaochun, and Li Junjie. 1994. *Xiangya chunqiu bashi nian* [Eighty-Year History of Xiangya Medical College]. Changsha: Zhongnan daxue chubanshe [Central South University Press].

Lockhart, William. 1861. *The Medical Missionary in China: A Narrative of Twenty Years' Experience*. London: Hurst and Blackett.

Ni Hong. "Minguo shiqi shanghai yiyuan guanli qingkuang jianjie" [Shanghai Hospital Management Briefing during the Period of the Republic of China]. Shanghai dang'an xinxi wang [Shanghai Archives Network]. http://www.archives.sh.cn/dazn/ztzn/201203/t20120313_5591.html.

Nihon Rikugun, Shinkoku Chūtongun, and Shireibu [Japanese Army, Qing Dynasty Army, and the Commanding Post]. 1986 [1909]. In *Ershi shiji chude tianjin gaikuang* [Overview of the Early Twentieth Century in Tianjin]. Translated by Hou Zhentong. Original title: *Tenshin shi* [Tianjin Annals]. Tianjin: Tianjin shi difang shizhi bianxiu weiyuanhui zongbianji shi [Tianjin City Local Records Compilation Committee Chief Editor's Office].

Renmin zhengxie wang [CPPCC Network]. 2009. *Woguo gudai de huimin yaoju* [Ancient Chinese Humanitarian Pharmacy]. http://epaper.rmzxb.com.cn/2009/20090811/t20090811_269070.htm.

Rockefeller Foundation. 1916. *China Medical Board: First Annual Report; December 11, 1914–December 31, 1915*. New York: Rockefeller Foundation.

Shandong daxue Qilu yiyuan zhi bianji weiyuan hui [History of Qilu Hospital at Shandong University Compilation Committee]. 2000. *Shandong daxue Qilu yiyuan zhi 1890–2000* [The History of Qilu Hospital at Shandong University, 1890–2000]. Dezhou: Shandong sheng neibu ziliaoxing chubanwu.

Shanghai tebie shi shehui ju [Shanghai Special Municipal Bureau of Social Affairs Report]. 1929. 301–307.

Shue, Vivienne. 1998. "State Power and the Philanthropic Impulse in China Today." In *Philanthropy in the World's Traditions*, edited by Warren F. Ilchman, Stanley N. Katz, and Edward L. Queen II, 332–354. Bloomington: Indiana University Press.

Tao Shuimu. 2004. "Beiyang zhengfu shiqi shanghai de cishan zuzhi yu cishan shiye" [Charity Organizations and Undertakings in Shanghai during the Period of the Northern Warlord Government]. In *Toushi lao Shanghai* [Perspectives of Old Shanghai], edited by Xiong Yuezhi and Takatsuna Hirobumi, 44–45. Shanghai: Shanghai shehui kexueyuan chubanshe [Shanghai Academy of Social Sciences Publishing House].

Tian Tao. 1995. "Qingmo minchu zai hua jidujiao yiliao weisheng shiye ji qi zhuanye hua" [Christian Medical Undertakings and Its Specialization in China during the End of Qing Dynasty and Beginning of the Republic of China Period]. *Jindai shi yanjiu* [Modern History Studies] 5:169–185.

Xu Yihua, and Han Xinchang. 2003. *Haishang Fanwangdu: Sheng Yuehan daxue* [St. John's College: Pope's Ferry Road by the Sea]. Shijiazhuang: Hebei jiaoyu chubanshe [Hebei Education Publishing House].

Yang Jingqiu. 1932. *Zhonghua jianli gonghui diyi ci da yihui jilu* [Minutes of the First General Assembly of China's Association of Supervision]. Quoted in Li Chuanbin. 2003. "Kangzhan qian nanjing guomin zhengfu dui jiaohui yiliao shiye de taidu he zhengce" [Attitude and Policies toward Missionary Medical Undertakings of the Nanjing Nationalist Government before the War against Japanese Invasion]. *Jiangsu shehui kexue* [Social Sciences of Jiangsu Province] 3:154–159.

Yu Xinzhong. 2003. *Qingdai jiangnan de wenyi yu shehui—yi xiang yiliao shehui shi de yanjiu* [Plague and the Society of Southern China during the Qing Dynasty: A Study of the History of Health and Society]. Beijing: Zhongguo renmin daxue chubanshe [Renmin University of China Press].

Zhang Daqing. 2009. "Zhongguo xiandai yixue chu jian shiqi de buju: Luokefeile jijinhui de yingxiang" [Structure of Early Period of China's Modern Medicine: Impact of the Rockefeller Foundation]. *Ziran kexue yanjiu* [Study of Natural Sciences History] 28 (2): 137–155.

Zhang Kaiyuan, ed. 1991. *Suzhou shanghui dang'an congbian (1905–1911)* [Suzhou Chamber of Commerce Archives Collection (1905–1911)]. Vol. 1. Wuchang: Huazhong shifan daxue chubanshe [Central China Normal University Press].

Zhang Yuzao, Weng Youcheng, and Gao Jinchang, eds. 1991 [1925]. "Renwu zhi—fu yiju" [Record of Famous Figures, with Benevolent Acts]. In *Minguo xu dantu xian zhi* [County Annals of Dantu in the Republic of China Period], Vol. 14, 332. Reprinted in *Jiangsu fu-xian zhiji* [Jiangsu Province Fuxian County Annals], Vol. 30, 679; ser. 8 of *Zhongguo difang zhi jicheng* [China Local Annals Collection]. Nanjing: Jiangsu guji chubanshe [Jiangsu Classics Publishing House]; Shanghai: Shanghai shu dian [Shanghai Bookstore]; Chengdu: Ba Shu shu she [Sichuan Book Society].

Zhou Licheng, and Wang Yongze, eds. 2007. *Waiguoren zai jiu Tianjin* [Foreigners in Old Tianjin]. Tianjin: Tianjin renmin chubanshe [Tianjin People's Publishing House].

Zhou Qingyun, ed. 1991 [1922]. "Yiju er" [Benevolent Acts II]. In *Nanxun zhi* [Nanxun Annals], Vol. 35, 3. Reprinted in *Xiang-zhen zhi zhuanji* [Special Issue of Township Annals], Vol. 22.1, 397; ser. 6 of *Zhongguo difang zhi jicheng* [China Local Annals Collection]. Nanjing: Jiangsu guji chubanshe [Jiangsu Classics Publishing House]; Shanghai: Shanghai shu dian [Shanghai Bookstore]; Chengdu: Ba Shu shu she [Sichuan Book Society].

Zhou Qiuguang, and Zeng Guilin. 2007. "Zhongguo jindai cishan shiye de neirong he tezheng tanxi" [Analysis of Contents and Features of Charities in Modern China]. *Hunan shifan daxue shehui kexue xuebao* [Hunan Normal University Social Sciences Journal] 36 (6): 121–127.

5 American Foundations in Twentieth-Century China

Zi Zhongyun and Mary Brown Bullock

AMERICAN FOUNDATIONS HAVE played a frequently constructive role in China, maintaining cross-cultural engagement amid the political and social upheavals of China's twentieth century and supporting the quest for modernization and reform. This engagement has significantly though by no means exclusively focused on philanthropy for health, with organizations such as the Rockefeller Foundation (RF) and the China Medical Board (CMB) meaningfully contributing to the spread of scientific medicine and the improvement of public health. As this paper will show, the history of American foundations' work in China during the twentieth century holds lessons for the twenty-first: as China emerges as a world power, striving to make its ongoing development sustainable and to grow its own philanthropic institutions, American foundations' successes and setbacks reveal the ability of philanthropic partnerships to transcend international differences and to make both China and the world a better, healthier place.

Historical Overview

Philanthropy for health has played an integral part in American foundations' activities in China from their earliest days: when the Rockefeller Foundation inaugurated its work in China in 1914, it sought to build on the work of earlier medical missionaries, who had introduced Western medical practice and training to Chinese hospitals. While these earlier missionary efforts had elements of both charity and philanthropy, the work of American foundations in China since the RF's arrival has been primarily philanthropic—that is, designed to address systemic health or social problems rather than exclusively focused on alleviating immediate human suffering. During the Republican era, for example, philanthropic strategies—training medical leaders and strengthening academic institutions—endeavored to complement Chinese efforts to create modern education and scientific infrastructure. The advent of the Sino-Japanese War reinforced American philanthropists' concern for China's medical and public health needs. But the establishment of the People's Republic of China and the eruption of the Korean War curtailed American engagement for a quarter of a century.

American foundations did not lose sight of China, but rather became fascinated with its developmental model in medicine, agriculture, and other fields. They also promoted the study of China and American China policy during the years of political estrangement during the Cold War. Not surprisingly, then, American foundations also took the lead in trying to encourage China's efforts to rejoin the community of nations, inviting scholars young and old, American and Chinese, to study abroad in an academic dialogue which continues today.

With the normalization of U.S.-Chinese political relations in 1979, the Chinese government—mindful of the devastation of China's higher education and research infrastructure during the Cultural Revolution—invited the resumption of American foundations' activity on the mainland. Organizations new and old played a major role in China's reintegration into the global community, and their number and range of work expanded. Many followed the Rockefeller model of focusing on professional and intellectual capacity building, with medicine once again a dominant field of interest. But while considerable attention was paid to medical education, biomedical research, and public health, foundations increasingly adopted a more holistic view, recognizing health's overlap with the social sciences, international relations, and environmental concerns. Against this backdrop, partnerships were forged with China's elite universities, as well as with relevant government institutes and research academies. Despite the Tiananmen crisis and its aftermath, American foundations have been able to continue their work in China, making adjustments according to the new situation by increasingly focusing on issues pertaining to law, governance, civil society, and environmental issues. They also started collaborating with emerging and fast-growing Chinese grassroots organizations and nongovernmental institutions. Still, with the recent arrival of the Bill & Melinda Gates Foundation and the continued work of CMB, philanthropy for health has remained the largest area of American engagement in the early years of the twenty-first century.

Two major case studies may serve to illustrate the developments discussed above. Moreover, they serve to underscore that American foundations had their own independent missions and did not necessarily follow U.S. government policies. The first—that of the Rockefeller Foundation and the China Medical Board—highlights the primacy of philanthropy for health in American foundations' engagement with China and its power, both past and present, to effect meaningful, positive change. The second—that of the Ford Foundation—illustrates the broader role of American philanthropy in China during the reform era, including concern for environmental and economic well-being, and highlights the potential of philanthropic organizations to transcend international differences. Particular attention is given to the early years of the Deng Xiaoping era because it was not a foregone conclusion that American philanthropies could successfully work in post-Mao China. These two case studies, along with a brief discussion of other organizations' work, reveal the powerful and usually nonpolitical role of cultural diplomacy in strengthening U.S.-China relations across a turbulent century. As will be seen in their leading role in the reopening to China in the 1970s, the persistence of their programs through the 1989 Tiananmen crisis, and the reimagining of priorities in the advent of China as a global power, the experiences of American foundations are as relevant today as they were in the twentieth century. The historical contributions of these philanthropic organizations to China's reform and modernization, as well as their motivations and means of achieving their goals, hold present-day potential as models for a China enjoying material wealth and increasingly eager to develop domestic philanthropy.

Looking across the century the question often asked by Chinese is: why do foundations come to China to conduct nonprofit work? The motivation of American foundations has often been suspect, in part because of cultural differences and the Cold War atmosphere that prevailed after 1949. Even at present, despite the positive results and thriving activities, such suspicion has not been completely dispelled. In the case studies which follow, five general philanthropic goals can be found: to reform China, to provide assistance to China as a developing country, to promote Chinese-American mutual understanding, to encourage Chinese philanthropy, and to promote sustainable development and thereby advance the cause of world peace and prosperity.

The Rockefeller Foundation

Both domestically and internationally, the great pioneer in American medical and public health philanthropy was the Rockefeller Foundation. Its major benefactor, John D. Rockefeller, had first steered its efforts toward medicine—specifically scientific medicine—at the turn of the twentieth century, and this interest endured: during the first half of the twentieth century China received the largest international disbursement of RF funds, and most of them went toward initiatives in medicine and public health. The RF's famous establishment of the Peking Union Medical College (PUMC) and its affiliated hospital, a transplantation of the Johns Hopkins model emphasizing scientific education, clinical experience, and research, stands as a particularly salient example of this dedication to philanthropy for health. PUMC not only was the earliest modern medical college and hospital in China, but it also trained many of the doctors and high-level medical professionals who would become the backbone of later medical development. PUMC's alumni were broadly humanistic but also versed in the latest scientific knowledge, setting them apart from the staff at missionary hospitals, whose expertise was more basic.[1]

While the RF's choice to focus on medical education was influenced by the medical work of missionary organizations, it had secular ambitions from the beginning, leading it to eschew the more potentially controversial project of creating a university. In the estimation of the Rockefeller philanthropic circle, health philanthropy could overcome all possible political obstacles, benefiting the people of all nations. This consideration did not mean that the RF avoided all risks: the fate of PUMC followed the vicissitudes of the Chinese situation. In the 1920s, it only partially complied with the Chinese government's policy of "sinicization," but by the late 1930s almost all of its faculty and administrative leaders were Chinese. During the Sino-Japanese War, PUMC was occupied and seriously damaged by Japanese troops; recovered in 1946 and nationalized after the outbreak of the Korean War by the newly founded PRC government (Rockefeller Foundation 1947), it would undergo several politically motivated name changes—including "Capital Hospital" and "Anti-Imperialist Hospital"—during the following three decades, before finally reverting to its original name amid more general "opening and reform" in 1986. It remains among the most prestigious medical institutions in China.

The RF's efforts during the Republican period were not, however, limited to explicitly medical education. The organization also helped develop the natural and social sciences, offering pioneering support for biology, chemistry, agricultural science, sociology, and economics. Yenching, Nankai, Nanjing, and National Central Universities each became preeminent in one or more of these fields due to RF support. One of the foundation's most famous initiatives, growing out of its support for paleontology, was financing the excavation and study of the "Peking Man" in Zhoukoudian; the specimen's skullcap was studied and certified jointly by Chinese and foreign scholars in the Department of Anatomy at PUMC. The RF model of targeted and sustained support for binational research collaboration in select disciplines established a model for Sino-American cultural relations which would be renewed in the 1980s (Rockefeller Foundation 1929; Bowers, Hess, and Sivin 1988, 3–29, 31–50, 81–82; Bullock 2011).

To complement its expensive, elite-focused PUMC initiatives, the RF also became involved with policy concerning public health and rural reconstruction. Public outreach in medicine came primarily from the faculty and graduates of PUMC's Department of Public Health, who became leaders in the national and provincial health administrations during the Republican period. The RF concurrently turned its attention to China's rural needs, establishing the North China Council for Rural Development to coordinate with James Y. C. Yen's Mass Education Movement in Ding County. This mainly grassroots work also exploited the RF's academic connections, involving sociology faculty from Yenching University and economics faculty and public health specialists from Nankai University. Although family planning was not officially part of its agenda, invitations to Margaret Sanger and staff reports stating that China's rural population would be open to birth control measures indicate that the RF's outlook on this issue was ahead of its time.[2]

In 1943–1944, the RF initiated a program to "rescue" Chinese intellectuals from the extremely difficult working conditions that accompanied the most desperate period of China's war of resistance against Japanese aggression when China's best professors and scholars persisted on pursuing their work, accepting suggestions from John K. Fairbank, who worked at the U.S. embassy, and Robert Winter, an American professor at Tsinghua University. The project consisted of sponsoring a year of study at American universities for a select group of Chinese scholars deemed crucial to postwar academic reconstruction. These top-ranking professors included the linguist Luo Changpei, the philosopher Feng Youlan, the architect Liang Sicheng, and the sociologist Fei Xiaotong. Their presence in the United States not only facilitated the publication in translation of their works, but also strengthened China studies in the United States, a long-term RF goal (Zi 2007, 169–171).

The work of the RF, combining health and medicine in elite institutions with grassroots work on rural reconstruction and support for the American study of China, established a framework for philanthropic support to China which would be emulated by itself and others when the United States and China reestablished relations in 1979. Perhaps the key to its success was its persistence, both in adapting to China's turbulent national conditions and—especially during the war of resistance against Japanese aggression—in enduring hardship alongside the Chinese people. At the same time, the foundation mainly avoided involvement in China's tumultuous politics, hoping to continue their work even after the Chinese Communist Party declared victory.

During the several decades of exclusion that followed the founding of the PRC, the Rockefeller family maintained its interest in China, and when American wariness began to relax during the Johnson administration, John D. Rockefeller III asked his employees to study ways to "break the ice" in U.S.-China relations. The RF also took the lead in making significant contributions to organizations endeavoring to reopen relations with China (Ensor and Johnson 1991, 47). It is thus not surprising that in 1979 the Rockefeller Foundation became the first foundation to restore its relationship with China. By this time medicine and public health were no longer explicit Rockefeller priorities, though other RF fields of interest with respect to China—such as the agricultural sciences, family planning, and the environment—retained an implicit connection to health. Beginning in the 1980s, the foundation went against mainstream opinion in the United States, providing moral and material help to China's family-planning endeavors; meanwhile, it continued to support China studies in the United States, and to sponsor American training of Chinese students and scholars in the agricultural and population sciences.

The RF focus has shifted over time. Total RF funding for China in the first half of the twentieth century was $54 million (approximately $600 million in 2000 currency), and from 1972 to 2005, $40 million. In 2005, the RF began to terminate many of its international programs, including those in China, focusing instead on a new global mission to impact poor and vulnerable people, with a particular emphasis on Africa (Bullock 2011, 161–171). But its legacy in China is still important: in January 2013 the Rockefeller Foundation celebrated its centennial anniversary at PUMC with an international conclave of public health and medical ministers.

Common to all RF programs had been the purposeful integration of Chinese scientists and research institutes into extensive international networks. At the beginning of this period, China's science was just beginning to emerge from isolation and the devastating Cultural Revolution. By the end of the twentieth century, China's scientific infrastructure had been reinvigorated and was well on its way to becoming integrated with world science; the country had established its own cutting-edge research and educational institutions and was poised for takeoff in the twenty-first century. A concern for health also proved to be an enduring feature of the RF's work in China—a legacy taken up by the China Medical Board.

The China Medical Board, Inc. (CMB)

Initially, the China Medical Board was the division of the Rockefeller Foundation responsible for the creation and management of the Peking Union Medical College. CMB was, however, fully endowed by the RF in 1947 and thereafter became an independent organization. During the Cold War era, it operated medical programs throughout Asia, having been excluded by the PRC, but after 1980 it also returned to China. Like the RF, CMB was invited back to China shortly after the normalization of diplomatic relations between the two countries. In consultation with the Ministry of Health, it was agreed that CMB would work with 7 key medical schools (later expanded to 13) rather than only with PUMC. Initially, its programs focused on faculty development, libraries, and research, in an effort to help rebuild China's core medical institutions after the ravages of the Cultural Revolution. Subsequent initiatives included medical research grants and the formation of national and regional networks, including networks for medical administrators and nurses. Although most of its focus in the 1980s and 1990s was on elite medical schools, CMB also began to work with Jiujiang Medical College, a three-year institution in Jiangxi Province tasked with developing a model curriculum for doctors practicing in rural areas. Beyond this partnership, CMB was also instrumental in the opening of a three-year medical college in Tibet. More broadly, reforms in medical education continued to be part of the CMB portfolio, evoking its earliest work at PUMC.

In 2006 CMB pivoted from a general focus on improving key medical universities, which are now well provided for by the Chinese government, to a tighter focus on ensuring equitable access to basic curative and preventive services. New objectives include establishing a network of rural medical schools and research and training centers for health policy science. CMB has also sought to bring the Chinese health system, including its recent reforms, to the attention of a broad international audience through a series of special issues of the *Lancet*. In 2009, it established a small office in Beijing primarily staffed by Chinese citizens, resuming a presence that had been disrupted in 1950. Between 1980 and 2008, CMB spent approximately $130 million in China—some three times the expenditure of its original parent organization, the RF. In 2010 its annual China program budget was approximately $8 million, third among international philanthropies with presences in China behind the Gates and Ford Foundations—a further testament to the prominence of health philanthropy in American foundations' work in China (Bullock 2011, 171–177, 193–196).

The Ford Foundation

The Ford Foundation (FF) began its work in China in 1978 and quickly became the preeminent American foundation working in reform-era China. Its early philanthropic strategy—focusing on institution building in key social science fields—echoed the Rockefeller Foundation's earlier pattern, but its early interest in strengthening economic and legal reforms and its subsequent attention to China's underprivileged populations have broken new ground in America's philanthropic engagement with China. The breadth of its activities suggests the many ways—some less direct than others—in which American foundations can impact Chinese public health, and its committed engagement with China demonstrates the potential of foundations to preserve international cultural ties even amid political turmoil.

The FF's role in China in the last quarter-century cannot be understood without recognition of its paramount role in supporting China studies during the Cold War era. When Ford funding started during the height of McCarthyism, when research on modern China was taboo, the foundation's leaders claimed that they were "moving against the wave."[3] Its earliest initiatives included a 1949 survey of intellectual refugees from mainland China residing in Hong Kong, and—more controversially—a grant of $28,600 to Zhang Guotao, a Chinese Communist Party "renegade" residing in Canada, to write his autobiography in English. The FF also inaugurated large-scale support for East Asian studies in the United States when it announced in 1953 a $488,150 scholarship fund to be given to 97 young Americans to pursue studies in Asia and the Middle East. This program expanded to include the study of China under a Communist regime, inviting famous China scholars like John King Fairbank, A. Doak Barnett, and George Taylor as advisors (Zi 2007, 178). The FF contributed a total of roughly $23 million to Chinese studies from 1959 to 1970, compared to the federal government's support of $15 million during the same period (Sutton 1987, 101). Beneficiaries included major universities and research institutes such as the Fairbank Center at Harvard University, founded in 1955 with Ford and Carnegie Endowment funding, and the American Council of Learned Societies.[4] At the beginning of the U.S.-China détente, the American journalist James Reston commented that a new generation of China experts had grown to meet the needs of the time and that the Ford Foundation had made a significant contribution to this.[5]

The Ford Foundation also played a pioneering role in changing rigid U.S. policy toward China during the 1960s. For example, it funded the collaborative work between the Council on Foreign Relations and the University of Michigan that ultimately yielded the eight-book series titled *The United States and China in World Affairs*. The series represented the first objective analysis of mainland China in American academia since the Korean War and was the first major study to call for a reexamination of American policy, concluding that the American public preferred a more flexible stance on China. Former CIA director Allen Dulles's chairmanship of the books' directing committee illustrates the indirect relationship between the Ford Foundation and American government diplomacy (Zi 2007, 180; Zi 1987).

This background of participation in policy debates explains why the FF was poised to support organizations involved with China during the 1970s and to initiate its own programs as soon as it political circumstances permitted. Following diplomatic renormalization, the foundation contributed $250,000 to the U.S. National Academy of Sciences' Committee on Scholarly Communication with the People's Republic of China, to Stanford University, and to other institutions for the purpose of conducting academic exchanges and international symposia on Northeast Asian security and China's economy and trade. Promising contacts were established between high-ranking FF officials—such as its director for international affairs, Marshall Robinson—and Chinese scholars and officials (Zi 2007, 182). Recognizing China's continued development and progress toward reform, the FF was ready by 1979 to commence direct assistance to China. While its general goals were similar to those of the RF, the FF saw its role in more comprehensive terms. By helping China to tackle its problems as a developing country—in particular, poverty and poor enterprise management—the foundation believed it would be supporting significant gains in human health and welfare, while indirectly contributing to the evolution of a more peaceful international community.

The FF's interest in facilitating academic dialogue persisted after the resumption of normal relations. In 1979, it negotiated a partnership with the newly independent Chinese Academy of Social Sciences (CASS), which it perceived to have great influence over policymaking in the reform era due to its membership of high-level scholars in the social sciences and humanities. More importantly, the CASS leadership—represented by Vice President Huan Xiang—looked favorably on international scholarly exchanges and funding. The collaborative agreement reached by the FF and CASS pledged to provide educational and research opportunities for Chinese and Americans that would "contribute to China's accomplishment of the four modernizations, to greater understanding by the world of China's development experience, and toward . . . knowledge and understanding as a contribution to the peaceful resolution of international issues." Initially the fields of economic management, law, and international relations were prioritized.[6]

From this modest starting point, the FF's activities rapidly expanded to include collaboration with other American organizations on managing extensive international training and research in these fields. For example, the foundation established the Committee for International Relations Studies with the PRC, which selected approximately 20 junior and senior scholars each year to study in the United States. Similar programs in law, economics, and other fields were established and continued for roughly 15 years, making a major contribution toward the establishment of these modern disciplines in China.

In 1987 these engagements led the FF to take the step—unprecedented for an American foundation since the founding of the PRC—of establishing an office in China. Only two years later, U.S.-Chinese relations would be shaken by the incident in Tiananmen Square, but Ford's active presence was not greatly affected. While some meetings were postponed or canceled, the director of the FF's office in China, Peter Geithner, and other leaders resisted pressure from the U.S. government to interrupt their work. Geithner insisted that the foundation should not abandon its Chinese partners during difficult times, and it would be easy to leave but difficult to return. The leadership at the foundation's headquarters was convinced: the FF's guiding principle would be to support China's reform and opening up, not a particular party or group. Geithner states that he did not receive any pressure from the Chinese side requesting Ford to leave and characterizes the 20 years of cooperation with China he witnessed as basically smooth.[7] Other foundations followed Ford's lead and continued their programs in China despite the political tumult, including the RF, the Rockefeller Brothers Fund (RBF), the China Medical Board, and the Henry Luce Foundation. This continuity attests to philanthropy's capacity to work as a form of cultural diplomacy and to preserve meaningful bilateral ties amid political crisis.

China's ongoing development and reform after Tiananmen created new problems that invited the FF to engage even more profoundly with social issues, many of them related to health. For example, in the 1990s the foundation added new programs focused on development, the environment, and reproductive health. (Chapter 9 in this section explores in detail the FF's contributions to gender and reproductive health.) Briefly, the FF—like the RF—maintained a positive disposition toward China's birth control program. The FF's efforts in this area included collaborative research with China's Population Information and Research Center on the impact of family planning across generations of women. After the 1994 International Conference on Population and Development in Cairo and the 1995 Beijing International Women's Conference, Ford strengthened its work in this area further. In recognition of the FF's contribution, the Chinese Family Planning Commission presented it with the Fourth Chinese Population—International Collaboration Award. FF president Susan Berresford made a special trip to China to receive this award, the first given by the Chinese government to a foreign foundation.[8]

In the first decade of the twenty-first century, the FF modified both its strategy and its tactics in China, increasing the breadth of its activities while simultaneously shifting its funding priorities from capacity building to direct action. Alongside new programs on the environment, culture, poverty alleviation, and education in remote areas, the foundation modified its grant-making to focus less on building the capacity of major academic institutions and more on specific localized projects and collaborative funding. Examples of this new approach include work on microloans with the Economic Cooperative for Poverty Alleviation and on specific activist projects pertaining to village elections, legacy advocacy, legal aid, and women's reproductive rights.[9] These shifts reflect the FF's changing global priorities; by 2010, the FF's China goal explicitly reflected society's need "to develop the social sector and help marginalized groups access opportunities and resources." By directly supporting "research entities, civil society organizations and government organizations that share in this goal [the FF seeks to] help disadvantaged people and communities participate as partners in China's development and help them gain essential resources to combat poverty, inequality and discrimination" (Ford Foundation 2010). Today Ford's activities fall into one or more of five program areas: democratic and accountable government; human rights; sustainable development; educational opportunities and scholarship; and sexuality and reproductive health and rights (Ford Foundation 2010; Ford Foundation n.d.).

The FF's China trajectory from the Cold War to active support of China's official reform and development policies and then extensive engagement with Chinese nongovernmental organizations illustrates a general trend in American philanthropic engagement in China. According to data from Ford's Beijing office, from January 1988 to 2010 the foundation provided $275 million to China. Although Ford's annual allocation for China has declined in the last decade, from roughly $16 million in the late 1990s to roughly $13 million in 2010, it still ranks as the largest American source of philanthropic funding in China.

Other American Foundations

Among American philanthropic institutions operating in China, the Rockefeller Foundation, China Medical Board, and Ford Foundation have had the longest history and made the largest financial contributions. Other organizations have also had significant presences, however, most notably the Rockefeller Brothers Fund, the Henry Luce Foundation, and the Asia Foundation. The Henry Luce Foundation and the Rockefeller Brothers Fund are of particular interest because they represent philanthropic legacies in China, while the Asia Foundation, with significant funding from the U.S. government, is more representative of the United States' foreign policy priorities.

The Henry Luce Foundation's engagement with China arose out of its benefactor's background. Luce, a media mogul and co-founder of *Time* magazine, had been raised in China by American missionaries and formed his foundation in 1936 to honor the work of his father, an educational missionary who had been one of the founders of Yenching University. From its inception, the Luce Foundation has promoted a deeper American understanding of China, with a particular interest in supporting the American China studies community and promoting collaboration between Chinese and American scholars (Guzzardi 1988).

The RBF also owes its interest in China to its founders' family background. Established in the 1940s by the five offspring of John D. Rockefeller Jr., the RBF has from its outset endeavored to play a different role from that of the RF and other earlier Rockefeller philanthropies. China emerged as one of its major focuses in the 1980s as it launched programs designed to address strategic issues in the Asia Pacific region in dialogue with China. In more recent years, the RBF has focused on environmental sustainability, with a particular focus on grassroots organizations in southern China. In the first decade of the twenty-first century, the RBF designated southern China as one of its four "pivotal places"; as of 2013, it is one of three such places, and has been the recipient of increasingly generous grants focusing on the environment, health, energy, and climate change. Empowering local civic organization has been an underlying goal of RBF's China philanthropy, and as such the RBF was one of the first major American foundations to embrace China's growing NGO community. Specifically, it uses the programmatic concept of "strengthening community leadership to support sustainable development" to encompass independent citizens' networks as well as local Chinese philanthropic organizations (Rockefeller Brothers Fund 2013).

The Asia Foundation represents another variety of American philanthropic engagement with China. Created in 1954 by act of the U.S. Congress, its original purpose was to support liberal democracies and market economies in Asia as bulwarks against communism. Over the years, however, the Asia Foundation became a more independent institution, drawing funding from private American sources as well as from technical assistance agencies in the United Kingdom, the

Netherlands, Canada, and Australia. In China it has worked on governance, law, and civil society with both national and regional organizations and with certain universities.

This is by no means an exhaustive survey. Many other smaller foundations, including the Kettering Foundation, the Maureen and Mike Mansfield Foundation, and the Carnegie Institute have overseen programs addressing specific issues. Of particular note is the Kettering Foundation, which has sponsored a U.S.-China Dialogue with CASS for twenty years. Modeled after the U.S.-Soviet Dartmouth Dialogue, this program has brought Chinese and American academics and political leaders together annually to explore sensitive issues of common concern. Still other foundations have newly established Chinese presences, including the Carnegie Foundation for International Peace, the Mellon Foundation, and—most recently—the Clinton Foundation. The largest new foundation to enter the China scene has been the Bill & Melinda Gates Foundation, which is significantly focused on health-related programs. (The Gates Foundation's work on HIV/AIDS in China is discussed in a later chapter in this section.) Taken as a whole, all of these foundations provide further evidence of the scope and variety of American philanthropic endeavors in China.

Reflections on American Philanthropy in China

Both continuity and change characterize American foundations' first century in China. Buffeted by sudden political shifts and gradual social ones, organizations have had to constantly adjust their goals and strategies; at the same time, however, certain enduring principles have provided them with the resolve needed to make such adjustments. Some are applicable to American philanthropy more broadly and have been discussed by the authors elsewhere—among them, American elites' *noblesse oblige* and their desire to mitigate capitalism's inevitable material inequities (Zi 2007)—but a consistent theme, echoing that of the missionaries, was the desire to reform the beneficiaries according to American standards. Throughout the twentieth century, as it struggled for its transformation into a modern country, China provided a perfect arena for American foundations. Chinese intellectuals in particular were ideal vehicles for introducing Western culture into their own as they sought to make their country healthy, prosperous, and modern.

During the Republican period, China's situation matched well with the Rockefeller Foundation's mission. China's unique standing as a large and populous country rich in culture and history but poor in wealth helped persuade the Rockefeller Foundation to make it an international priority. Moreover, Chinese society was in the midst of a dramatic historical change, opening itself to the West and to new ideas. The intellectual elites of the time, deeply cultivated in traditional Chinese culture but at the same time open-minded and eager to modernize China, were ideal conduits for Western ideas, which attracted American philanthropists like the RF. Since modern medicine and public health were relatively uncontroversial aspects of Western culture, they were ideal philanthropic projects, benefiting all peoples. An undated letter preserved in the RF's archive written by an American teacher at the Union Medical College—the predecessor to PUMC—notes the eagerness with which Chinese students wanted to learn Western medicine and reveals the kind of thinking inherent in the RF's initial mission to China, which also applied to other American foundations throughout the century:

> The century for us to help China has come, because China has realized its needs. Chinese young people are eager to learn western medicine. But what we can accomplish is far beyond establishing the medical foundation for this great country. We have much more opportunities: we could form the character of future Chinese doctors, who can be transformed to human being [*sic*] touched by Chinese holy spirit. Everything is experiencing dramatic change. . . . Chinese are eager to accept whatever we can give. There are many indications that China will not be so willing to learn from foreigners. But at present we can influence China. Chinese would like to listen to us, to be influenced, and do so under the theory of our framework.[10]

During this initial phase of American philanthropies' work in China, there was certainly a desire to help a poor country develop, but there was an interest—often motivated by appreciation of China's rich cultural heritage, and of the bravery and spirit of its people—in helping China in particular. The RF's staff expressed admiration for Chinese bravery and took pride in sustaining its work in China during the Sino-Japanese War, for instance, and in 1944, its president wrote,

> The war is bringing China into the forefront among the nations. A long and distinguished civilization and a great people are at last about to take their place among the leading forces of the world. Their heroic services in this war have earned the gratitude and admiration of the world, and the contributions which their great native abilities and inherent friendliness are bound to make to an advancing civilization entitle them to every consideration in the difficult days ahead. (Fosdick 1944, 17)

In the last decades of the century, this special sympathy for China from the first half of the century reappeared, easing the return of American foundations to China after a 30-year hiatus and mitigating some American political constraints on assistance to Communist countries. Indeed, especially since the U.S. government did not sanction developmental assistance funding for China until very recently, American private foundations truly played a distinct role. Foundations such as the Ford Foundation, for example, held a long-term view of their work in China, which was not easily dissuaded by the Chinese political situation.

This second phase in U.S.-China cultural relations began with China's re-opening in the late 1970s and continued through the first decade of the twenty-first century. During this period, health philanthropy, the avant-garde of Republican-era reform, remained important, but many foundations followed Ford's lead and sought to more directly promote reform, democratization, and modernization. This phase took on a different tone thanks to added communication channels and more comprehensive programmatic initiatives. Moreover, with China having a far stronger government than it did during the Republican era, American foundations often found themselves compelled to pursue reform jointly with national or regional agencies and think tanks. At the same time, the proliferation of Chinese nongovernmental organizations as reform agents led other foundations to concentrate on supporting grassroots activities. Different foundations developed different views on how best to promote reform, and focused their work accordingly. These reforms often involved changing government policies, some of which were critical of international involvement. Foundation staff had to cope with these fluctuations and sometimes adjust priorities in order to be effective. The persistence of foundation visions, however, illustrates that foundations usually made policies and decisions independently, free from either Chinese or American government intervention.

Promoting American understanding of China was another rationale for American engagement with China and also a way to influence U.S. policymaking, especially after 1949. Philanthropic relationships between American foundations and their Chinese collaborators made tremendous strides in this regard. Foundation-supported research played a role in policy changes, especially in the 1960s. Foundation officials believed that helping Chinese understand Americans would also reduce animosity, thus generating a positive impact on bilateral relations.

In addition to promoting mutual understanding, and hoping to reform China in ways that would benefit the people of China, during both of these phases American foundations provided assistance to China as a developing country, particularly in health and education. Yet, by the early twenty-first century, it became more difficult for Americans to see China as a developing country, thus altering the premise for previous philanthropic work. Recognizing the strides China had made, the Rockefeller Foundation ended its formal work there, shifting to focus on Africa and other less-developed regions, while the Ford Foundation reduced its China funding and refocused much of what remained on marginalized people and institutions within China. Other foundations sought a new rationale for promoting philanthropic work in an increasingly wealthy country, and placed greater emphasis on such issues of common global concern as the environment and emergent civil society, frequently in collaboration with nascent Chinese organizations.

In summary, through long-term interaction with the Chinese, American foundations developed a better understanding of Chinese culture. While not abandoning their own values, for over one hundred years they have adapted their work to China's conditions. American foundations have also possessed a kind of endurance and resilience in the face of instability and fluctuating situations. They have learned to work with many different levels of Chinese government and society—from national institutes to key universities to grassroots organizations—and their activities in China have had a broad geographical sweep, from Yunnan to Beijing. They have assisted in building Chinese intellectual capital in many fields and observed successive generations taking over the reins of institutional leadership. At the same time, they have strengthened American understanding of China's reform process at both the national and local levels.

The Future of U.S. Philanthropic Foundations in China

With China having become an emerging world power, no longer "poor and backward" in the eyes of foreign observers, some may question whether its philanthropic partnership with American foundations even merits continuation. As noted above, some foundations have already begun to focus on less-developed countries where the impact of philanthropic work is more visible. Moreover, if one accepts that philanthropic foundations' original *raison d'être* was to help the disadvantaged and promote social progress, such a shift in focus may appear warranted. Reflecting on the motivations of the American-Chinese philanthropic partnership and on the current state of Chinese society demonstrates, however, that far from ending their mission in China, foreign foundations—and American foundations in particular—are still very much needed, and can play an important role in helping to further develop Chinese civil society.

As described above and demonstrated through the case studies, five underlying philanthropic goals can be ascribed to American foundations' work in China: to reform China, to provide assistance to China as a developing country, to promote Chinese-American mutual understanding, to encourage Chinese philanthropy, and to promote sustainable development and thereby advance the cause of world peace and prosperity. The first two goals predominated during the first phase of American foundation work in China, and the third during the political tumult of the second phase—while American Sinology had been sponsored by the RF in the early days, promoting mutual understanding underpinned the Ford Foundation's support for China studies in the 1950s, for instance, and continues with the Luce Foundation's ongoing support of Chinese and American scholarship.

During the first two decades of the twenty-first century, one sees the continuation of American interest in promoting reforms, assisting development, and promoting mutual understanding. But as China has emerged as a global power, the last two goals—encouraging Chinese philanthropy and promoting sustainable development—are especially salient today. With many NGOs within China emerging to fulfill social welfare functions not performed by the state, the availability of American foundations as role models and partners is crucial for the further development of a distinctly Chinese philanthropic culture.

It should be noted that the encouragement of Chinese philanthropy by American foundations is quite new. As Chinese NGOs and foundations proliferate, international foundations now find themselves in a complementary rather than dominant role. American foundations are now not only contributing to the work of the Chinese NGO community but are also assisting in providing leadership training for China's nascent but burgeoning philanthropic community. As is evident from the chapters in this volume, this community draws inspiration and lessons from a century of American philanthropic work, but it is simultaneously creating a distinctly Chinese modern philanthropic culture. Beyond providing leadership training, American organizations can effect change by spreading their values and culture to Chinese organizations, including their ideals, spirit, ethics, and their experiences in management. Under the present new circumstances in China, the following are areas in which American foundations can play a role in encouraging Chinese philanthropy:

Burgeoning Foundations and NGOs

- Form partnerships with relatively advanced and mature Chinese foundations to carry out joint programs and share mutually helpful experiences
- Support capacity building through various programs in NGOs throughout the sector, including training courses, publications, and support for the establishment of centers and faculties in educational institutions

Potential Donors

- Encourage the growth of the sector by educating potential donors through sharing knowledge and experiences. In China, donors consist mainly of affluent entrepreneurs or the super-rich, in contrast to the United States, where people of different socioeconomic statuses give large and small donations to causes that are important to them. The emerging wealthy class in China does not lack the will to make philanthropic contributions, and the concept of corporate social responsibility (CSR) has become quite popular. However, many of these potential donors lack the knowledge of how to best engage in philanthropy, and they do not know how to contribute effectively to benefit both the needy and society at large.

Lawmakers

- Engage in dialogues with Chinese lawmakers to help build a more hospitable legal framework. The main obstructions to philanthropic work in China at present stem from the legal and regulation system. Representatives of U.S. foundations could find and create opportunities to interact with Chinese officials who are concerned with promoting the growth of philanthropy within China.

Needy Grassroots NGOs

- Assist grassroots NGOs suffering from a lack of funding and facing oner-ous registration requirements. So far, many grassroots NGOs have relied on foreign support to continue their work. Here, the direct assistance of U.S. foundations is still crucial.

Beyond encouraging and enabling Chinese philanthropy, American founda-tions can also play a significant part in promoting sustainable development, and thereby contributing to the cause of world peace and prosperity. While China is perhaps not a "developing" country, its economy is still not as developed as that of the United States and other Western nations, and its ongoing development has taken a heavy toll on the health of its environment and people. That this toll has implications for international peace has been acknowledged by the Carnegie Foundation, which seeks to strengthen U.S.-China strategic dialogue on issues ranging from nuclear proliferation and regional security to climate change pol-icy. Thus, American philanthropic motives to promote world peace and sustain-able development, and health philanthropy in particular, remain significant.

In conclusion, American philanthropy in China has a long and venerable history and has proved resilient and adaptable to changing conditions in both countries over a long century. Moving into the twenty-first century, there are many opportunities for new forms of partnership between American philan-thropy and China's own national, and perhaps global, philanthropy.

Notes

This paper has been adapted from Zi (2007), modified and updated by the author. It has been further revised and updated by Mary Brown Bullock. For an earlier article on the Rockefeller Foundation see Zi (1996); for an English version of the same, see Zi (1995).

    1. Articles and books on the Rockefeller Foundation and the Peking Union Medical Col-lege are numerous. For reference, see Ferguson (1973); Bullock (1980); Bowers (1972); and Wang (1991).

    2. "Microfilm Series 1.1 (Project)—China, Introduction," n.d., Rockefeller Foundation Ar-chives, Rockefeller Archive Center, Sleepy Hollow, NY.

    3. Joseph Slater, n.d., oral history, Ford Foundation Archives, Rockefeller Archive Center, Sleepy Hollow, NY.

    4. "Report of the Director, Harvard University, East Asian Research Center," December 1965, R. 1601, 67–166, Ford Foundation Archives.

5. "Responding to opportunities related to the People's Republic of China," n.d., International Division (Asia and the Pacific), FF 0331119, Box #16599, Ford Foundation Archives.

6. "Information Paper—Next Steps for the Foundation Concerning China, Asia and Pacific Program," June 1979, FF 033119, Box 16599, Ford Foundation Archives; "General Terms of Agreement Between the Chinese Academy of Social Sciences and the Ford Foundation," March 23, 1983, attachment to "Discussion Paper, The Ford Foundation and China," for discussion at the meeting of the Trustees' Human Rights, Governance and International Affairs Committee, FF 033119, Box #16599, Ford Foundation Archives.

7. Peter Geithner, former director of Asia Programs, Ford Foundation, in discussions with Zi Zhongyun, 1990–2000.

8. The Chinese Population Award is China's highest family-planning award.

9. Tony Saich, former representative of the Ford Foundation in China, in discussion with Zi Zhongyun, 1997.

10. Also RG 4, S1, Box 11, File 50, Rockefeller Foundation Archives. The letter is undated, but according to its contents, it is estimated to have been written between 1915 and 1916.

References

Bowers, John Z. 1972. *Western Medicine in a Chinese Palace: Peking Union Medical College, 1917–1951.* New York: Josiah Macy Jr. Foundation.

Bowers, John Z., J. William Hess, and Nathan Sivin, eds. 1988. *Science and Medicine in Twentieth-Century China: Research and Education.* Ann Arbor: Center for Chinese Studies, University of Michigan.

Bullock, Mary Brown. 1980. *An American Transplant: The Rockefeller Foundation and Peking Union Medical College.* Berkeley: University of California Press.

———. 2011. *The Oil Prince's Legacy: Rockefeller Philanthropy in China.* Washington, DC: Woodrow Wilson Center and Stanford University Press.

Ensor, John H., and Peter Johnson. 1991. *The Rockefeller Conscience.* New York: Macmillan.

Ferguson, Mary E. 1973. *China Medical Board and Peking Union Medical College: A Chronicle of Fruitful Collaboration.* New York: China Medical Board.

Ford Foundation. 2010. *Annual Report 2010.* http://www.fordfoundation.org/about-us/2010-annual-report.

———. n.d. "China: Overview." Accessed December 2013. http://www.fordfoundation.org/regions/china/.

Fosdick, Raymond B. 1944. "The President's Review for 1944." In *The Rockefeller Foundation, Annual Report 1944*, 1–40. New York: Rockefeller Foundation. http://www.rockefellerfoundation.org/uploads/files/d336704a-253d-45da-8572-5c98bcd65801-1944.pdf.

Guzzardi, Walter, Jr. 1988. *The Henry Luce Foundation, A History: 1930–1989.* Chapel Hill: University of North Carolina Press.

Rockefeller Brothers Fund. 2013. "Pivotal Place: Southern China Guidelines." http://www.rbf.org/program/pivotal-place-southern-china/guidelines.

Rockefeller Foundation. 1929. *Annual Report—1929.* New York: Rockefeller Foundation.

———. 1947. *Annual Report—1947.* New York: Rockefeller Foundation.

Sutton, Francis S. 1987. "American Philanthropy in Educational and Cultural Exchanges with the PRC." In *Educational Exchanges: Essays on the Sino-American Experience*, edited by Joyce Kalgren and Dennis Simon, 96–118. Berkeley, CA: Institute of East Asian Studies.

Wang Ning. 1991. "Peking Union Medical College: The Rockefeller Foundation's Contribution to the Progress of Chinese Medicine." In *Zhongxi wenhua yu Jiaohui daxue* [Christian Universities and Chinese-Western Cultures], edited by Zhang Kaiyuan and Lin Wei, 271–300. Hankou: Hubei jiaoyu chubanshe.

Zi Zhongyun. 1987. "Huanman de jiedong—Zhong-Mei guanxi dakai zhi qian shi ji nian jian Meiguo dui Hua yulun de zhuanbian guocheng" [Slow Détente: The Process of Change in American Public Opinions During the Decade Prior to the Normalization of China-U.S. Relations]. *Meiguo yanjiu*, no. 2: 7–35.

——. 1995. "The Rockefeller Foundation and China." *American Studies in China*, no. 2: 84–121.

——. 1996. "Luokefeile jijinhui yu Zhongguo" [The Rockefeller Foundation and China]. *Meiguo yanjiu*, no. 1: 58–89.

——. 2007. *The Destiny of Wealth: An Analysis of American Philanthropic Foundations From a Chinese Perspective.* Dayton, OH: Kettering Foundation.

6 Connecting Philanthropy with Innovation

China in the First Half of the Twentieth Century

Darwin H. Stapleton

THE HISTORICAL RELATIONSHIP between modern American philanthropy and modern technology is deep and multifaceted. By examining that history through case studies in China in the first half of the twentieth century, this chapter will examine that relationship as a means of better understanding how modern philanthropy not only has attempted to realize its goals through technological innovation, but in some cases has also chosen distinct goals incorporating technological innovations.

Modern American philanthropy is rooted in the great wealth created by the American industrialization of the latter nineteenth and early twentieth centuries. The exemplars are Andrew Carnegie and John D. Rockefeller, each of whom accumulated enormous resources rapidly (and in ways that forced the rethinking of government regulation of business), and who believed that with wealth came social responsibility for its disposition. Both men (and others, such as Olivia Sage and Julius Rosenwald) chose the organizational format they were familiar with—the corporation (albeit the nonprofit form of a philanthropic foundation)—as a means of disposing of the greatest portion of their wealth, thus giving us the shape of modern organized philanthropy. Many of those who became the trustees of those first great foundations were schooled in the industrial world, and we should not be surprised that they often displayed a technological bent as they innovated the programmatic means of spending previously unheard of sums of money for philanthropic ends.

It is necessary to say a few words here about the use of the term "technology." Today, the term is often used to refer to the synergy of digital computers and the internet. A recent informative work that engages current trends in philanthropy is titled *Disrupting Philanthropy: Technology and the Future of the Social Sector.* While the text could have referred to technologies in medicine or agriculture or literacy, it is solely interested in digital technologies, as shown in this passage: "Information networks—the Internet primarily, and the increasingly SMS (text-messaging) and 3G (smart-phone) cell phone technologies—are overturning core practices of philanthropic foundations and individuals" (Bernholz 2010, 4).

Instead, within this chapter the term "technology" refers broadly to human-created material products, and the means of creating those products, and particularly to innovations. The chapter draws liberally on works in the history of technology, a field of study that (like the formal study of philanthropy) is little more than a half-century old.

It is also worth noting that in popular culture there is confusion between what is science and what is technological innovation. That confusion is well-founded because of the increasing interrelationship and interdependence of science and technological innovation in the last 150 years. Generally, "science" refers to theoretical and experimental approaches to knowledge creation, with close affiliations to philosophy, while "technological innovation" refers, again, to significantly new human productions in the material world. The intersection of science and technology occurs in such areas of human creation as industrial research and laboratory instrumentation—which derive from overlapping scientific and technological insights (Stapleton 2008b, 217–230).

Contexts

The Technological Environment

Modern philanthropy has depended heavily on technology for communications and management. The archives of the Rockefeller Foundation document the use of an array of innovative transportation and communications technologies available at the beginning of the twentieth century—telephone, telegraph, railroads, ocean liners, and, increasingly, the automobile and the airplane—to maintain the foundation's global reach and operations. Many Rockefeller officers were almost constantly on the move, crossing oceans and continents, while remaining fully in contact with the foundation's headquarters in New York, and often with regional and national offices as well.

An important tool of the philanthropic trade was the diary that recorded meetings, conversations, and events, which was often spiced with pungent observations of people and institutions. A time-honored form when handwritten in the original, it became a modern form when transcribed and typed in several duplicate copies and distributed to superior and collateral staff within the foundation. Diaries that recorded trips often were accompanied by black-and-white photographs of the locales and individuals encountered—taken with Kodak cameras that appear to have been standard equipment. (It has been remarked that the basics for Rockefeller officers—who were often physicians—when they went into the field were a typewriter, a camera, and a stethoscope.)

An American Predilection

It is not difficult to argue that historically Americans have tended to seek techno-logical solutions to social, economic, health, and even political problems. At least from the time of the American Revolution others have commented on that pre-dilection, and one can see that it remains an American passion today (Stapleton 1986, 21–34). Whether we look at the adoption of the railroad in the nineteenth century, the adoption of the automobile in the twentieth century, or today's fasci-nation with digital electronics, Americans have looked to technology as a means of accomplishing their goals.

As an example, one could look at the Century of Progress World's Fair held in Chicago in 1933—at the depth of a global economic depression. A dazzling array of buildings and events were intended to demonstrate that the American future lay in continuing growth in material culture and continuing technologi-cal innovation. The Century of Progress's motto was "Science Finds, Industry Applies, Man Conforms." That is a neat summary of the American technological imagination for the first half of the twentieth century.

It is not surprising, then, that the great American philanthropies have en-thusiastically selected technological innovation as providing solutions to the problems they have identified, and they have even tended to address problems based on whether there were available or emerging technological solutions. For example, the Rockefeller Foundation, and its coordinate body the International Health Board, chose to attack the global malaria problem primarily through in-secticidal technologies, rather than through viable alternatives, such as long-term environmental amelioration, or the wider distribution of drugs.[1] The Rockefeller choice was consequential, in that the foundation trained a global generation of public health officials to take that perspective, deeply influencing the latter twen-tieth-century strategies of the World Health Organization and the Pan American Health Organization.

Perhaps the best expression of the Rockefeller Foundation's enthusiasm for technological solutions (particularly in the health sciences) was a passage in Ray-mond Fosdick's 1947 "President's Review":

> In no area of knowledge and practice are changes occurring more rapidly than in medicine and public health. We seem to be on the threshold of an era more promising than any we have known. The sulfonamides, penicillin, radioac-tive isotopes, DDT—to mention only a few new instruments which have been placed in our hands—foreshadow a new move forward, a new renaissance, a new period in human development when the imagination is endowed with

wings. If only we can be freed from the shrieking insanity of another war, it does not seem impossible to believe that within a period of no unreasonable duration we shall be able to limit the ravages of diseases like cancer, tuberculosis, infantile paralysis and perhaps some of the degenerative disorders and even the common cold. (Fosdick 1948, 25)

I quote this at length because it is a summation of what might be described as the "technological sublime" in philanthropy in the first half of the twentieth century.

China Medical Board

The China Medical Board is usually thought of as the medical-scientific organization that founded and sustained the Peking Union Medical College, intended to be the "Johns Hopkins of China." Scholarship generally has supported the view that, in the first thirty years after its founding, PUMC trained physicians and medical researchers at the highest levels and made significant contributions to the operations and planning of a Chinese health infrastructure. The Rockefeller philanthropic style permeated the China Medical Board and PUMC, and technological approaches were deeply embedded in PUMC's response to the medical and public health problems of China.

The Physical Plant of Peking Union Medical College

The greatest technological achievement of the China Medical Board is hidden right before our eyes, historically speaking: it is the magnificent physical plant of the Peking Union Medical College, built between 1917 and 1921—at a final cost of $7,552,839 (Ferguson 1970, 34). The architect of the complex of buildings dedicated in 1921, Charles Coolidge, was the same one who designed medical complexes for Harvard Medical School, Western Reserve University, and the original buildings for the Rockefeller Institute (now Rockefeller University). Nothing was spared in the layout and furnishings of the laboratories, classrooms, offices, and hospital. As the China Medical Board's annual report for 1921 put it:

> It is hoped that it may serve as a model for other medical schools, not in the sense that it necessarily represents the ideal in all matters of organization and construction, nor that it is as yet complete in every respect as a few of the largest institutions in other countries may be said to be complete, but that it presents, in China, a demonstration more nearly adequate than any that has preceded it, of the essential elements of a modern medical school. (Greene 1922, 247)

Moreover, while the PUMC campus had the veneer of Chinese architectural style (Greene 1922, 263), its underpinning was an infrastructure of modern utilities that were then unavailable in Beijing, making it "inevitably much larger and more complicated than would be necessary for a medical school of the same size in any large city of the Western world" (Greene 1922, 275–276).

PUMC represented a quantum leap in Western-style Chinese medical education simply in the facilities it afforded the staff, and it introduced Chinese medical educators and practitioners to innovations and techniques that were hardly available elsewhere in China. Thus, the physical presence of PUMC made a powerful technological statement, on par with the science and medicine its staff were teaching and promoting.

It should be noted that the Rockefeller philanthropies had a fascination with laboratory and research instrumentation, and supported technological innovations on a global basis, notably in the development of the cyclotron, the centrifuge, the Tiselius apparatus, the electron microscope, and computing (Kohler 1991; Farley 2004, ch. 10; Stapleton 2008b).

X-ray Technology as a Case Study

An early statement of PUMC's mission to diffuse knowledge and skills is useful to consider:

> The College seeks to point the way by which the future system of Chinese medical education may be adapted as well as possible to the actual conditions in the country. If the hopes of its founders are realized, it will graduate a select group of leaders in medical education, in research, and in public health administration, and a larger number of useful practitioners of medicine and surgery. In addition it will offer to men and women who have graduated from other schools, further training and experience to fit them for posts of greater responsibility in Peking or elsewhere. Organizations engaged in the great work of medical education in China may be interested in watching the progress of the school, and in observing, with profit to themselves, those features of its work which experience shows to have been wisely or unwisely adopted. (Greene 1922, 247–248)

The working out of this mission may be seen in the early years of the roentgenology department of PUMC. Today, we would call this the radiology department, or even the X-ray department, returning to Röntgen's original term for his discovery in 1896 (Röntgen 1896, 726–729). X-ray technology developed rapidly in the early twentieth century, becoming both a tool for scientific investigation and an incredibly valuable addition to the diagnostic capabilities of medicine (Richtmyer 1926, 550–554; Richtmyer 1931, 454–457). It is not surprising that it became a standard part of PUMC's equipment and program.

The roentgenology unit initially (1919–1927) was headed by Paul C. Hodges.[2] He was, according to one historian, "a recognized master of radiological instrumentation" who made an "enduring contribution to the introduction of diagnostic radiology to China" (Bowers 1972, 142–143).[3] The roentgenology unit was one of the first places at PUMC to make a commitment to Chinese leadership. This occurred in the person of Dr. Chih-kuang Hsieh, who graduated from the Hunan

Yale College of Medicine in 1922 and became an assistant resident in PUMC's roentgenology unit the same year.[4] He already had taken a special X-ray course at PUMC in 1921 under Hodges, who apparently identified Hsieh as a potential future leader.

In 1925, Hseih was awarded a China Medical Board fellowship for study at the University of Michigan, where he went for a year, enrolling in a master's program and immediately engaging in both scientific and clinical work with X-rays. At Christmas time, he visited leading hospitals in Michigan, including the Henry Ford Hospital. In January, he reported to the China Medical Board that he was

> having a very enjoyable time in Ann Arbor. . . . [He was] going through different divisions of [the] Department of Roentgenology— . . . bone and joint, gastro-intestine, therapy and interpretation. For the past 2 months [he has been] working in the gastric room with another junior man. [He is] much pleased with good varieties of conditions seen here in the department. [He] feels that [his] views have broadened in many ways.[5]

After subsequent travel in the United States and Europe, Hseih returned to Beijing in September 1927 when he was wanted by Hodges to teach the fall term at PUMC.[6] In the next year, he took over as head of PUMC's roentgenology unit, and served there for the next 20 years. In 1931, he oversaw the purchase of new diagnostic X-ray machines for PUMC.[7] It is appropriate to note that this transfer of knowledge continued to another generation. Fang Hsien-chih, a PUMC graduate of 1933, became head of the radiology department at the China Union Medical College, the renamed PUMC, in the mid-1950s (Bullock 1980, 222).

Returning to Paul Hodges, it is important to note that he was active in transferring X-ray technology to other institutions in China through the actual provision of equipment. Beginning in 1922, he turned his laboratory into a factory for the production of inexpensive, portable X-ray devices after an experience he had that year in assisting a military medical team. In Hodges's own report, written in 1922, he described his experience and efforts:

> About two years ago, following a trip to Changsha, I conceived the idea of attempting to assemble in China an X-ray machine designed so that it would operate on any of the various electrical supplies that are met with in China, and able to compensate for the hourly variations in a given supply. Several mission hospitals, including Changsha, Nigpo, and Shoahsing . . . placed orders for these specially constructed machines. . . .
>
> By March, 1922, the ultimate design was practically decided upon and work was actually begun on winding the auto-transformers, the part of the machines particularly adapting them to use in China. . . . By the beginning of the X-ray summer course, June 18, 1922, a sample machine had been completed. . . . By this time there were nine orders from mission hospitals. It was decided to fill these nine orders, make a 10th for use in teaching and demon-

stration at the P.U.M.C. and make an 11th . . . for sale to some station where it seemed particularly needed.[8]

Hodges also supervised the installation of each of these units, and summarized their cost as about three thousand dollars at an "absolute minimum," but with the costs of "tube stands, tubes, tables, fluoroscopes, stereoscopes and dark room equipment" still to be covered for each machine.[9]

According to one account:

> With a grant of $15,000 from the [China Medical Board], Hodges . . . [had] develop[ed] a simple, inexpensive machine that was able to withstand . . . sharp fluctuations in voltage. The relatively low cost of the units was in part attributable to the fact that it was necessary to import only a few components from the United States. (Bowers 1972, 142–143)

The China Medical Board also made grants directly to several Chinese hospitals for the purchase of X-ray equipment.[10] Documentation suggests that the operators of those units routinely received training from Hodges.[11]

In 1923, Hodges visited universities in Germany to observe the teaching of X-ray technology to medical students and the use of X-rays for scientific research. He then spent the next academic year in Madison, Wisconsin, working on new trends in medical therapy using X-rays.[12] He persuaded the PUMC administration to add deep X-ray therapy to its medical treatment program, although it took some years to purchase the proper equipment and Hseih had to complete the negotiations with German and American manufacturers.[13]

Thus, we see in the roentgenology unit that technological innovation at PUMC was expressed not only in the buildings, but, in one department, in the practice and education processes themselves.

The Peking First Health Station

The technological impulse did not reside in the roentgenology unit alone: it was broadly evident in PUMC's public health training. Interestingly, in line with the initial concept of PUMC as a laboratory-based medical school, PUMC did not open with public health in its curriculum; it was somewhat of an afterthought in response to pressing needs in China that quickly became obvious to the faculty and administration of PUMC. The Department of Hygiene and Public Health was initiated only in 1924 when John B. Grant joined the faculty as the founding chair.[14] Short of hiring a qualified Chinese educator to head the department, Grant was an ideal choice: he had been born and raised in China and spoke Mandarin; he was a graduate of Johns Hopkins' School of Public Health; he had been working as a field officer of the International Health Board, a Rockefeller philanthropy, since 1917; he had carried out a "General Health Survey of Peking, China" in 1922;[15] and he had a confident and outgoing personality.[16]

In short order, Grant proposed to PUMC and the Rockefeller hierarchy that the students in public health needed practical experience and that PUMC should set up a fieldwork unit in a poverty-ridden district of Beijing. In September 1925, the Peking Health Demonstration Station was in operation. While in the global operations of the Rockefeller philanthropies local health units had become part of their public health programs, this unit was the only one in a major city, and it served a much larger population than the rural units (an area with an estimated population of 56,000 when it opened, and 100,000 when its catchment area was enlarged in 1928).[17]

The station had a broad program, including the control of communicable diseases such as smallpox, typhus, and the plague; the licensing of food purveyors; inspection of nuisances; a testing laboratory; a pre- and postnatal clinic, including midwifery; school inspections and visits, and public health education; sewage control and inspection; and the collection of vital statistics. One can see in this list the technological slant of many elements of the program. In the view of the Rockefeller officials, these functions were almost completely neglected by the Chinese government: in his report of 1922, Grant stated that "public health activities of an official nature may be said to be almost totally absent in Peking,"[18] and in Grant's view, little had changed by 1927 when he reported that "there has been in the past practically no effective health administration in Peking city."[19]

The Health Demonstration Station was just that: a demonstration of what could be done to improve the health of the people. One might say that it was being carried out with the exceptional Rockefeller resources behind it—but part of Grant's strategy in setting up the station was to carefully record expenses and results, and to show over time that relatively modest expenditures could have significant results.[20] In one of the few references to the implementation of technology, Grant drew on the spirit of the roentgenology department when he stated, in regard to the equipment of the station, that "in so far as it is compatible with teaching requirements the station is run on as nearly local standards as is practicable" (Grant 1929, 114). At another point he stated,

> The raison d'etre of the Health Station is to afford comparable facilities in preventive medicine as is already secured to [PUMC students in] curative medicine through the hospital, i.e., to provide for project method teaching and material for research.[21]

In any case, the station immediately became a field-practice arm of PUMC's public health education, with Grant's public health students taking over the functional work of the station, spending months to a year or more at their posts. (Formally, the station was headed by the director of the National Epidemic Prevention Bureau in Beijing in its first year, then by the Chinese surgeon general for two years, and then in 1928 it became a division of the new Municipal Health

Department of Beijing—but in practical terms it remained under the direction of John Grant and his students.) Beginning in 1928, with the station well-established, all medical students at PUMC—regardless of whether or not they were focusing on public health—were required to have a three-week internship at the station. Grant (and one of his students) promoted the station as a place where PUMC students could learn not only public health techniques, but also the practice of the relatively neglected field of preventive medicine.[22] It was claimed that "some of the best of the [early] graduates" of PUMC were those who had been "attracted" to public health work, presumably through their exposure to the field at the station.[23]

The influence of practice at the station on the subsequent leaders of medicine and public health in China was substantial: many who held positions there as students, or went there after graduation, occupied leading public health posts from the 1930s into the era of the People's Republic, including national and regional positions, and professorships. (This phenomenon was not limited to the field of public health: one observer commented that "many of the great minds in China [in 1989] are Western-trained senior scientists whose data bases still largely rest on pre-1949 experience" [Donald 1989, xxix].)

Dingxian and the Mass Education Movement

Moreover, the experience of the PUMC students in the Peking Health Demonstration Station was transferred to another important public health initiative, the public health arm of the Mass Education Movement at Dingxian, a rural site southeast of Beijing containing four hundred thousand residents in four hundred villages. The brainchild of John Grant and Yan Yangchu (also known as Jimmy Yen), the Mass Education Movement was an attempt to create a self-replicating uplift movement among rural Chinese, combining education, self-government, and basic health services. The Rockefeller Foundation began funding the Mass Education Movement in 1935, taking a particular interest in the public health work that the movement had initiated in 1929.[24] A further connection with Rockefeller philanthropy was that two alumni of PUMC and the Peking Health Demonstration Station became successive directors of the public health service at the Dingxian unit. Other PUMC students served in other capacities.

Although short-lived as a major program (its operations were limited after the beginning of the Sino-Japanese War), the Mass Education Movement's Dingxian model had a long-term influence on public health in China. Arguably, the well-known "barefoot doctors" campaign of the People's Republic stemmed in large part from what transpired at Dingxian and, by extension, at PUMC's Peking Health Demonstration Station (Bullock 1980, 166, 189). Dingxian also influenced public health in other countries because global public health leaders came there to observe, and, in some cases, the Rockefeller philanthropies sent their trainees to Dingxian.

As I noted at the beginning of this chapter, my investigation of the technological aspects of public health education at PUMC, and training at the Peking Health Demonstration Station and at Dingxian, is continuing. It is difficult to identify the role of technological diffusion, innovation, and adaptation in documentation created largely by a scientific and medical staff who thought and wrote in scientific and medical terms, and the historical literature also has approached the Peking and Dingxian stories largely as triumphs of scientific medicine. Yet the Health Demonstration Station's equipment was expected to "be as simple as possible," and an account by one of the Dingxian directors states clearly that work undertaken there utilized "locally manufactured equipment and locally constructed facilities," suggesting that the approach to technological innovation taken by the roentgenology department permeated the PUMC graduates who worked at both places (Chen 1989, 96–97).[25]

An American commercial attaché to the American embassy in Beijing who visited Dingxian in 1937 was fascinated by the technological innovations there, and he gives us some specifics regarding the "locally manufactured equipment and . . . facilities." He reported the following:

> A central hospital is functioning at Tingcheng [*sic*] and workers are there trained for duty in various parts of the district. Each village is furnished with a small box of ten simple remedies among which are copper sulphate for treating trachoma common throughout North China, aspirin, iodine, Vaseline, etc., the whole kit costing but one dollar in local currency, or 25 cents U.S. gold. . . . In this district, as throughout North China, windlasses are commonly used for drawing water from wells for irrigation purposes. These are generally operated by two men but a device has been invented by one of Jimmie Yen's co-workers which costs $2.00 less than the windlass in common use and can by operated by one man and pump more water in the same length of time. . . . A new [chicken] coop has been devised, also made of sunburnt clay bricks, but with ventilation secured by a window made of willow sticks. The coop is larger and costs no more but assures of better health conditions among the poultry. . . . Experiments are being conducted in a laboratory by special workers for devising a simple and inexpensive radio for broadcasting purposes throughout the villages of this district.[26]

A few weeks later a Rockefeller Foundation officer visiting Dingxian commented in his diary,

> Visited health stations and farm experiments [at Dingxian]. . . . Improving the breed of hogs and the strains of cotton proving the most successful on the agricultural side. In medical work, obstetrics and ophthalmological care most successful, also excellent work in cholera control. The sight of a small broadcasting station fitted up in what was not long ago a provincial examination hall is a remarkable sight. Yen has tried to study the Chinese rural conditions to see what can be done and what is simple and cheap enough and useful enough to be spread successfully by a much less talented crowd than the present group.[27]

Although the influence of the work at Dingxian cannot easily be estimated, it is worthwhile to note that the site was reportedly "swamped with visitors."[28] It is also apparent that MEM's "remarkable results" were well-known throughout the Chinese government.[29]

The Rockefeller Foundation

Suffice it to say that the Rockefeller Foundation's global programs in the first half of the twentieth century were suffused with technological inclinations. Its public health programs (insecticides and sanitary engineering), agricultural and scientific programs (promoting laboratory instrumentation), and even its humanities programs (promoting the use of microfilm, radio, and television) all drew on modern technologies for programmatic innovations.

Hookworm Disease

In China, as in much of the rest of the world, the opening wedge for Rockefeller philanthropies was its hookworm control program. Drawing on the visible nature of the infection (hookworms, unlike bacteria and viruses, could be seen with the naked eye, or observed with a simple lens), and its particular virulence in industrial and plantation settings, Rockefeller operatives were able to convince national and local authorities to combat hookworm in selected demonstration sites.

Anti-hookworm measures that were first developed in the southern United States included sampling and testing methodologies, curative methods (killing hookworms by having infected persons swallow chenopodium or carbon tetrachloride, followed by an Epsom salts purgative), and preventative strategies (building sanitary privies [or latrines] and improving sewerage). This package of technologies, which was adapted to local conditions by the Rockefeller officials, often had dramatic short-term results in terms of lowered infections, but equally importantly, it was a powerful demonstration of a systematic intervention to deal with a public health problem. Rockefeller operatives expected rapid changes in health, and technological approaches were their primary means to realize those changes.

In China, the earliest Rockefeller project for hookworm control, begun in 1917, was at the Pingxiang coal mines in Jiangxi Province. It was frankly reported "as a means of entering the public health field in China" (Rockefeller Foundation 1920, 73–74). At those mines, an initial survey reported an infection rate of 85 percent among the workers in the mine itself, and the main Rockefeller response was to initiate the construction of sanitary latrines that would keep human waste from the water supplies and from direct contact with the miners. After two years the infection rate was reported to have been reduced to 35 percent (Rockefeller Foundation 1918, 154–156; Rockefeller Foundation 1919, 175–176). Perhaps as important in the long run for Chinese public health was that the Pingxiang mines, along with early experiences with Rockefeller hookworm projects in the American south, were John Grant's introduction to public health work in China. Grant, who had grown up in China, obtained his medical degree from the University of Michigan in 1917 and soon thereafter joined the Rockefeller project at Pingxiang. According to historian Liping Bu, "Grant's early working experience in rural North Carolina . . . and in the Pingxiang coal mines of central China deepened his understanding of the social causation of epidemic diseases with first-hand observations" (Bu 2012, 132).

Grant became the first director of the public health curriculum at the Peking Union Medical College, so it is no surprise that his students' work had a technological orientation.

Malaria

One of the major public health problems attacked by the Rockefeller philanthropies was malaria, a disease active in every inhabited continent. Although quinine had been recognized since the 1600s as a potent means of suppressing malaria, the Rockefeller approach from 1916 onward was to interrupt transmission of the disease by control of the anopheles mosquito, the disease vector. Almost all of the first means of mosquito control were technological—such as screening windows to keep the mosquitoes out of residences, particularly at night; draining swamps by ditching and pumping; and oiling the surfaces of pools of water to suffocate the mosquito larvae. In the 1920s, to these strategies was joined a powerful new tool—an insecticide, Paris Green, that was particularly effective in killing mosquito larvae.

The best-known and most visible Rockefeller anti-malaria activity was in Italy, beginning in 1924. Disdaining the long-term ameliorative programs of the Italian government, which included the gradual filling of swamps and river estuaries, and the free distribution of quinine in areas of high malaria incidence, the Rockefeller approach was to identify the habits and environments of the malaria-carrying mosquitoes and to liberally spray Paris Green on all water surfaces where those mosquitoes were found. The ten-year Rockefeller program in Italy influenced a generation of public health workers around the world, many of whom visited the program's demonstration sites (Stapleton 2008a).

Rockefeller's anti-malaria work came to China in 1939–1940, at which time it was noted that approximately 30 percent of Chinese soldiers were malaria-infected. The Rockefeller project was headed by a Peking Union Medical College parasitologist, L. C. Feng, who initiated studies of the mosquito vector, and by 1943 there were trials of Paris Green for larval control. The training of public health officers for malaria control began the next year, and in 1945–1946, a malaria laboratory was established in Nanjing to expand studies. The testing of DDT, the wartime innovation in mosquito control, began at that time, although the collapse of the Chinese central government soon after meant that all Rockefeller anti-malaria activity was soon relocated to Taiwan.[30]

Conclusion

Technological innovations, particularly in public health, characterized Rockefeller and other global philanthropic strategies in the first half of the twentieth century. Arguably, that tendency continued in the latter half of the century, when philanthropic approaches to such widely divergent areas of activity as agricultural improvement, population control, and literacy also embraced technological means. Why were technological solutions so appealing?

First, technological approaches to problems seemed "neutral," in that political and social changes—while hoped for—were not immediate and foremost. While it can be argued that the choice of one technology may imply elite control, and another may promise universality of access, those implications often are not apparent at the time of selection. In the case of the Rockefeller anti-malaria program, for example, the choice of vector control through the use of insecticides may have seemed to avoid the messy problems of forcing people to take quinine, or of relocating them from malarious areas—both of which were potentially effective choices.

Second, the continuing industrialization of the world in the first half of the twentieth century seemed to provide an ever-growing array of technological possibilities. Raymond Fosdick's rapturous comment that he foresaw "a new period in human development when the imagination is endowed with wings," and the Chicago World's Fair slogan, cited earlier in this chapter, are illustrations of the positivist, optimistic view of technology that permeated the Western world in the twentieth century, and not incidentally also reverberated with Marxist ideology.

Finally, the backgrounds and training of many of the Rockefeller personnel gave them experiences and skills that befitted technological choices. Some had backgrounds in industry or commerce that made them familiar with the potential of new technologies, as well as knowledge of the excitement of technological innovation and change. Some had university training in the sciences and medicine, fields which since the latter part of the nineteenth century had embraced the laboratory with its ever-increasing equipment as the proper location for investigation and discovery. Others, I believe, simply imbibed the era's progressive, technology-loving environment, particularly in the United States. While the horrors of modern technological warfare created some qualms (particularly noticeable in the scientists who created the atomic bomb), almost all of those who emerged from the university laboratory had a faith in technology.

In all, technological innovation was central to the programs and policies of the China Medical Board and the Rockefeller Foundation in China.

Notes

1. For commentary on the American fascination with technology in the early nineteenth century, see Stapleton (1986).

2. Biographical information on Paul C. Hodges can be found in his personnel record at the Peking Union Medical College Archives (hereafter cited as PUMCA), Beijing (copy in possession of the author).

3. Bowers, a physician with extensive experience in the Far East, wrote by far the most technically informed study of PUMC, and these two pages are the only substantial commentary I have located on Hodges and X-ray technology at PUMC. A better-known and still-standard account of the history of PUMC is Mary Brown Bullock's *An American Transplant.* Another important rendering of PUMC's history, by a participant, is Ferguson (1970). For valuable recent essays, see also Marilyn Bailey Ogilvie, "The Rockefeller Foundation, China, Western Medicine, and PUMC," in *Philanthropy and Cultural Context: Western Philanthropy in South, East, and Southeast Asia in the 20th Century,* ed. Soma Hewa and Philo Hove (Lanham, MD: University Press of America, 1997), 21–38; and Ma Quisha, "The Peking Union Medical College and the Rockefeller Foundation's Medical Programs in China," in *Rockefeller Philanthropy and Modern Biomedicine: International Initiatives from World War I to the Cold War,* ed. William H. Schneider (Bloomington: Indiana University Press, 2002), 159–183.

4. "Hseih, Chih-Kuang," n.d., fellowship recorder cards, China Medical Board fellowships, Rockefeller Foundation Archives, Rockefeller Archive Center, Sleepy Hollow, NY (hereafter cited as RAC). Much of the biographical information on Hseih is derived from these three cards, because the more detailed fellowship files of the Rockefeller Foundation were destroyed in the 1960s.

5. "Hseih, Chih-Kuang," n.d., RAC. I have expanded abbreviations and added text as required for oral coherence.

6. "Hseih, Chih-Kuang," n.d., RAC.

7. C. K. Hsieh to Roger S. Greene, February 27, 1931, folder 979, box 136, China Medical Board Archives, RAC.

8. Paul C. Hodges to L. C. Goodrich, September 11, 1922, attached to L. C. Goodrich to R. S. Greene, September 13, 1922, folder 968, box 134, China Medical Board Archives, RAC. Documentation of the acquisition of X-ray equipment by some of these institutions is in folder 1784, box 76, China Medical Board Archives, RAC.

9. Ibid.

10. Summary of cable, September 16, 1922, folder 1814, box 78, China Medical Board Archives, RAC.

11. L. C. Goodrich to R. S. Greene, October 18, 1922, folder 1784, box 76, China Medical Board Archives, RAC; L. C. Goodrich to R. S. Greene, December 22, 1922, folder 1814, box 78, China Medical Board Archives, RAC.

12. Paul C. Hodges to Roger S. Greene, June 10, 1923; June 22, 1923; January 31, 1924; February 9, 1924, folder 968, box 134, China Medical Board Archives, RAC; Paul C. Hodges to H. S. Houghton, October 24, 1923, attached to Paul C. Hodges to Margery K. Eggleston, October 26, 1923, folder 968, box 134, China Medical Board Archives, RAC.

13. Memorandum, "X-Ray treatment machine," November 17, 1930, folder 978, box 136, China Medical Board Archives, RAC; R. S. Greene to M. K. Eggleston, November 25, 1930, folder 978, box 136, China Medical Board Archives, RAC.

14. Much of this essay's discussion of PUMC's public health training, the Peking Health Demonstration Station, and the Dingxian health unit is derived from chapters by Darwin H.

Stapleton, Liping Bu, and Bridie Andrews in *Science, Public Health and the State in Modern Asia*, eds. Liping Bu, Darwin H. Stapleton, and Ka-che Yip (New York: Routledge, 2012).

15. John B. Grant, "Report on a General Health Survey of Peking, China," February 1922, vol. 393, PUMCA. This is the original report, with photographs; a copy of the report without photographs is in box 55, Record Group 5.2, RAC.

16. Roger S. Greene to Max Mason, March 13, 1930, John B. Grant personnel file, Record Group 9, Rockefeller Foundation Archives, RAC. See also Jim Duffy, "John Black Grant: A Revolutionary in China," Prologues of Public Health, 2005, http://www.jhsph.edu/publichealthnews/magazine/archive/mag_spring05/; and But and Fee (2008).

17. On health units, see Bu, Stapleton, and Yip, eds., *Science, Public Health and the State in Modern Asia*, chaps. 3, 4, and 5; and Darwin H. Stapleton, "Malaria Eradication and the Technological Model," in *Disease, Colonialism, and the State: Malaria in Modern East Asian History*, ed. Ka-che Yip (Hong Kong: Hong Kong University Press, 2009), 71–84.

18. John B. Grant, "Report on a General Health Survey of Peking, China," PUMCA.

19. A graduate of PUMC writing in 1935 stated that "previous to . . . 1927, no adequate attention was paid to public health in this country" (I-Chin Yuan, "Progress of State Medicine in China," 1, PUMCA, reprinted from *Chinese Recorder*, January 1935, vol. 3632).

20. A report on the first seven years of the Health Demonstration Station noted that "the Station is rendering a large volume of work at a reasonably low cost" (Li Ting-an, "A Critical Study of the Work of the Health Station, First Health Area Department of Public Safety, Peiping, for the years 1925–1932, with Suggestions for Improvement," vol. 387, 10, PUMCA). At about the same time a visiting Rockefeller Foundation officer reported that Dr. Li Ting-an gave him a "good exposition of the organization [of the Health Station] . . . 120,000 people in this area or ward of Peiping. The services must always keep costs in view" ("Dr. Alan Gregg's diary while in China," September 15, 1932, folder 465, box 66, China Medical Board Archives, RAC). Li Ting-an, a graduate of PUMC, was then the director of the Peking Health Demonstration Station (*Chinese Medical Directory, 1941.* [Nanking?]: Chinese Medical Association, 1941), 143.

21. "Dr. Grant to Budget Committee—re: Health Station budget," February 4, 1926, folder 465, China Medical Board Archives, RAC.

22. John B. Grant and Y. C. Yuan, "Permeation of the Curriculum with a Preventive Viewpoint," March 30, 1928, folder 370, box 45, series 601, RG 1.1, RAC.

23. Roger S. Greene to George E. Vincent, December 27, 1927, folder 366, box 44, series 601, RG 1.1, RAC.

24. "Jimmy Yen Revisits America," October 1, 1943, folder 69, box 7, series 601, RG 1.1, Rockefeller Foundation Archives, RAC; C. C. Ch'en, "Public Health in Rural Reconstruction at Tinghsien," 1934, a publication of the Chinese National Association of the Mass Education Movement, vol. 354, PUMCA; H. Y. Yeo, "Department of Public Health of the Chinese National Association of the Mass Education Movement," December 1929, folder 69, box 7, series 601, RG 1.1., Rockefeller Foundation Archives, RAC. A valuable report on a demonstration health unit near Nanking that was inspired by Dingxian notes the important function of the "public health engineer" in sanitation work from 1933 to 1937 (S. C. Hsu and L. S. Ma, "Kiangning Hsien Rural Health Program," c. 1947, folder 365, box 44, series 601, RG 1.1, Rockefeller Foundation Archives, RAC).

25. See also Li Ting-an, "A Critical Study of the Work of the Health Station, First Health Area Department of Public Safety, Peiping, for the years 1925–1932, with Suggestions for Improvement," vol. 387, 10, PUMCA.

26. Julean Arnold, "The Mass Education Movement in China," June 20, 1932, folder 70, box 7, series 601, RG 1.1, RAC.

27. Allan Gregg, diary entries, September 30, 1932–October 2, 1932, folder 70a, box 7, series 601, RG 1.1, RAC.

28. G. E. Hodgman to M. Beard, June 23, 1931, extract, folder 60, box 7, series 601, RG 1.1, RAC.

29. Selksar M. Gunn to TBK, July 4, 1939, extract, folder 71, box 7, series 601, RG 1.1, RAC.

30. This section is based on the author's passages in Yip, ed., *Disease, Colonialism, and the State*, 79–82.

References

Bernholz, Lucy, Edward Skloot, and Barry Varela. 2010. *Disrupting Philanthropy: Technology and the Future of the Social Sector.* Chapel Hill, NC: Center for Strategic Philanthropy and Civil Society, Duke University.

Bowers, John Z. 1972. *Western Medicine in a Chinese Palace: Peking Union Medical College, 1917–1951.* Philadelphia: Josiah Macy Jr. Foundation.

Bu, Liping. 2012. "Beijing First Health Station: Innovative Public Health Education and Influence on China's Health Profession." In *Science, Public Health and the State in Modern Asia*, edited by Liping Bu, Darwin H. Stapleton, and Ka-che Yip, 129–143. New York: Routledge.

Bu, Liping, and Elizabeth Fee. 2008. "John B. Grant: International Statesman of Public Health." *American Journal of Public Health* 98 (April): 626–629.

Chen, C. C. 1989. *Medicine in Rural China: A Personal Account.* Berkeley: University of California Press.

Farley, John. 2004. *To Cast Out Disease: A History of the International Health Division of the Rockefeller Foundation (1913–1951).* Oxford: Oxford University Press.

Ferguson, Mary E. 1970. *China Medical Board and Peking Union Medical College: A Chronicle of Fruitful Collaboration.* New York: China Medical Board.

Fosdick, Raymond. 1948. "President's Review." In *Annual Report for 1947*, Rockefeller Foundation, 1–48. New York: Rockefeller Foundation.

Grant, John B. 1929. "Department of Public Health and Preventive Medicine: Peking Union Medical College." In *Methods and Principles of Medical Education.* 14th series. New York: Rockefeller Foundation.

Greene, Roger S. 1922. "China Medical Board: Report of the Director." In *Annual Report for 1921*, Rockefeller Foundation, 243–310. New York: Rockefeller Foundation.

Kohler, Robert. 1991. *Partners in Science: Foundations and Natural Scientists, 1900–1945.* Chicago: University of Chicago Press.

McDonald, T. David. 1989. *The Technological Transformation of China.* Washington, DC: National Defense University Press.

Richtmyer, F. K. 1926. "'Seeing' with X-rays." *Scientific Monthly* 22 (June): 550–554.

———. 1931. "X-rays and Their Uses." *Scientific Monthly* 32 (May): 454–457.

Rockefeller Foundation. 1918. *Annual Report for 1917.* New York: Rockefeller Foundation.

———. 1919. *Annual Report for 1918.* New York: Rockefeller Foundation.

———. 1920. *Annual Report for 1919.* New York: Rockefeller Foundation.

Röntgen, W. K. 1896. "A New Form of Radiation." *Science,* new series 3 (May 15): 726–729.

Stapleton, Darwin H. 1986. "Neither Tocqueville Nor Trollope: Michel Chevalier and the Industrialization of the United States and Europe." In *The World of the Industrial Revolution: Comparative and International Aspects of Industrialization*, edited by Robert Weible, 21–34. North Andover, MA: Museum of American Textile History.

———. 2008a. "Technological Solutions: The Rockefeller Foundation and the Insecticidal Approach to Malaria Control." Paper presented at the conference "The Global Crisis of Malaria: Lessons of the Past and Future Prospects," Yale University School of Medicine, New Haven, CT, November 7–9.

———. 2008b. "The Critical Role of Laboratory Instruments at the Rockefeller: Biomedicine as Biotechnology." In *Biomedicine in the 20th Century*, edited by Caroline Hannaway, 217–230. Amsterdam: IOS Press.

———. 2009. "Malaria Eradication and the Technological Model: The Rockefeller Foundation and Public Health in East Asia." In *Disease, Colonialism, and the State: Malaria in Modern East Asian History*, edited by Ka-che Yip, 71–84. Hong Kong: Hong Kong University Press.

7 International Philanthropic Engagement in Three Stages of China's Response to HIV/AIDS

Ray Yip

Introduction

Since the start of the first outbreak of the HIV epidemic in 1989, China has come a long way in its response to this global pandemic—from total denial to now a strong response. In many ways, the real response came relatively late, around 2003, but the response was by far one of the strongest among developing countries. Throughout this journey, both from denial to awakening and from a weak to a strong response, international partners have played an important role. The complex nature of the HIV/AIDS epidemic, particularly regarding cultural and behavioral factors that result in intense stigma and discrimination, have made the response very challenging worldwide and even more so in China. Additionally, China's health system has undergone tremendous changes in the past three decades, which have contributed to challenges in effective HIV prevention and care beyond social and culture factors. The nature of the management structure of the system, exacerbated by inefficient financing mechanisms, has resulted in reduced access to and quality of service, especially for those with challenging or costly conditions. For these reasons, international efforts have played an important role in assisting China in confronting these challenges. The purpose of this chapter is to recount the contributions of international philanthropy, broadly defined, to China's HIV/AIDS response in the context of sociocultural, political, and health system constraints. This review is not intended to be exhaustive, but rather to highlight the roles of different organizations that, during various time periods, have made significant contributions to addressing specific aspects of the HIV/AIDS epidemic in China.

China's Evolving Health System and the Implications for HIV/AIDS Prevention and Care

A Health System with Distorted Financing Affecting Access and Quality of Medical Service

In parallel with the shift from collective socialism to a market economy that started in the late 1970s, China's health system has also experienced a dramatic shift over the past three decades. Unlike the economy, which has soared with marked improvement of living standards, especially for the urban population, China's health system has undergone a long decline in every aspect of key measures—performance, cost efficiency, and, worst of all, equity (WHO 2001). Beginning in the mid-2000s, a meaningful effort toward reforming the health system was started in an attempt to reverse this dangerous trend, and the process is still ongoing.

The main reasons for the devolution of China's health system can best be summarized as the result of a transition failure with the change of economic management systems—central planning with excessive control coupled with inappropriate use of market practices for health care financing when health care is a known area of market failure. Under the economic reforms, China's health system continued to be entirely managed by its central planning mechanism with strict price controls for all chargeable items such as fees for clinic visits, surgery, and the use of hospital rooms. Perplexingly, this fee schedule has been frozen at an early-1980s level, which is grossly undervalued today. The most notable change since 1980 is that health care and preventive service facilities have been classified as "business" or "enterprise" units instead of government units because of their income-generating capacity. In doing so, the facilities and workers receive only partial funding or salary, often below 50 percent of what was determined as the full allocation. But as a government-owned enterprise unit, the facility can generate and retain income to make up for the shortfall in official allocation. This partial funding with a severe limitation on charging market value for service created a much-distorted financing model for the health system—with the majority of income coming from the profits of consumables, mainly drugs and diagnostics. This model has encouraged providers to use more drugs or more expensive drugs and resulted in greater utilization of diagnostics and procedures. Over time this evolved into a pattern of overutilization, often not in the best interest of the patients. The long-term consequences of this distorted financing model are:

- Much higher overall cost even though service fees are very low because of the leverage effect of drugs—average profit margin for the providers is 15–20 percent, but the patient has to pay 100 percent of the cost

- Reduced access to care for those who are poor or do not have medical insurance
- Decline in service quality and professionalism—direct financial incentives from drugs and procedures influencing the decision and behavior of service providers

Ongoing health reform measures try to address these issues, including low medical insurance coverage. Before the reform process started in 2006, medical coverage extended to about 50 percent of urban residents and less than 15 percent of rural residents. The high cost for medical care and inadequate coverage, especially for the rural population, almost reached crisis proportions by the mid-2000s, leading to an ongoing comprehensive reform effort. Reflecting the commitment for this effort, by 2011 rural health insurance coverage reached over 95 percent. Starting that same year, the reform process began to address the dangerous model of financing through drug profits. This is a more challenging task because of the entrenched interest from those who continue to benefit from overutilization and the need to define alternative sources of funding.

The Preventive Service Arm of the Health System with the Mandate for HIV Prevention and Control

China's preventive health service system, known as the Center for Disease Control (CDC), is charged with the mandate of HIV prevention together with other prevention-oriented functions such as immunization and tuberculosis (TB) controls. This mandate and CDC's position as serving as the holder of the budget for HIV prevention is both a strength and a weakness of China's response to AIDS. As a dedicated agency for preventative health services with a network from national to township levels, the CDC is very capable of implementing surveillance, health education, and laboratory-related services—all essential components of a strong AIDS response program. However, the AIDS response also requires the contribution of social and psychological support and care, medical treatment for those with HIV, and intervention among high-risk groups such as injection drug users (IDU) and men who have sex with men (MSM), all of which are outside the normal function of the CDC system.

Prior to 2004, there was very limited funding from the central government earmarked for HIV prevention, and the majority of the HIV funding came from international donors as special projects managed by the CDC system. After the SARS epidemic in 2003, the government paid much greater attention to public health, and HIV funding began to steadily increase. Around the same time, the Global Fund also started to provide sizable support. By 2011, the CDC system across China was able to receive adequate funding for general operations, and today HIV is by far the best-funded program area, with combined national and international inputs.

Challenges in Care and Treatment for HIV/AIDS Related to the Health System Structure and Function

A substantial part of the post-SARS increases in funding for HIV were for antiretroviral (ARV) treatment, but this part of the clinically oriented program was administered by the CDC system even though it does not provide the full range of clinical services outside of ARV drug distribution. Without meaningful participation of the medical service arm of the health system, adequate treatment and care for HIV/AIDS remains a challenge today. This is an area in which a number of international organizations have been assisting by setting up clinics or training centers for physicians. But without the funding and training of HIV/AIDS care and treatment's being directly linked to the CDC's medical service, this problem will not be fully resolved. In theory, the rural health insurance scheme's expansion in coverage should improve access for AIDS treatment, but HIV funding has been allocated through the CDC system and is one of the disease conditions excluded by the insurance scheme. Through the advocacy effort of some international organizations, AIDS care has been added as part of the rural insurance scheme and is now being piloted in selected provinces.

The History and Status of the HIV Epidemic of China

Because the diagnosis of the first case of AIDS in 1985 was a foreign tourist, the prevailing view throughout the 1990s was that HIV/AIDS was a foreigner's disease related to sex and drugs, which implied that Chinese people were "immune" due to their conservative culture and social norms. Even though that myth ended with the discovery of the first wave of China's HIV/AIDS epidemic due to injection drug use in Yunnan Province in 1989, general perception did not change for some time due to lack of recognition of the significance of this epidemic for another decade (Yan 2007).

Unlike the sub-Saharan African HIV epidemic, which is a generalized one mainly among heterosexuals, China's pattern is mainly concentrated among high-risk groups—IDU and MSM—similar to epidemics in Western countries. Unlike concentrated epidemics in Southeast Asia and India, where a major component has been the epidemic among commercial sex workers (CSW), China's overall prevalence for CSW has been relatively low and has remained stable at near or below 1 percent since surveillance began in 1996. What is unique for China was that a major concentrated epidemic started in the early 1990s due to unsafe plasma collection. In the mid-2000s, a new MSM-based epidemic started, and it remains the most pressing challenge of China's AIDS response today. The three distinct waves of HIV epidemics are discussed in brief below.

The First Wave: The IDU-Driven Epidemic, 1989 Onward

The first recognized HIV epidemic was discovered in an area on the border of China and Myanmar in Yunnan Province's Dehong prefecture. This is an area where opium use was common because of its proximity to the Golden Triangle. The switch from smoking opium to injecting heroin was an unintended consequence of increased international pressure and effort against narcotic trafficking in the 1980s. Because heroin is much easier to traffic than opium, about one-tenth in weight, it resulted in a switch to heroin, which is mainly administered intravenously. The needle-sharing among heroin injection users was the main reason for HIV transmission.

After the discovery of the IDU-based HIV epidemic in one location in Yunnan, the Chinese government's main focus was on epidemiological surveillance, and, in terms of policy and funding support, it took no real action to address the epidemic until 2004. During these 15 years of inaction, the IDU epidemic spread across all of Yunnan Province and into surrounding provinces (Guangxi, Guizhou, and Sichuan), and to a lesser extent to many of the southern provinces. The notable exception is Xinjiang in the northwestern part of China, mainly among the Uyghur minority there, but the source of their HIV epidemic is also linked to Yunnan.

Unlike Western countries and Australia, where IDU-based HIV epidemics have been urban-based, with the exception of Xinjiang, China's epidemic was predominately a rural one that mainly affected minority populations, which made it a highly stigmatized disease for mainstream Chinese society to address. Overall, the prevalence among IDU has been stable, with some modest decline in recent years. The most notable effort to develop a model of intervention for the IDU-based epidemic prior to the national response was the China-UK project funded by DFID (the Department for International Development, United Kingdom), to be detailed later. After China started to respond to AIDS in 2004, harm reduction programs including methadone maintenance treatment were introduced, and now China has the largest state-funded methadone maintenance treatment program in the world. In the last few years, the IDU-based epidemic appears to have been brought under control, and the estimated number of newly infected IDU is declining. This is due in part to the meaningful AIDS response, but more importantly, it can be attributed to the decline of heroin use across China, as evidenced by the public security system's data on drug-related arrests.

The Second Wave: The Epidemic Due to Unsafe
Plasma Collection, 1991–Mid-2000s

Among the number of epidemics related to poor blood safety practices throughout the global history of the HIV/AIDS pandemic, one that stands out is the large epidemic in central China during the early 1990s resulting from unhygienic commercial plasma collection, during which an estimated 250,000 people, mainly rural peasants, were infected with HIV. The five most heavily affected provinces were Henan, Anhui, Shanxi, Hubei, and Shandong (Mastro and Yip 2006).

Starting in the early 1990s, many rural commercial plasma collection centers were established in central China to supply a booming industry of blood products. The market was poorly regulated and some of the blood centers combined the blood from multiple ABO-matched plasma donors in order to conduct more efficient, large-volume plasma separation. The pooled cell fraction was then returned to the original donors. Unfortunately, this practice of the reinfusion of pooled blood cells is also the most efficient way to transmit hepatitis and HIV. This plasma-based HIV epidemic was first detected in 1992 during a survey for hepatitis among plasma donors in Henan, but the local government suppressed the information. The practice of plasma collection was not banned until 1995 after mounting evidence of HIV infections was documented in multiple locations.

The unsafe plasma–based epidemic only became obvious in the summer months of 2000 when a number of highly affected villages in Henan Province's Zhumadian area suffered from a high incidence of severe illness and death, which were then diagnosed to be AIDS. The local government again suppressed the information and kept journalists away. Through the actions of Gao Yaojie in Henan and Gui Xian in Hubei, two outspoken doctors who were taking care of a large number of AIDS patients, and some persistent journalists, eventually the news got out and in 2002 it reached the top leadership in Beijing. Around the same time, Vice Premier Madame Wu Yi, known as the "Iron Lady," became the minister of health after the firing of the previous minister for holding back information about the SARS outbreak, which had contributed to the spread of the disease. Her leadership signified the beginning of China's taking the AIDS epidemic seriously and turning its response to AIDS from denial to action (Kaufman 2010). In contrast to the sex- and drug-related HIV epidemics, this HIV epidemic with "Chinese characteristics," which mainly affected poor and rural peasants, helped make the high-level response politically feasible because victims were viewed as having been undeserving. The formal response to AIDS from the highest level of the Chinese leadership took place on International AIDS Day (December 1) in 2003, when Premier Wen Jiabao and Vice Premier Wu Yi visited the Ditan Infectious Disease Hospital and shook hands with two AIDS patients, which attracted nation-wide media coverage.

In 2004, Henan, the province with the majority of HIV infections due to unsafe plasma collection, conducted mandatory HIV screening in villages known to have had plasma collection activities and started a comprehensive relief program for those found to be HIV-positive. The mandatory nature of the screening program received strong criticism from a number of international agencies. In retrospect, although this program failed to meet the strict standard for Voluntary Counseling and Testing (VCT), it demonstrated the feasibility of preventing new HIV infections within a given community through a combination of testing and ARV treatment, so that those who are HIV-positive learn their positive status and those who test positive receive treatment, which reduces their viral load and transmutability. This strategy, now known as "treatment for prevention," has started to gain momentum globally over the past two years.

After the 2004 screening effort, Henan Province reported a total of 35,000 people living with HIV, and the average prevalence from this mass screening was 8.9 percent (Li et al. 2010). Depending on the estimated number of people who had already died, the overall estimate of those infected with HIV through unsafe plasma collection is probably in the range of 150,000 to 350,000. The China CDC estimated that over 90 percent of those infected with HIV in Henan in the early 1990s due to unsafe plasma collection were detected and received care and treatment such that there was very little further transmission.

Before the central government fully began to confront this epidemic by the end of 2003, local governments made every effort to keep outsiders out of the affected areas, so international philanthropic organizations were minimally engaged, with two notable exceptions. The Hong Kong–based Chi Heng Foundation was able to work under the radar to provide schooling and nutrition programs in a few villages for children orphaned or affected by HIV/AIDS, and UNICEF was officially invited by the Henan government in 2001 to develop a Prevention for Mother to Child Transmission (PMTCT) program. This program, which began in 2002, is now funded fully by the central government in all provinces.

The Third Wave: The Epidemic among Men Who Have Sex with Men (MSM), 2005–Today

By the mid-2000s, with the IDU-driven epidemic showing signs of receding and the epidemic due to unsafe plasma collection almost totally controlled, China was near being able to declare that its HIV epidemic was under control (declining HIV incidence, or number of new cases). But a new epidemic emerged among men who have sex with men (Gao, Zhang, and Jin 2009) more than twenty years after the initial epidemic in the United States and Western Europe. The sociodemographic pattern is very similar to the original epidemic in the West, which was concentrated in large urban centers where sexual networking is fueled more easily by venues that can facilitate encounters (gay bars, clubs, and bathhouses). As in the pattern in the West in recent years, the internet is also becoming a major means of finding partners. Why is China's HIV epidemic among MSM lagging twenty years behind those of Western countries? The best plausible explanation is that with the economic transformations that started in the 1980s came a loosening of social controls in the 1990s, including the lifting of restrictions on the country's internal migration policy, and this mass migration to the cities reached a critical mass for gay men to have a strong underground network in large cities by the 2000s.

The limited surveillance of the MSM population that has taken place since 1995 did not note any trend of increase in HIV prevalence until 2004. More in-depth surveillance in Beijing and Shenzhen sponsored by the U.S. Centers for Disease Control and Prevention as part of the Global AIDS Program (GAP) in China detected an alarming trend: HIV prevalence in the MSM population doubled from 2004 onward. By 2006 there was sufficient information to conclude that there was a rising epidemic among MSM in a number of very large cities across China. The first formal assessment was a national HIV prevalence survey for MSM in 61 cities in 2008, and the findings were sobering. Even though the overall prevalence of 4.9 percent may not seem high from an international perspective, the prevalence in the top 20 biggest cities by population was much higher. On average, most large cities in the northeast and coastal provinces had a prevalence ranging from 5 to 10 percent, and the cities in the southeast like Chongqing and Chengdu had a prevalence of over 15 percent. What was disconcerting was not the prevalence, but the speed by which the prevalence increased in a short period of time. Based on limited data from various studies, none of these cities had a rate of more than 1 or 2 percent a few years before. Epidemiological data clearly showed that by the late 2000s an explosive epidemic among MSM, like that of United States in the 1980s, was taking place in China.

Currently this latest epidemic is still raging, with no sign of abating, mainly because the nature of prevention work for MSM is very different from that of the epidemics due to IDU or sex workers. The existing AIDS response mechanism by and large lacks the ability to reach the MSM community. As in many countries, homosexuality is taboo in China, and perhaps even more extremely so because, in a traditional Chinese view, it is a grave sin for a man not to produce offspring to continue the family line. Many workers in the preventive health services and medical fields also hold conventional views toward members of this community, making interaction difficult, particularly in working with nongovernmental organizations (NGOs) which can reach out to gay men. Several international organizations, particularly the Bill & Melinda Gates Foundation, have been focusing their work in China on bridging the government HIV response, the MSM community, and organizations that can reach out and support them.

National Response to HIV/AIDS

Political Commitment

As discussed, along with SARS, the second wave of the HIV epidemic among poor peasants in central provinces due to unsafe plasma collection precipitated a high-level government response in 2003. This represented a transformation from denial of the epidemic, with minimal resources provided for it, to a strong commitment to providing free treatment and prevention services. Beyond adequate resources, commitment also came in the form of the establishment of the State Council AIDS Working Committee, chaired by the Vice Premier, with members from all 31 ministries and all provinces significantly affected by AIDS (Wu et al. 2007). The Ministry of Health's Disease Control Bureau serves as the secretariat for the State Council AIDS Working Committee; therefore, funding for HIV response still mainly flows through their subsidiary, the CDC system. Unfortunately, the CDC does not have significant reach into areas such as medical service or the ability to effectively partner with NGOs that are also vital in contributing to the efforts. In essence, the overall effort has been concentrated in the CDC arm of the Health Ministry and is not truly multisectoral.

The only part of China where a strong multi-agency effort took place in response to HIV was in Henan Province, where the current premier, then party secretary Li Keqiang, mobilized the Communist Party to mount a comprehensive program to control the epidemic due to unsafe plasma collection. This effort involved a number of key ministries beyond health, such as civil affairs, education, and finance, and was largely successful in bringing the epidemic under control and creating a sound support program for all affected individuals and their families. In contrast to many Chinese leaders' traditional approach of looking at how much money is spent on what, Li has paid great attention to key result indicators such as the number of people newly found to be HIV-positive and number of people on ARV treatment.

By 2011, China's annual earmarked central budget for AIDS response reached 1.9 billion RMB (the equivalent of $300 million), a huge increase from the $20 million allocated in 2003 prior to the start of a meaningful national response.

The Role of International Philanthropy in the HIV Response

For the purpose of reviewing the contribution of international philanthropy to China's HIV/AIDS response, a broader definition is adopted to define such organizations. Beyond the traditional nonprofit private foundations or NGOs that meet the standard definition of international philanthropy, bilateral and multilateral aid agencies are also being included to build a complete picture of the external contributions to this effort.

Over the past 20 years, a large number of international organizations have contributed to the AIDS response in China. This review is not exhaustive, and the work of only a subset of these organizations is presented by highlighting those that made significant contributions at critical times or were pioneers in a particular area. By not describing the work of some other organizations, this review is by no means suggesting that their contributions were not important. The organizations highlighted below are listed based on their starting time in China, from early to recent.

Barry & Martin's Trust, United Kingdom

Barry & Martin's Trust is a British philanthropic organization founded by Gordon Barry that since 1996 has been active in China in AIDS education, prevention, and care. Although the trust's giving is modest, approximately $150,000 a year, its influence has been impressive. This is due in part to the trust's being the first organization actively engaged in and giving sustained support to medical care for AIDS and mobilizing HIV prevention for the gay community. The catalytic effect of the trust has been particularly effective in mobilizing leadership for AIDS prevention for the gay community through an annual prize by recognizing those who made special contributions in the service of HIV prevention or care. The trust is best known for its flexibility and deep engagement with its partners in China. In essence, it is a good model for catalytic philanthropy.

The trust was the earliest supporter of HIV/AIDS treatment and care in leading hospitals in China. Presently it supports projects at leading national hospitals for AIDS care in Beijing and Yunnan. The trust also supports the MSM community in China through strategic grant-making to grassroots organizations, especially through Qingdao Medical College's sexual health center, the Red Ribbon Centre at Beijing Ditan Hospital, and the Quiet Garden project at Beijing You'an Hospital. These centers have become models for psychosocial support and have served as models and resources for the development of similar centers in other cities.

HIV/AIDS Prevention and Care Project, Funded by the Department for International Development (DFID), United Kingdom

The United Kingdom's HIV/AIDS Prevention and Care Project (HAPAC) started in 2000 as the first large-scale HIV/AIDS cooperation program in China and focused on developing replicable models for prevention and care for high-risk groups in order to inform government policy. HAPAC became the first program to make a serious effort in establishing prevention efforts targeting IDUs and CSWs.

HAPAC supported the development of large-scale models for high-risk and vulnerable groups in order to gain policy support based on evidence and experience obtained. From 2000 to 2006, through HAPAC's £20 million project, pilot programs based in Sichuan and Yunnan focused on social marketing of condoms and needle exchange and were centered on the following objectives:

- Improving HIV/AIDS awareness and knowledge of AIDS prevention, and reducing the stigma against people with AIDS by the general population

- Improving the development and delivery of services to high-risk groups, including CSWs, IDUs, and MSM through the engagement of "peer workers" who are members of the high-risk communities
- Establishing management systems and personnel that effectively support program activities

HAPAC undertook trailblazing work prior to 2003, before the national response to AIDS occurred. According to an independent external review of the project, HAPAC led to "significantly increased condom use; significant reduction in needle-sharing amongst IDUs; changes in gender power relationships, enabling sex workers to negotiate 100% condom use; and a reduction in stigma" (DFID China 2008). More importantly HAPAC pilot programs were adopted by and scaled up in China's first national HIV/AIDS program, known as the Demonstration County Project (2001), and later the Global Fund Round 4 project for IDU intervention (2005). HAPAC's needle exchange program was also very useful in demonstrating the usefulness of "peer workers," current and past drug users working for the local CDC to provide outreach services. In short, HAPAC broke new ground with a number of meaningful measures for HIV prevention by targeting two high-risk groups, and provided China with strategic assistance at a critical time.

United Nations Children's Fund (UNICEF)

In 1997 UNICEF established an HIV/AIDS program focused on health education and promotion, mainly targeting youth. In 2001 the Henan government invited UNICEF to establish a Prevention of Mother to Child Transmission (PMTCT) program in communities heavily affected by AIDS due to unsafe plasma collection. This cooperation was significant because at that time information about the epidemic due to poor blood safety practices was still being suppressed while there was increasing local pressure to provide care for affected individuals and their families. UNICEF's commencement of PMTCT to prevent further HIV transmission to infants signaled the beginning of a meaningful response to the legacy of unsafe plasma collection. The PMTCT program began in 2002 with imported Neverapin, the first officially sanctioned AIDS drug in China. The engagement of the Henan government with UNICEF also represented the first official program targeting prevention efforts for people living with HIV/AIDS, in contrast to all previous efforts, which had targeted high-risk groups for behavioral change. Since the national response to HIV began in 2003, the PMTCT program has been scaled up to over half the counties in China and is a major part of the national program.

The Joint United Nations Programme on HIV/AIDS (UNAIDS)

As the coordinating office for all United Nation (UN) agencies' AIDS work, UNAIDS has consistently played an important advocacy role in China. Prior to the

2003 turnaround when the strong national response started, the UN's principle effort was to urge the Chinese government to change its approach toward the disease from denial to an active response. During UN Secretary-General Kofi Annan's multiple visits to China, he consistently raised with senior leaders the need to confront AIDS. In 2001, the UNAIDS Beijing Office issued a report entitled *HIV/AIDS: China's Titanic Peril*, which suggested that if no meaningful response was put forth, China's HIV caseload would increase from estimated 650,000 at that time to over 10 million by 2010 (United Nations Theme Group for HIV/AIDS 2002). Although the projected figure was not based on any epidemiological model, and was clearly an excessive one (it turned out to be off by 10 times, as China's HIV burden was estimated to be approximately 780,000 in 2011), it raised substantial international and local attention and debate. In retrospect, it can be argued that it was useful in raising the awareness that may have contributed to a quicker turnaround from denial to response.

Since the start of the national response in 2003, UNAIDS' advocacy role has focused on promoting the inclusion of civil society in China's AIDS response, particularly in working with hard-to-reach groups such as drug users and MSM. The lack of civil society's participation is a major weakness of the current national program administered by the CDC system, which has limited experience and capacity in reaching these populations. The effort to promote greater inclusion of civil society partners will continue to be an important mission of UNAIDS.

Doctors Without Borders/Médecins Sans Frontières (MSF), France

In 2003 MSF started the first dedicated AIDS facility in a rural area in Xiangfan, Hubei Province, where many people had been infected due to unsafe plasma collection. MSF imported ARV drugs and made a determined effort to maintain the same level of care at this rural treatment center as existed in Western countries. The project was managed in cooperation with the local CDC, and the center was turned over to local government in 2008. The Xiangfan center proved that quality AIDS care can be delivered in rural China.

Another MSF-supported project on AIDS treatment also began in 2003 in Nanning, the capital of Guangxi Province, where rates of HIV transmission through intravenous drug use were high. At the time, government funded treatment programs were still restricted to those infected due to plasma donation, and this center, housed within the Guangxi CDC, became the first to treat a substantial number of AIDS patients who had become infected through sexual transmission or drug use. Additionally, MSF supported the development and operation of a quality counseling service both for VCT (Voluntary Counseling and Testing) and for ARV adherence (both are done poorly in most other facilities). In this particularly underdeveloped region of China, a functional model was very useful and the Guangxi CDC rolled it out in dozens of counties across the province.

Overall, MSF's work demonstrated a strong partnership with local health authorities and introduced best practices that were later scaled up.

The Chi Heng Foundation, Hong Kong

The Chi Heng Foundation (CHF), founded by Cheung To, began providing assistance to AIDS orphans in some of Henan's most affected villages in 2002. At that time, the local government was still trying to keep the AIDS epidemic under wraps, so CHF's work there was an underground operation. CHF primarily focused on paying for the AIDS-affected children's education and living expenses, transmitting all funds directly to schools and families. CHF does not operate orphanages or foster homes. Instead, it supports local relatives who take the children in, allowing them to continue to grow up in their home villages. To further decrease the children's sense of social stigma and isolation, CHF places them in schools that purposely integrate the orphans with children not affected by HIV/AIDS, contrary to the government policy of keeping HIV-infected children out of regular schools. CHF and To are pioneers in caring for AIDS-affected children in China. In 2004, after the start of the national response, local governments established orphanages and unfortunately made the effort of keeping children within their communities difficult, at times outlawing it.

CHF also has been active in supporting HIV prevention work among the gay community in several large cities and promoting the rights of sexual minorities. In addition to working directly with these communities, CHF educates the owners of saunas and brothels. CHF attracted notice in China in 2004 when it helped organize a graduate-level class at Shanghai's Fudan University on the subject of homosexuality, the first such class in the country.

Global AIDS Program of the United States Centers for Disease Control and Prevention (U.S. CDC)

The Global AIDS Program (GAP) was started in China in early 2003 on the basis of a cooperative agreement with the China CDC to establish a comprehensive model of HIV prevention in 15 provinces, focused on a "prevention for positives" strategy. This strategy was adopted because at the time China had yet to actively respond to AIDS. The limited government resources devoted to HIV/AIDS were mainly focused on behavior improvement and self-protection of the general public through health education, and to a lesser extent behavior-based interventions with high-risk groups such as IDU and CSW. Most of these investments had proven ineffective at slowing the spread of the epidemic in other countries. The program aimed to fill a gap by targeting those people already infected with HIV and developed the cooperative agreement to strengthen this approach.

The overall program framework, based on the "prevention for positives" strategy, put HIV testing at the center of an effort with the following components:

- Improving surveillance via greater HIV testing among high-risk groups such as IDU or MSM, while at the same time ensuring follow-up care and intervention for those found to be HIV-positive (testing for surveillance also contributing to intervention)
- Encouraging the scale-up of HIV testing sites for high-risk groups and adding these sites to expand the national sentinel surveillance system (HIV-testing effort also contributing to surveillance)
- Assuring follow-up for all those found to be HIV-positive regardless of where they were found—beyond VCT site (surveillance sites, hospitals, and prisons) to create linkages between intervention, care, and treatment in order to reduce secondary transmission to others

Because the U.S. CDC is a technical agency, the above framework was implemented as technical assistance in the form of capacity building for laboratory testing, epidemiological surveillance, and treatment-capacity building through the key divisions of the National AIDS Center of China CDC. The initiation of a meaningful national response to AIDS by 2004, with a commitment to ARV treatment, contributed a great deal to moving this strategy forward. To a large extent, "prevention for positives" now is the central aspect of the national strategy and policy, and its introduction to China can be attributed to the effort of GAP.

One specific contribution of GAP to the expansion of AIDS treatment has been its joint program with the Clinton Foundation, which established a rural training program in Lixin county, Anhui Province, one of the most severely affected areas due to unsafe plasma collection. Begun in 2005, this program provided training for lower-level (county and township) doctors to provide routine AIDS care and ARV management. This created an alternative to the existing model of only infectious disease specialists in large hospitals in provincial capitals providing for AIDS medical care, which precluded the access of many patients because they lived in rural areas and lacked the financial means to go to more expensive institutions farther away.

The Clinton Foundation China HIV/AIDS Initiative (CHAI), United States

CHAI ran from 2004 to 2011 and focused completely on improving the quality of treatment for people living with AIDS and increasing their access to quality care. It was by far the largest international philanthropic program dedicated to AIDS treatment. The Rural AIDS Training Centre at Lixin county, Anhui Province, was the first program launched by CHAI in 2005, in partnership with GAP. CHAI's second AIDS treatment program was started in 2005, based in Kunming, Yunnan Province, and focused on clinical training as well as ARV treatment. Begun in 2006 with funding from the Australian Agency for International Development (AusAID), CHAI started a third program in Xinjiang Province which was designed to improve access to AIDS care and ARV treatment for those infected due to injection drug use. In both the Yunnan and Xinjiang treatment programs, the U.S. standard laboratory monitoring practice of using both CD4 counts and viral loads was adopted. CHAI provided technical assistance to the National Center for AIDS, part of the China CDC, in order to accelerate access to CD4 and viral load testing, which are essential in quality AIDS care.

Another important CHAI contribution to China's AIDS response was the introduction of pediatric AIDS treatment into the country. Starting in 2004 through special arrangement with the Ministry of Health, CHAI provided imported ARV drugs for children infected through maternal transmission in Henan Province.

The Bill & Melinda Gates Foundation, United States

The China-Gates Cooperation AIDS Program funded by the Gates Foundation was planned in 2006. It was the foundation's first major program in China as part of the global strategy to improve HIV prevention effectiveness. The program was designed at a time when there was early indication that the MSM-based epidemic was starting. Another area of the program's focus was to address an underdeveloped area of the national program: the prevention aspect for those already living with HIV/AIDS. The five-year program began in late 2007 with two strategies:

1. Prevention for high-risk groups, particularly MSM, with two major areas of focus:
    - Supporting the mobilization of grassroots-level NGOs in working with local CDC systems for outreach work with high-risk group communities
    - Adding HIV testing as part of the prevention outreach effort (beyond condom promotion)
2. Prevention for positives, also with two areas of focus:
    - Ensuring the linkage of those tested positive by the CDC system with hospitals for follow-up prevention and treatment services
    - Improving the working relationship between CDC, hospitals, and NGOs as partners for HIV/AIDS service

These two program strategies nowadays are becoming better known as a form of "treatment for prevention," or more accurately as "seek-test-link-treat" (Dieffenbach and Fauci 2009). In 2006, the existing national program clearly supported testing and treatment, but it was weak on the seeking and linking aspects. The program is focused on a response to the emerging MSM epidemic and operates in 15 large cities. In order to ensure NGO participation, funding was distributed through two channels: the China CDC and two national-level government-operated nongovernmental organizations (GONGOs), the China STD & AIDS Association and the Chinese Preventive Medicine Association, which distribute funding at the local level to community-based organizations. Coverage for both MSM and people living with HIV reached over 25 percent in some of the project cities. The key challenge remaining is whether coverage can be brought to a scale high enough to control the epidemic (according to modeling using China data, such a target would mean reaching more than 60 percent of the MSM community or finding more than 60 percent of all people with HIV in a given community).

The Gates program played an instrumental role in shifting the national focus to the MSM epidemic and prevention for high-risk groups, and enforced the role of prevention for positives as a key strategy of AIDS response. The key program indicators became what has been defined as the Five-Year National HIV/AIDS Strategy issued by China's State Council in 2011, which focuses on increasing testing for high-risk groups, expanding follow-up and treatment for eligible HIV-positive people, and using hard targets for evaluation. The national HIV/AIDS program is also building on the Gates program's models for government procurement of NGO services in order to address issues of HIV prevention and control among the MSM population.

Outlook and Recommended Model for International Philanthropic Engagement

International assistance has always played a major role in China's AIDS response, but the last two years have seen the winding down of a period of substantial foreign financial assistance for HIV/AIDS. In financial terms, the Global Fund has been the largest contributor since 2004, with support totaling almost $600 million. In 2011, because of organizational funding shortfalls, the Global Fund made China ineligible to receive new funding by invoking a new rule that disqualified G20 countries as recipients, except for South Africa. Also in the last two years, most major bilateral programs such as DFID and AusAID terminated their assistance to China. By 2012, UN programs, the U.S. CDC, the MSD Foundation, and the Gates Foundation were the only international organizations with significant HIV/AIDS programs in various part of China. Based on an analysis of the effectiveness of the Chinese government's HIV/AIDS strategy and program, there are still areas in which China can benefit from international cooperation even though from a financial point of view China is doing well.

From the global experience and program management points of view, the Chinese government's response still has room for improvement and can benefit from engaging international organizations in the following areas:

- Establishing a response mechanism that goes beyond the preventive health (CDC) system and includes engagement of the medical service system and civil society
- Formalizing a multisectoral response, beyond the Ministry of Health

- Improving the HIV-positive case-finding system: liberalizing HIV testing to all interested parties beyond the CDC and adopting more cost-efficient approaches such as using rapid tests for screening and confirmation
- Improving access to ARV treatment by allowing drugs to be obtained beyond the patients' official location of residence and their local CDC
- Shifting from input-based program management to output-based or result-based programs to assure that coverage for prevention and treatment can be scaled up
- Fully and candidly confronting the epidemic among the MSM population
- Taking measures to decrease social discrimination against high-risk groups, particularly the MSM population

In conclusion, further engagement of international philanthropic organizations would be beneficial in addressing these more difficult issues and supporting policy changes to capitalize on the Chinese government's high level of political commitment and financial support.

Acknowledgment

The author wishes to thank Lani Marsden for research and editing assistance and thoughtful feedback.

References

DFID (Department for International Development) China. 2008. "Briefing Paper: HIV/AIDS." Beijing: DFID China.

Dieffenbach, Carl W., and Anthoney S. Fauci. 2009. "Universal Voluntary Testing and Treatment for Prevention of HIV Transmission." *Journal of the American Medical Association (JAMA)* 301 (22): 2380–2382.

Gao Lei, Zhang Li, and Jin Qi. 2009. "Meta-Analysis: Prevalence of HIV Infection and Syphilis among MSM in China." *Sexually Transmitted Infections* 85 (5): 354–358.

Kaufman, Joan. 2010. "Turning Points in China's AIDS Response." *China: An International Journal* 8 (1): 63–84.

Li Ning, Wang Zhe, Sun Dingyong, Zhu Qian, Sun Guoqing, Yang Wenjie, Wang Qi, Nie Yugang, Wu Zunyou 2010. "HIV among Plasma Donors and Other High-Risk Groups in Henan, China." *Journal of Acquired Immune Deficiency Syndromes (JAIDS)* 53 (suppl. 1): S41–S47.

Mastro, Timothy D., and Ray Yip. 2006. "The Legacy of Unhygienic Plasma Collection in China." *AIDS* 20 (10): 1451–1452.

United Nations Theme Group for HIV/AIDS in China. 2002. *HIV/AIDS: China's Titanic Peril—2001 Update of the AIDS Situation and Needs Assessment Report.* http://www.hivpolicy.org/Library/HPP000056.pdf.

WHO (World Health Organization). *2001*. The World Health Report *2000*: Health Systems; Improving Performance. http://www.who.int/whr/2000/en/whr00_en.pdf.

Wu Zunyou, Sheena G Sullivan, Yu Wang, Mary Jane Rotheram-Borus, and Roger Detels. 2007. "Evolution of China's Response to HIV/AIDS." *Lancet* 369 (9562): 679–690.

Yan Xiao, Sibylle Kristensen, Jiangping Sun, Lin Lu, and Sten H. Vermund. 2007. "Expansion of HIV/AIDS in China: Lessons from Yunnan Province." *Social Science & Medicine* 64 (3): 665–675.

8 Gender and Reproductive Health in China

Partnership with Foundations and the United Nations

Joan Kaufman, Mary Ann Burris,
Eve W. Lee, and Susan Jolly

Introduction

China's sexual and reproductive health and rights story has a mixed history. On the one hand, huge improvements in basic health care since 1949, including access to and promotion of family planning and facility-based birth delivery and the legalization of abortion since the 1970s, have led to impressive reductions in maternal mortality and child survival (Fang and Kaufman 2008; Xing et al. 2011). On the other hand, the imposition of a strict birth control policy has led to major violations of reproductive rights and a highly distorted sex ratio at birth in favor of boys (Hvistendahl 2009). Activism by women's groups and human rights advocates on reproductive rights is constrained by the uncompromising nature of the top-down population policy. A large youth population with rapidly changing sexual attitudes, identities, and behaviors (Zheng et al. 2010) has come of age in the last decade. These youth require information and services even while government services continue to focus on married couples and promote youth abstinence. An escalating AIDS epidemic (Ministry of Health, Joint United Nations Programme on HIV/AIDS, and World Health Organization 2010) is challenged by the restrictions on civil society organizations that can best reach groups at risk and affected by the disease, and by continuing stigma.

Two international donors, the United Nations Population Fund (UNFPA) and the Ford Foundation, have been actively engaged in China since the 1980s, promoting and supporting policy change and program development aimed at improving reproductive and sexual health and rights. While both organizations have shared some core goals and initiatives related to the promotion of international norms and practices agreed to at the International Conference on Population and Development (ICPD) (UNFPA 1994), each organization has unique features and ways of working, using different strategies, approaches, and its place at the table to achieve its goals, at times working in tandem to leverage institutional advantages on common areas of work. We review each organization's work in China, focusing on contextual factors, such as the domestic context of China's one-child policy, international human rights movements, and the implications for philanthropy strategies and operations in these contexts. While a number of other donors have supported projects on gender and reproductive health in China in the last 30 years, including AusAid (the Australian bilateral assistance agency), the Rockefeller Foundation, PATH, the International Planned Parenthood Foundation, Family Health International, the Department for International Development (the UK bilateral assistance agency), and the Swedish International Development Cooperation Agency (SIDA, the Swedish bilateral assistance agency), we focus on UNFPA and the Ford Foundation as the two organizations with in-country offices and dedicated China programs supporting work on gender and reproductive health improvement over the entire three decades.

We examine several issues that have spanned UNFPA's three decades of programming and the Ford Foundation's more than two decades of grant-making in China, reviewing progress in improvements in quality of care in the family planning program and contraceptive choice, acknowledgement and action on domestic violence, improvement in HIV prevention and treatment through support to civil society organizations, and support for sexuality research that has contributed to the sexual health of youths and has improved HIV prevention. We examine how these organizations have carried out their role as donors, particularly the ways in which they intervened in sensitive areas like reproductive rights, sexual rights, and supporting civil society.

Background on China's Reproductive and Sexual Health and Rights

Both the Ford Foundation and UNFPA have been working in China in a context dominated by China's one-child policy, the most draconian population policy in history and one posing significant challenges to reproductive and women's rights. In addition to the pressures on women for mandatory contraceptive use and involuntary abortions, the policy has exacerbated son preference and led to a skewed sex ratio at birth in favor of males, largely attributed to sex-selective abortion. China's last official intercensus survey in 2005 reported a national sex ratio at birth figure of 120.5:100 in favor of males, but when examined by parity, the distortion reaches 143.2:100 for the second birth and 156.4:100 for the third birth (National Bureau of Statistics 2007; Census of China 1982, 1993).

China's one-child policy has contributed to the drop in maternal mortality through the large reduction in the number of births and sped up China's demographic transition to a low-fertility country. China's average maternal mortality rate is 38 per 100,000 live births, but rates can be four times higher in poorer areas (Fang 2004). The lifetime risk of maternal death in China is 1 in 1,500 compared to 1 in 140 in India (Asian-Pacific Resource & Research Centre for Women 2010). With current trends, China's population will halve in about 30 years. A number of recent surveys document that fertility desires are low and unlikely to change even if the policy is lifted (Zheng 2010). The size of China's elderly population aged 60 and above will increase to two hundred million by 2015, and to over three hundred million by 2030 (Wan, Muenchrath, and Kowal 2012).

China's youth, many born since 1980, are delaying or not marrying, reaching puberty earlier, and are more sexually active than in the past. In urban areas, they are often only children, well educated, and with disposable income and regular access to the internet and social media. Rural youths typically migrate to the cities for work before marriage where they are exposed to more modern ideas about gender and childbearing. Among youth in urban areas there is a social and sexual networking culture facilitated by the internet. Internet usage in China has exploded, with estimates that 420 million Chinese are currently online (Jing 2010). A recent survey of teenagers 14 to 17 years old found that at least 80 percent had some kind of internet access and 30 percent had viewed pornography (Pan and Huang 2011). The commercialization of sexuality has influenced social norms, especially for youth, and there is increasing acceptance of sexual relations outside of marriage as well as of homosexuality.

But because the family planning program mainly targets married women, these youths lack access to contraceptive services and sexual health information, as evidenced by the high rates of abortion among unmarried youths. In 2008, abortion rates increased in China to 9 percent (16.15 million) (Gu 2009) from 6 percent in 2001, with most of the increase among unmarried youth. A nationwide survey in 2010 found that among rural female youth who are sexually active, nearly 24 percent of 15–24-year-olds have become pregnant, 6 percent with repeat pregnancies and 86 percent ending in abortion, with repeat abortions accounting for 19 percent (Zheng et al. 2010). Youth obtain abortions at urban hospitals or private clinics, where the procedure is provided with anonymity.

China's HIV epidemic also continues to expand, even though it is considered low by international standards (national prevalence is under 0.5 percent). The government and UNAIDS estimate that 780,000 persons are HIV-infected. The epidemic is becoming a sexually transmitted one—of the new infections in 2011, 81.6 percent were sexually transmitted (UNAIDS 2008), including among men who have sex with men (new infections in 2011 accounted for 29.4 percent of the total) (UNAIDS 2008). The percentage of women among the infected is increasing, from 19.4 percent in 2000 to 28.6 percent in 2011 (UNAIDS 2008), with spousal transmission increasing as well. Condom use rates have increased in many populations including sexually active youth and urban businessmen, but at the same time both formal and informal sex work has had a resurgence in China. There are ubiquitous entertainment venues, staffed by young male and female migrants, where sexual services are available, even in rural cities and towns. Increasing HIV rates among lower-level sex workers in southern China are a big concern for the national AIDS prevention program.

Historical Context of UNFPA and the Ford Foundation in China

When Deng Xiaoping was launching China's market reforms in 1979, he invited the United Nations Development Programme (UNDP), UNFPA, and a few other UN agencies to work in China and assist in China's "Four Modernizations."[1] In the late 1970s, population control was seen as a critical potential drag on economic development and a goal was set to cap China's population at 1.2 billion by 2000. Population control through family planning service provision was a major component of development assistance and was a major aspect of UNFPA's mandate, along with support for population data collection and analysis.

In 1988, the Ford Foundation established an office in China, and in 1991 it launched a reproductive health portfolio.[2] The foundation's China reproductive health work began at a time when reproductive health was just entering the international population and health discourse and was still a virtually unknown concept in China. Work both globally and in China included efforts to strengthen women's movements as a means of fostering more dialogue, debate, and changes in the areas of reproductive rights and health, which has been a key feature of such change in Europe, the United States, Brazil, Mexico, and India. Links between international feminists and women's studies scholars and Chinese women activists were developed to coordinate efforts to strategize for greater gender equity and gender awareness in China.

The International Conference on Population and Development (ICPD) in Cairo in 1994 and the Fourth World Conference on Women in Beijing in 1995 provided unique opportunities for both UNFPA and the Ford Foundation to promote reproductive health concepts and commitment in China. Following the ICPD, the Chinese government began to explore ways to shift its target-driven population policy toward a more rights-based approach, albeit within the limits of a population stabilization strategy, and this opened the door for both UNFPA and the Ford Foundation to help shape this effort.

The ICPD changed the public discourse on family planning programs by introducing stronger considerations of reproductive rights and women's empowerment into the population control field. It also stressed important linkages to women's health and sexual health services for youths and for sexually transmitted diseases including HIV/AIDS, as well as violence against women. International donors adopted the new approach, with UNFPA taking a lead role in the implementation for the UN System. The Ford Foundation's New York–based Reproductive Health Program led the paradigm shift and joined with other large private philanthropies to support the emphasis on rights and empowerment at the global policy level and through its regional and country programs. The foundation also promoted the importance of social science research on sexuality and the inclusion of sexual health and rights in the new global agenda (Ford Foundation 1991).

In 1995, the Fourth World Conference on Women in Beijing solidified commitments on reproductive and sexual health and rights and made further connections between women's rights and reproductive health organizations funded by donor organizations. This common agenda for action very much characterized the decade of the 1990s. Growing concern about the global AIDS epidemic in the later 1990s and the discovery of an effective treatment for AIDS increased donor attention and resources for AIDS programs in the following decade.

China is a signatory to all of the major conferences and action plans concerned with reproductive health and gender equity,[3] as well as all three political declarations resulting from the UN General Assembly special sessions on AIDS (UNAIDS and UNIGASS 2006). But at the same time, China's one-child policy has been criticized for its focus on numbers over reproductive rights, its AIDS response characterized by crackdowns on risk groups such as sex workers (Branigan 2010), and its violating the rights of women, youth, and sexual minorities. Both UNFPA and the Ford Foundation have been engaged in efforts to reform the population policy, mitigate some of its worst impacts on women, and bring China's AIDS response into line with international best practices.

Strategic Philanthropy: UNFPA and the Ford Foundation

In the 30 years since the UN System began working in China and the Ford Foundation set up its China office, both China and the world have changed enormously. China has moved from an isolated and closed state to a major player in the global economy, and the world is increasingly globalized through the mechanisms of global finance, the internet, and regional and global geopolitical governance mechanisms like the Association of Southeast Asian Nations (ASEAN). UN agencies have been partners and contributors to China's 30-year economic and social transformation from an isolated developing country in 1980 to the world's second-leading economy after the United States in 2010. Unlike bilateral donors, the Chinese government regards UN support as neutral and without a political or hidden agenda. UNFPA's decision to not stop working in China in the face of U.S. pressure and budget cuts has solidified a strong relationship of trust with the government of China, affording UNFPA an important place at the table and the ear of leaders. UNFPA has used this access to advise on needed policy modifications.

The UN System works almost exclusively through government. From the inception of UN's China country programs, UN agencies have provided technical assistance and umbrella coordination mechanisms, partnered with Chinese Ministries in development planning, and linked international NGOs and other organizations to the government. For work on reproductive health in China, UN-FPA has been primarily engaged with China's National Population and Family Planning Commission (NPFPC), while at the same time coordinating its global agenda.

Unlike UNFPA, the Ford Foundation, was the only nonbilateral or multilateral (UN) donor based in China in the 1990s working on reproductive health (and, until the early 2000s, on HIV/AIDS) that was not obliged to work exclusively through government. Although both UN agencies and the UK-based Department for International Development (DFID) have worked with NGOs and academic institutions since the late 1990s, most such funding is controlled by government partners.

Because of its relative autonomy, Ford has been able to develop new talent and organizations through supporting different types of actors, including the NGO community and academic researchers. Ford has also engaged in sensitive issues regarded as too risky by government and bilateral donors. The Chinese government has often explicitly supported Ford's engagement in new and controversial areas as a way to test out this kind of work without doing the work itself—reform of the population program, clean needle programs for injecting drug users, HIV prevention for sex workers, support for LGBT communities, advocacy for the rights of HIV-positive persons, and prevention of sex-selective abortion and rural female suicide. For the improvement of sexual and reproductive health, the foundation has focused on building movements for social change: increasing the capacity of champions and organizations working on new or previously unaddressed issues, supporting pilot projects, linking key actors to transnational movements and global norms, and supporting their participation in the policy process. This work has resulted in issues becoming institutionalized in social and policy dialogues and debates as well as scaling up to policy change and implementation.

UNFPA's Assistance to China

UNFPA has had seven five-year country programs in China since 1980.[4] The largest set of projects was China's State Statistical Bureau conducting the 1982 census, still regarded as the best head count in China to date and the basis for many subsequent demographic projections. The training and equipment provided created a human and technological infrastructure that continues to act as the backbone of the rural statistics system to this day. A second major contribution was the training of four hundred young demographers abroad at the PhD level and support of population research centers at leading universities around China.

These demographers form the pillar of China's social science and economics research intelligentsia and play a major role in social policy research throughout the country.

Other projects built up the contraceptive production capacity of China, leading to contraceptive self-sufficiency and a network of key contraceptive research institutions. A new population information and policy research institution, the China Population Information and Research Center, was established in affiliation with the State Family Planning Commission. From 1990 to 1994, $57 million was provided to support rural family planning service improvement, including improving its integration with the Ministry of Health's maternal and child health services in 305 rural counties.

One of UNFPA's major efforts during this period was advocacy for reproductive rights. After ten years of the one-child policy and increasing international criticism of coercion in its implementation, UNFPA stepped up efforts to engage the Chinese government on the human rights dimensions of this policy and the need for voluntarism. UNFPA made it clear that its projects in China would need to strictly adhere to ICPD principles and criteria, making approval of its next phase of support conditional on the removal of birth targets in project-supported counties. It took until 1998 for the Chinese government to agree. The quality-of-care approach was initially launched in 32 rural counties where birth targets and quotas had been lifted. This approach of integrated family planning and maternal and child health services was later expanded to 62 counties. Further efforts were made to institutionalize the ICPD principles through extensive work with the National Population and Family Planning Commission (formerly known as the State Family Planning Commission) to revise standards of care, harmonize them with Ministry of Health maternal and child health standards, and remove birth targets and birth spacing requirements from national policy guidelines.

UNFPA's sixth country program, with a budget of $27 million, continued the client-oriented and gender-sensitive reproductive health program in project-supported counties. HIV/AIDS prevention activities and projects focused on youths, migrants, and commercial sex workers. There was increased collaboration with like-minded donors, including the Ford Foundation. UNFPA's current program is budgeted at $22 million and will run from 2011 to 2015 in parallel with China's 12th Five-Year Plan. It continues efforts to institutionalize the reproductive health and rights paradigm developed at ICPD and to work increasingly at a subnational level. An expanded focus of the program is to link HIV and reproductive health services for vulnerable populations, especially commercial sex workers.

Ford Foundation's China Program

The Ford Foundation's reproductive health program in China has had four phases. Initiatives have been based on a strategic analysis of challenges, input from a wide range of stakeholders, and the potential for impact. During the first phase (1991–1995), Ford promoted intersectoral and social science approaches for improving Chinese women's reproductive health, including community-based, participatory approaches for identifying needs and programming strategies, such as seeding newly emerging social organizations and quasi-governmental groups working on reproductive health problems that were not being addressed by regular government programs or services. These included sexual education for youth; the needs of divorced women, single parents, and urban migrant women; reproductive tract infections; domestic violence; and suicide of young rural women. Public education efforts were focused on sexual and reproductive health awareness while policy-focused research and symposia extended to the ethical dimension of reproductive health policies, including the impact of the population policy on women.

Program work in Yunnan Province focused on building understanding of reproductive health through research on a range of issues, such as the impact of health privatization on access to basic reproductive health services for poor women and the prevalence of undiagnosed reproductive tract infections in rural women (Yan, Wang, and Kaufman 1997). Other projects during this period included a series of national-level, ethics-focused, closed-door dialogues on a broad range of issues related to reproductive rights, homosexuality, and local feminism which linked China with global discussions (Qiu 1996); support of the creation of domestic NGOs such as the Yunnan Reproductive Health Research Association, which conducted research on a range of issues; the fostering of important links between government agencies; and helping to link a newly emerging set of Chinese women's activist NGOs with global feminist organizations working on women's rights. Many of these organizations have become the core women's rights NGOs in China (Hsiung, Jaschok, and Milwertz 2001; Jolly forthcoming; Kaufman 2012).[5] The early program also established a social science research institute at Renmin University on gender and sexuality that conducted sexual behavior research. It also funded research at Xi'an Jiaotong University on the impact of the family planning policy, which became the core of government efforts to address son preference and the distorted sex ratio at birth (Zhu et al. 1997).

In the next phase (1996–2001), pilot projects were launched to foster global connections with international reproductive health organizations such as the Population Council and the International Women's Health Coalition. Reform of family planning services was supported to bring them into line with international practices (Kaufman, Zhang, and Xie 2006). Support was continued for research and advocacy on the negative gender impacts of the population policy, while a new initiative brought together the Yunnan Reproductive Health Research Association and the Ministry of Health to ensure that reproductive health services were included in China's rural health service reform pilots. Another effort focused on China's emerging AIDS epidemic, at that point still unacknowledged, supporting newly emerging AIDS nongovernmental organizations working with gay men and commercial sex workers, such as the Friends Exchange group, Aizhixing, and Ziteng. During this period, the Ford Foundation worked closely with UNAIDS and other early AIDS donors to marshal an urgent policy response. Many projects aimed to raise awareness of HIV risks to women and youth, the sexual and reproductive health needs of youths, the unrecognized problem of women's reproductive tract infections, and the conditions of and people involved in commercial sex work (Pan 1999). In collaboration with other donors, support was provided to an alliance of women's NGOs working on raising attention and taking action against domestic violence.

From 2001 to 2010, the program strengthened its efforts to reorient the population control program toward reproductive health and rights, scaling up new quality-of-care approaches and institutionalizing innovative practices, and integrating gender equality and male participation. Ford and UNFPA worked together to raise attention to the distorted sex ratio at birth. Another initiative aimed to reduce AIDS and related stigma through education, advocacy, and activism. A group of activist AIDS NGOs representing HIV-positive persons was supported and now forms the backbone of China's AIDS NGO community—AIDS Care China, Mangrove Support Group, and Positive Art—many of which are linked to international advocacy groups. The Chinese Alliance of People Living with HIV/AIDS (CAP+) was launched, forming a coalition for grassroots groups, bringing together diverse groups, such as rural women and young men living with HIV, and linking them to the Global Network of People Living with AIDS (GNP+). Funding was also given for a special global initiative on sexuality, aimed at building capacity for sexual behavior research, which helped to establish and maintain the National Sexuality Resource Center at Renmin University.

The current program, since 2010, has narrowed the portfolio's focus to one main line of work: youth sexuality and reproductive health and rights, with an emphasis on sexuality and reproductive health education. The program is supporting efforts to shift sexual and reproductive health education toward more progressive and positive content, to expand its reach, and to increase leadership in this area by young and marginalized people themselves.

Case Studies of Social Change for Health and Rights

The following case studies illustrate how Ford Foundation support for key Chinese actors and institutions has contributed to change on some critical issues affecting the health of the Chinese population. The cases also serve to highlight UNFPA's contributions to advancing these issues and how the two organizations have leveraged each other's efforts.

Quality of Care in Family Planning and Reproductive Rights

Beginning in the early 1990s, both the Ford Foundation and UNFPA supported activities to reach the Chinese government, leading up to the ICPD in 1994 when

China's participation in that conference provided an opening to reform the highly criticized population program. A series of high-level closed-door workshops supported by the Ford Foundation explored sensitive issues like reproductive rights and ethics. Senior leaders participated in seminars outside China led by well-known leaders in reproductive health that introduced similar themes. In Yunnan, the aforementioned YRHA, a reproductive health NGO, was formed and supported with both domestic and international linkages.

UNFPA's strong advocacy for reproductive rights, including conditional support based on the removal of birth targets in project-supported counties, was an important effort to lessen overt local targets and their associated coercion. Chinese internal reformers initiated a pilot project to explore alternatives to their coercive family planning service delivery approaches, modeled on the quality-of-care approach that offered counseling and contraceptive choice to couples. The Ford Foundation provided funding for these early pilots, linked in external technical assistance, and supported its network of grantees in Yunnan to expand experimentation and scale up the model (Kaufman, Zhang, and Xie 2006). Visits by leaders to India provided examples of how other countries were reforming their service delivery in line with ICPD principles.

In 1988, when the UNFPA program resumed, in cooperation with the State Family Planning Commission, the quality-of-care approach provided the basis for scaling up the model as the modus operandi of the national program. Moving forward, the Ford Foundation, in close collaboration with UNFPA, continued and broadened support for the scaling-up and expansion of the project. Both organizations also supported efforts to bring attention to one of the most troubling impacts of the population policy: the skewed sex ratio at birth in favor of boys, resulting from son preference and the easy availability of ultrasound (to determine the sex) and abortion. A Ford Foundation–supported pilot program in Anhui in the 1990s with Xi'an Jiaotong University, aimed at changing traditional values and raising the value of girls in rural China, became the major vehicle for the NPFPC's own "Caring for Girls" campaign, while more recently, both organizations have been involved in workshops for government and international conferences, sharing the experiences of China's Asian neighbors such as South Korea and bringing together sexual rights advocates with people working on sex ratio imbalance, respectively.

Domestic Violence

Domestic violence was one of the topics discussed in grantee-organized high-level closed-door meetings during the early days of the Ford Foundation. Moreover, violence against women was one of four major themes of the Women's Conference held in Beijing in 1995. But there was minimal discussion of the issue on the China side (except for the director of the Women's Hotline, who reported on calls to her hotline). Efforts by the Ford Foundation to call attention to domestic violence—both through legal and health channels—were met with resistance by the government and the claim that it was not a serious issue in China. "Wife beating" was considered a private family matter and was rarely dealt with by the police, courts, or medical system. Shelters and other places of refuge for battered women did not exist.

The issue of domestic violence as a public health and women's rights issue became a significant area of work for the Ford Foundation globally, and in Asia in particular. In 1997, the foundation's five regional Asia offices organized a regional meeting in India titled "Violence against Women as a Public Health Issue," combining grantees from the law and rights and reproductive health programs. Individuals from organizations starting work on domestic violence in China were invited to attend.[6] Representatives of NGOs working on domestic violence in India, the Philippines, Indonesia, and Malaysia discussed advocacy and services for domestic violence in their countries.

Following participation in the India workshop, discussions continued through the Gender and Development Forum. A nucleus of organizations, including government officials and NGO professionals working in journalism, law, health, hotlines, and other fields, came together to form a domestic violence network. Ford mobilized co-funding and in 1998 launched the China Domestic Violence Network. It has become a vibrant engine for advocacy, legal reform, and government action on domestic violence in China. Numerous smaller projects have supported the actions of the network: training for police and health professionals from the Family Violence Prevention Network, support for county level legal initiatives, pilot special courts to hear domestic violence cases in Tianjin, and judges training, work with a district in Beijing to train marriage counselors at local women's federations to recognize and refer cases of domestic violence, and support to the Women's Law Center at Beijing University to provide legal aid and publicize particularly heinous cases of domestic abuse. These efforts were augmented by UNDP's efforts on gender training and the publication of a gender-training manual which was adopted by the network to help government officials change their understanding of domestic violence. In 2001, the revised Marriage Law adopted the term "domestic violence." In 2005, an amendment to the Law on the Guarantee of the Rights and Interests of Women further prohibited domestic violence and provided remedial mechanisms. The China Domestic Violence Network began drafting and proposing a new law on the prevention and prohibition of domestic violence in 2007 (Lin and China Women's University 2009). In 2008, a new guide was developed by the Supreme People's Court for nine pilot courts trying cases of domestic violence, which clarified what constitutes domestic violence (physical violence, sexual violence, mental violence, economic control) and established protection orders for women who have been threatened (Li and Center for Women's Law Studies and Legal Services of Peking University 2009). Strong resistance has, however, prevented the establishment of shelters.

HIV/AIDS

There has been significant donor support for HIV prevention and treatment programs in China in the last decade (as detailed by Ray Yip in the preceding chapter), but during the 1990s, before the Chinese government acknowledged the extent of the epidemic, there were few programs and little funding. During this period, the Ford Foundation played an important role, working on sensitive issues and building civil society groups. It initiated and piloted approaches to HIV prevention and stakeholder participation processes and then served as a safe mechanism for trying out new and politically sensitive ideas, often with government support and endorsement. Moreover, the Ford Foundation was an early partner in the UNAIDS effort in China, organizing a meeting in Yunnan in the early 1990s to promote multisectoral responses. Later in the 1990s, Ford supported a training workshop in Yunnan, a closed-door meeting with health and public security officials in Beijing, and a pilot project in Guangxi that introduced HIV harm-reduction approaches for intravenous drug users—needle exchange and methadone—both strongly opposed by public security officials at that time, but now embraced by the government. Education, training, advocacy, and experimentation were supported for interventions and projects with commercial sex workers and homosexual or bisexual men. The foundation also provided financial support to newly emerging organizations working at local levels, such as Aizhixing in Beijing (aiding homosexual men in the prevention of HIV/AIDs), Ziteng (promoting sex workers' legal rights and HIV prevention in Hong Kong and southern China), and Friends Exchange in Qingdao (an organization reaching many hidden homosexual men with AIDS prevention information). In the last decade, support to AIDS NGOs has also helped to build a network of domestic grassroots, international, and transnational organizations representing people living with HIV and AIDS (such as the Mangrove Support Group, the Ark of Love, Positive Art, AIDS Care China, CAP+, and GNP+). UNFPA's work on HIV/AIDS supported youth sex education programs and HIV education through rural reproductive health service projects during the 1990s. More recently, UNFPA has assumed responsibility for outreach and education to low-level commercial sex workers. The newest UNFPA country program (2011–2015) includes funding for HIV prevention and linked SRH services in four counties in Hainan, Guizhou, and Jiangxi Provinces.

Sexual Health and Rights

No other donor has worked as much to build the field of sexuality and sexual health research in China as the Ford Foundation. The benefits of the research on sexual behavior have extended to the HIV prevention field and programs for youth. It has also helped to document the rapid changes in Chinese society in the 30-year period of economic reforms and the initiation of the one-child policy. The support for social science research on sexuality and for the inclusion of sexual rights in reproductive health and rights discourse was a foundational principle of the foundation's work on reproductive health (Ford Foundation 1991). One of the program's earliest grants was to help establish a new research center on gender and sexuality at People's University, led by Pan Suiming, China's preeminent sociologist studying sexual behavior. With continuous grants over 20 years of the program, the center has conducted numerous studies on the sexual behavior of college students, Chinese businessmen and married couples, sex workers and their clients, and homosexual men, as well as elucidated values and norms related to gender and sexuality. These studies have contributed in innumerable ways to HIV and STI prevention programs and trained a new generation of sexuality researchers. They have crucially gone beyond a disease framework to look at sexuality as a broader social and political issue. The center has become an active part of a global network of sexuality researchers supported by the Ford Foundation in the last 10 years.

The foundation has also supported efforts to promote positive and safe sexuality for youth since it began work in China, and this is a major focus for the current program. Despite numerous pilot projects supported by donors including the Ford Foundation, UNFPA, UNESCO, SIDA, and others, there remains strong reluctance toward discussing sexual matters with youth in schools, which have retained educational messages mainly promoting abstinence. This is in sharp contrast to rapidly changing behaviors and earlier sexual initiation, especially for urban youths, the exposure to media including social media, and experimentation with new definitions of gender and sexual identity. The commercial marketing of sexual imagery and stereotypes has a bigger impact on youth attitudes, knowledge, and behaviors toward sex than official government or family dictates. Therefore, the Ford Foundation's current focus on sexuality education includes work with media, new media, activists, and researchers as well as educational authorities, recognizing that young people get their information on sexuality as much from the internet, peers, and media as from school. One of the largest-scale studies on youth SRH, which gathered data from over 22,000 unmarried young people aged 15–24 in 30 provinces in China (Zheng et al. 2010) found that 22.4 percent had had penetrative sex of one kind or another, and that the median age of first sex was 20, with boys having sex slightly earlier than girls. Of those sexually active, 20 percent had more than one partner in the past year and 20 percent of sexually active girls had been pregnant, with over 90 percent of the pregnancies ending in abortion. Among the sexually active group, 15–19-year-olds were more likely to have multiple partners and more likely to have repeat abortions than the 20–24-year-olds. A recent survey reported that over 50 percent of young people think homosexuals and heterosexuals should be treated equally (Pan and Huang 2011).

Reproductive Tract Infections

A number of projects since the early 1990s have contributed to raising awareness of reproductive tract infections as a serious health problem needing medical attention and to developing simple diagnosis and treatment services for rural women. Early qualitative research as part of the Yunnan Reproductive Health and Development Project flagged the problem as one which plagued many rural women. But they were too embarrassed to seek care from mostly male doctors. A study by researchers at Kunming Medical College supported by international experts documented the extent of the problem in rural Yunnan, using laboratory diagnostics for over two thousand women, and contributed to the acknowledgement during the 1990s that sexually transmitted diseases were having a resurgence in China (Kaufman et al. 1999). The Ford Foundation then supported revisions to medical school manuals, training for field-based diagnosis, and treatment as well as advocacy about the "silent epidemic" among rural women by Yunnan Reproductive Health Research Association (YRHRA). A reproductive health improvement project from 1998 to 2002 with the Ministry of Health and YRHRA drew attention to the issue as a needed service for basic rural primary health services being developed in collaboration with a large World Bank loan in seven provinces, and it was scaled up to routine services through that larger program.

Perspectives from Grantees and Partners

The writing of this chapter involved vibrant exchanges among the authors and interviews with former and current grantees, as well as key leaders in the areas of work reviewed. Their perspectives on the positive and negative aspects of donor funding provide commentary on the power dynamics and the role of funders in catalyzing work on new ideas and giving legitimacy to certain issues. Some of the main threads that have spanned the 20 years of Ford Foundation grantmaking in China include work on rights as a means to improve health; connecting researchers and activists inside and outside China through the foundation's global networks; flexibility to work with all actors—activists, researchers, government—and to bring them together, often behind closed doors for needed dialogues; support for experimental (radical, sensitive) new organizations as they have come together; and relatively light reporting requirements relative to other donors and reliance on narrative reports that allowed the organizations to focus mainly on the work.

One interviewee thought the biggest impact of the Ford Foundation program in China was that Chinese women's NGOs had been integrated into the international women's movement. Another interviewee discussed how consensus building, the convening of different disciplines and stakeholders, and early discussions on human rights led to policy change and law reform in several areas, including HIV/AIDS, legal rights, and domestic violence. Interviews with several of the leading internal reformers spoke to the importance of early Ford Foundation funding for the quality-of-care project and funding to support internal dialogue on population policy reform. Rather than pushing human rights early on, the foundation provided initial funding to enable the reformers to do what they thought would be successful to push reform inside the government. Another interviewee said that working with the Ford Foundation had led him from "flying a kite to riding a bicycle," a metaphor for working on practical problems on the ground, which showed him the importance of cooperating with scholars from other disciplines. Other interviewees highlighted how important it was that the Ford Foundation gave money to do what grantees thought was right and didn't direct them. They appreciated the lack of bureaucracy and that there were no burdensome reporting requirements. Longer-term grants which were broader and not so specific or task-based gave them greater flexibility and independence. On the other hand, one interviewee stressed that the Ford Foundation was less accountable compared to other donors because it undertook little formal impact evaluation or monitoring, while other interviewees felt the recent focus on benchmarks actually hamstrung efforts to work toward bringing about a long-term impact and that small amounts of funding continually restricted the scaling-up of efforts as initiatives matured. Some felt that new restrictions on using funds for research limited the ability of grantees to do what they thought was required to make an impact or add depth to the work.

Other insights highlighted the importance of long-term strategies not tied to short-term impact evaluation. A number of grantees noted that early funding for social change did not contribute to major impact until after a decade or more. Finally, mention was made of how power relations, including headquarters-driven priorities and dynamics between donor and grantee, especially by an American foundation, at times can negatively influence movements for social change, which are at the heart of grant-making intentions.

Discussion and Conclusion

Both the Ford Foundation and UNFPA have been working in China in the context of the one-child policy, which has shaped the nature and, to some degree, the impact of both organizations' programs. Even while heavily criticized by the international community for its population policy, the Chinese government has resisted doing away with it, defended its necessity, and strictly limited internal dissent. The first steps toward relaxing the policy were announced in November 2013, permitting more couples to have a second child. Both organizations operate at the will of the Chinese government and therefore tread a difficult line between constructive engagement on policy reform and accountability to the international community as well as Chinese human rights activists on global human rights norms. This has been particularly difficult for UNFPA, as it is the main UN agency engaged with China's National Population and Family Planning Commission and it is tasked with the implementation of the ICPD Platform for Action. Nevertheless, UNFPA's continued presence in China despite strong criticism and defunding from the United States, and its continuing dialogue with the Chinese government on the need for policy reform, has perhaps been the most important countervailing force against targets and coercion in the 30 years of the policy.

UNFPA's long-term engagement on so many issues has contributed to China's social and economic progress in the last three decades, helping to identify and initiate work on important problems. A few contributions stand out, including the support for the first and subsequent censuses and the capacity it created for basic population statistics generation; the human resource capacity built up through the demographic training and research support; the technical assistance that established China's contraceptive variety and self-sufficiency; and the persistent and long-term efforts to reorient family planning at the grassroots level toward a more client-oriented approach, including holding the line on the removal of targets and quotas in pilot counties.

Changing the context both within China and within the Ford Foundation in China has impacted the foundation's approach and style and created limits at times. For example, fear about Ford's influence and perceived agenda on civil society activism has intersected with the political climate in China at regular intervals. This has affected the way Ford is perceived by the government. On the foundation's side, it has resulted in more caution in choosing partners and funding certain types of work and organizations, and it has caused worry on the part of some Chinese organizations about the risk of being too closely associated with Ford. Depending on how open the political space is for civil society, the foundation's support for work on sensitive issues is seen either as positive or as interference by an American foundation. Sensitivities about the role of donors and their power dynamics with grantees and the role of American foundations intervening in sensitive areas and insufficiently funding grassroots NGOs have been the subject of both a recent Chinese NGO report on donors and a recent journal article (Busgen 2010; Spires 2011). However, many current political leaders in China have benefited from Ford's early funding for economic and legal training and reform and provide an important source of support and counsel. On the other hand, the power of the New York–based global reproductive health program has waned, both at the Ford Foundation and worldwide.

The Ford Foundation's engagement in China has been more focused on building internal social movements for change, engaging with internal reformers and activists, and connecting them to global movements. The strong focus on rights—reproductive rights, women's rights, and sexual rights—has been supported through grants to civil society groups and academics who then often link their work to government for scaling up to policy and programs. Early issue identification and dialogues on HIV and reproductive rights begun at that time eventually progressed to legal reform on HIV discrimination and to less of a stigma toward homosexuality. The strong focus of work on women's rights and the facilitation of connections between China's women's rights activists and global feminists have been important mechanisms for building internal movements for women's rights, such as work on domestic violence.

Would these developments have occurred without both organizations providing funding, support for policy research and data collection, policy engagement and advice, and the facilitation of global connections? How have the different institutional cultures of the Ford Foundation and UNFPA influenced the depth and impact of funding and engagement? Within each organization, how has the domestic Chinese political climate and the personalities of organizations' representatives and their supervisors influenced risk-taking and the latitude to work on sensitive but critically important issues? Private foundations and the UN System work with different actors and under different types of political, organizational, and financial constraints, which limit their spheres of action. But they can be complementary in crucial ways, as described in the case studies. Internal and external power dynamics limit or enable funders' ability to catalyze work on new or sensitive ideas, in China and elsewhere. The implication for philanthropic actors is clear: social change is a long-term process that requires internal champions. It is often impossible to create an impact in one grant cycle, and any benchmarks and indicators, especially those used to assess the efficacy of funding and its continuation, should assess the context, the need, the stage, and the long-term prospects for lasting policy reform and the change of norms required for social progress.

Notes

1. The "Four Modernizations" launched by Deng Xiaoping in 1978—in agriculture, industry, defense, and science and technology—were aimed at quadrupling China's GDP and per capita income by the year 2000.

2. Following a needs assessment in 1989 by foundation staff and consultants Lincoln Chen, Jose Barzelatto, Peter Geithner, and Joan Kaufman.

3. These include the ICPD Program of Action (UNFPA 1994), the Beijing Platform of Action ("Platform for Action and the Beijing Declaration"), the Millennium Development Goals (MDGs), and the Convention on the Elimination of Discrimination Against Women (CEDAW).

4. The first two country programs, from 1980 to 1989, each for $50 million, involved 64 projects covering a wide range of government institutions and technical assistance areas.

5. These include the Maple Women's Hotline, Rural Women Knowing All, the Beijing University Women's Law Center (now Beijing Zhongze Women Legal Consultant & Service Center), and the China Women's Health Network, which translated and adapted *Our Bodies, Ourselves.*

6. These included the Women's Hotline, the Jinglun Family Center, the Law Institute of the Chinese Academy of Social Sciences, and Rural Women Knowing All.

References

Asian-Pacific Resource & Research Centre for Women. 2010. "MDG 5 in Asia: Progress, Gaps and Challenges, 2000–2010." http://www.mdg5watch.org/Regional/MDG5 RegionalBrief.pdf.

Branigan, Tania. 2010. "Chinese Sex Workers Protest against Crackdown." *Guardian* (London), August 3. http://www.guardian.co.uk/world/2010/aug/03/china-prostitution-sex -workers-protest.

Busgen, Michael. 2010. *Same Bed, Different Dreams? How Chinese NGOs View Their Cooperation with Foreign Institutional Donors.* In cooperation with the Institute for Civil Society (ICS) of Sun Yat-sen University and the Capacity Building and Assessment Center (Beijing), and in partnership with NGO.cn (Yunnan) and the Social Resource Institute (Beijing). Unpublished China Donor Assessment Research Report, Beijing.

Census of China. 1982. *1982 Population Census of China One Percent Household Sampling.* Vols. 1–4. Beijing: Department of Population Statistics, State Statistical Bureau of China.

———. 1993. *Tabulations on the 1990 Population Census of the People's Republic of China.* Vols. 1–4. Edited by the Population Census Office under the State Council and Department of Population Statistics, State Statistical Bureau. Beijing: China Statistical Publishing House.

Fang Jing. 2004. "Health Sector Reform and Reproductive Health Service in Poor Rural China." *Health Policy and Planning* 19 (suppl. 1): 40–49.

Fang Jing, and Joan Kaufman. 2008. "Reproductive Health in China: Improve the Means to the End." *Lancet* 372 (9650): 1619–1620.

Ford Foundation. 1991. *Reproductive Health: A Strategy for the 1990s.* New York: Ford Foundation.

Gu Baochang. 2009. *Induced Abortion in China.* Beijing: Center for Population and Development Studies, Renmin University of China.

Hsiung Pingchun, Maria Jaschok, and Cecilia Milwertz. 2001. *Chinese Women Organizing.* Oxford, NY: Berg.

Hvistendahl, Mara. 2009. "Making Every Baby Girl Count." *Science* 232:1164–1166.

Jing Jun. 2010. "Red Light Districts in Chinese Cyberspace." Paper presented at the conference "Sex Work in Asia," Harvard University, Cambridge, MA, October 3–4.

Jolly, Susan. Forthcoming. "Gender and Sexuality Activism in Beijing: Negotiating International Influences, National and Local Processes." In *Changing Narratives of Sexuality: Contestation, Compliance and Women's Empowerment,* edited by Charmaine Pereira. London: Zed Books.

Kaufman, Joan. 2012. "The Global Women's Movement and Chinese Women's Rights." *Journal of Contemporary China* 21 (76): 585–602.

Kaufman, Joan, Zhang Erli, and Xie Zhenming. 2006. "Family Planning Quality of Care in China: Scaling Up a Pilot Project into a National Reform Program." *Studies in Family Planning* 37 (1): 17–28.

Kaufman, Joan, Yan Liqin, Wang Tongyin, and Anne Faulkner. 1999. "A Study of Field-Based Methods for Diagnosing Reproductive Tract Infections in Rural Yunnan Province, China." *Studies in Family Planning* 30 (2): 112–119.

Li Ying and Center for Women's Law Studies and Legal Services of Peking University. 2009. "New Developments in Prevention and Prohibition of Domestic Violence in China." Unpublished paper.

Lin Jianjun, and China Women's University. 2009. "Anti-Domestic Violence Law in China." Unpublished paper.

Ministry of Health, Joint United Nations Programme on HIV/AIDS, and World Health Organization. 2010. "2009 Estimates for the HIV/AIDS Epidemic in China." http://www.unaids.org.cn/en/index/Document_view.asp?id=413.

National Bureau of Statistics, Department of Population and Employment Statistics. 2007. *Tabulation on the 2005 National One Percent Population Sample Survey.* Beijing: China Statistics Press.

Pan Suiming. 1999. *Zhongguo guodi xiaxing chanye kaoke* [Three Red Light Districts in China]. Beijing: Qunyan Publishing House.

Pan Suiming, and Yingying Huang. 2011. *Chinese Sexuality Random Sampling Survey, 2010.* Beijing: Institute of Sociology, Renmin University of China.

Population and Economics Editorial Office, ed. 1983. "An Analysis of a National One-per-Thousand-Population Sample Survey in Birth Rate." Special issue, *Population and Economics.*

Qiu Renzong. 1996. *Reproductive Health and Ethical Considerations.* Beijing: Chinese Xiehe Medical University Press.

Spires, Anthony J. 2011. "Organizational Homophily in International Grantmaking: US-Based Foundations and Their Grantees in China." *Journal of Civil Society* 7 (3): 305–331.

State Family Planning Commission, ed. 1984. "Chart for One-per-Thousand-Population Fertility Sampling Survey in China." Special issue, *Population and Economics.*

UNAIDS (Joint United Nations Programme on HIV/AIDS). 2008. "China: Key Data." http://www.unaids.org.cn/en/index/page.asp?id=178&class=2&classname=Key+Data.

UNAIDS (Joint United Nations Programme on HIV/AIDS), and UNIGASS (UN General Assembly Special Session on AIDS). 2006. "High-Level Meeting on AIDS Uniting the World against AIDS." http://www.un.org/ga/aidsmeeting2006/declaration.htm.

UNFPA (United Nations Population Fund). 1994. *Report of the International Conference on Population and Development.* http://www.un.org/popin/icpd/conference/offeng/poa.html.

Wan He, Mark Muenchrath, and Paul Kowal. 2012. *Shades of Gray: A Cross-Country Study of Health and Well-Being of the Older Populations in SAGE Countries, 2007–2010.* U.S. Census Bureau. http://www.census.gov/prod/2012pubs/p95-12-01.pdf.

Xing Linfeng, Guo Sufang, David Hipgrave, Zhu Jun, Zhang Lingli, Song Li, Yang Qing, Guo Yan, and Caraine Ronsmans. 2011. "China's Facility-Based Birth Strategy and Neonatal Mortality: A Population-Based Epidemiological Study." *Lancet* 378 (9801): 1493–1500.

Yan Liqin, Wang Tongyin, and Joan Kaufman. 1997. "A Community Study of Women's Reproductive Infections and Related Morbidity, Risk Factors in Rural Yunnan Province, China." *Modern Preventive Medicine* 24 (3): 269–272.

Zheng Xiaoying, Chen Gong, Han Youli, Chen He, Lin Ting, Qiu Yue, Yang Rongrong et al. 2010. *Survey of Youth Access to Reproductive Health in China.* Beijing: Institute for Population Research, Peking University; National Working Committee on Children and Women; United Nations Population Fund.

Zheng Zhenzhen. 2010. "Below Replacement Fertility and Childbearing Intention, Findings from the Jiangsu Fertility Intention and Behavior Survey." Paper presented at the Population Association of America meeting "China's One Child Policy after 30 Years: Time for a Change?" Dallas, TX, April.

Zhu Chuzhu, Li Shuzhuo, Qiu Changrong, Hu Ping, and Jing Anrong. 1997. *The Dual Effects of the Family Planning Program on Chinese Women.* Xi'an: Xi'an Jiaotong University Press.

9 Foreign Philanthropic Initiatives for Tobacco Control in China

Jeffrey P. Koplan and Pamela Redmon

Introduction

Tobacco has nearly as long a history in China as it does in the West. First introduced from the New World via European trading networks in the late sixteenth century, it quickly entered domestic cultivation in the southeastern coastal areas of Fujian and Guangdong. By the time of its earliest extant reference in 1611—when Yao Lü (d. 1622) wrote of it in his *Book of Dew*—it had begun to spread throughout the country, from the Lower Yangzi Delta to Manchuria in the northeast (Benedict 2011a, 7). Smoked by everyone from elite literati to poor peasants, tobacco became a prominent part of Chinese culture, serving as both an everyday luxury and—uniquely—as a common token in social reciprocity and exchange (Redmon et al. 2013). It has remained so to the present: China now produces more tobacco, more cigarettes, and more smokers than any other country in the world.

The history of the state's involvement in tobacco's cultivation, marketing, and control is also long. Already by the 1630s, the government had issued laws threatening those who cultivated, consumed, or sold tobacco with corporal punishment or stiff fines. Such laws were, however, typically short-lived, and were primarily aimed at asserting state control over a valuable economic resource rather than improving public health (Benedict 2011b, 35). Today, the government-owned China National Tobacco Corporation is the largest tobacco company in the world, with privileged access to China's more than three hundred million, disproportionately male smokers: 53 percent of Chinese men smoke (Giovino et al. 2012) versus roughly 3 percent of women, and tobacco is considered responsible for 1 in 8 male deaths versus 1 in 33 female deaths (Benedict 2011a, 241). By 2020, it is projected that China will suffer two million deaths annually due to tobacco use (Gan et al. 2007). While the government regards tobacco as an aspect of Chinese culture and tradition and a crucial element of the economy, generating roughly 8 percent of the central government's total revenues (Benedict 2011a, 253), it increasingly recognizes it as a pernicious health threat exacting an ongoing and increasing toll in diseases and premature deaths.

The government is not the only entity to have this insight, however. While the government's health imperative has not yet overcome its commercial interests in tobacco, in recent years tobacco control has become a topic of foreign philanthropic interest in China as donors have recognized the impending health threat resulting from the epidemic of tobacco use and exposure to secondhand smoke. The international philanthropic community has a long history of supporting advances in medicine and public health in China, dating back to the mid-eighteenth century. It was not until 1996, however, that the World Bank became the earliest donor to provide significant fiscal support to China's tobacco control efforts. Numerous donations from international donors totaling millions of dollars followed, and these donations helped to elevate tobacco control to a prominent national public health issue. Philanthropic donors that have contributed to China's tobacco control efforts include the World Health Organization (WHO), the World Bank, the American Cancer Society (ACS), the John E. Fogarty International Center (FIC), the Bloomberg Initiative, the China Medical Board (CMB), and the Bill & Melinda Gates Foundation (BMGF) (Redmon et al. 2013).

As of 2012, four philanthropies continue to provide support for tobacco control in China: BI, WHO, BMGF, and CMB. BI supports China's efforts through partner organizations including WHO, the International Union Against Tuberculosis and Lung Disease, the Johns Hopkins Bloomberg School of Public Health (JHSPH), the World Lung Foundation (WLF), the Centers for Disease Prevention and Control Foundation (CDC Foundation), and the Campaign for Tobacco-Free Kids (CTFK). BMGF continues to provide support for tobacco control in China through grants to the Emory Global Health Institute (EGHI), the China Red Cross (CRC), and CTFK. CMB also continues to provide financial support to tobacco control research efforts (Redmon et al. 2013).

International philanthropies have provided funds and technical support to national, city, and provincial government organizations, nongovernment organizations, universities, and health care organizations throughout China since 1986. The funds have been used to increase the organizations' capacity to develop and deliver effective tobacco control interventions, support national and local governments in adopting and enforcing smoke-free policies, provide cessation services, deliver effective media campaigns, and conduct important tobacco control research. The funding support has also been used to establish centers and organizations devoted to promoting tobacco control, to support conferences and workshops, and to create educational products and tools.

This chapter identifies the international philanthropies that have invested in tobacco control in China and describes their role and strategies in changing the social norms of tobacco use. Information on the philanthropies' program goals, activities, and outcomes was not readily available, and either specific investments or outcomes were not publicly available or it was still too early to assess their ultimate impact. The information was gathered from multiple sources including organizational websites, key informant interviews and e-mails with project officers, and published research papers and reports.

Philanthropic Organizations, Strategies, and Outcomes

The World Health Organization (WHO)

In 1986, WHO established the WHO Collaborating Center for Tobacco or Health. The first few years were dedicated to conducting tobacco surveys to determine smoking habits and attitudes among medical students in Beijing, Zhejiang, and the Capital University of Medical Science (1989, 1999), middle school teachers in Beijing and Liaoning Province (1990), and female factory workers in Beijing (1991), and the smoking prevalence among armed police (1992). In 1996 it conducted a national survey of smoking prevalence among the general population, and in 1998 it conducted a survey to determine smoking prevalence among medical personnel of 10 hospitals in Beijing. The results of the study of the Beijing medical professionals were used as the basic reference for establishing smoke-free hospitals in China. Other efforts have involved the establishment of quit lines and cessation clinics (1996–2010) and general mass education activities (Redmon et al. 2013). In 2011, WHO provided support to implement a smoke-free policy in all Chinese Traditional Medicine hospitals.[1]

The center has organized and participated in various large-scale antismoking education activities, such as World No Tobacco Day, annually since 1988. Highlights include smoking cessation consulting clinics set up in 30 hospitals in Beijing in 1999 and a large-scale internet promotion campaign in 2001 on a popular website, sohu.com, on the harms of secondhand smoke. In addition, the center holds tobacco control training sessions and lectures for schools, hospitals, and businesses. It has also conducted a wide range of tobacco control research, smoking cessation research, and clinical trials.[2]

The center focuses much of its efforts on cessation. China's first smoking cessation clinic and the national quitline were set up by the center in 1996 and 2004, respectively. In 2010, it provided grant funds to continue the national quitline, developed an online course for a clinical smoking intervention, and delivered a certified training program for tobacco treatment specialists.[3]

From 2008 to 2009, the center played an important role in organizing participants from eight ministries such as the Ministry of Industry and Information Technology, the Ministry of Health, the Ministry of Foreign Affairs, and the Ministry of Finance, to develop the China Tobacco Control Action Plan. Beginning in September 2011, the center partnered with the Ministry of Health (MoH) to produce a white paper on the harms of smoking and secondhand smoke, analogous to the U.S. Surgeon General's report. According to WHO, the objective of the paper was to "provide the Chinese senior leadership with credible, authoritative Chinese evidence of the harms of tobacco as part of the briefing package for the UN Summit on NCDs, and to follow with a full length publication quality document" (WHO 2012a). The MoH published *China's Report on the Health Hazards of Smoking* on May 30, 2012. Management, technical assistance, and overall guidance for the report was provided by multiple national and international organizations, including Chaoyang Hospital, the MoH, WHO, JHSPH, and the U.S. CDC, among others. In addition to WHO funding, the project received funds from AusAID (Ministry of Health 2007; Beijing Institute of Respiratory Medicine 2012).

World Bank Health Loan VII

While not a traditional philanthropy, the World Bank provided a series of loans to China throughout the 1980s and 1990s, with the goal of assisting economic development by improving the health status of the Chinese population. The first formal consultation and externally supported tobacco control effort in China is found in the health promotion component of Health Loan VII, conducted from 1996 to 2004. The health promotion component of the loan largely focused on tobacco control efforts. It was funded at $10.9 million, with project cities and provinces matching their financial support. The Chinese MoH was the implementing agency, with the project goals—including a decrease in the overall smoking rate via Quit2Win competitions, an increase in knowledge of the harms of tobacco use, improved training in health promotion, prohibitions on outdoor advertising and cigarette sales to minors, implementation of warning labels, and the enactment of smoke-free policies for public places—pursued in seven cities: Beijing, Chengdu, Liuzhou, Luoyang, Shanghai, Tianjin, and Weihai (World Bank 2005; Redmon et al. 2013).

The project employed multiple health education and promotion interventions aimed at increasing knowledge of tobacco hazards and changing population attitudes toward smoking and smokers' behaviors. Both internal and external evaluations of the tobacco component of Health VII were largely very favorable, and attributed its success to "its multi-pronged approach which included city-wide strategies and strategies for neighborhoods, schools, hospitals, and workplaces" (World Bank 2005).

The World Bank named five primary lessons learned (External Evaluation Panel for Health VII Project of World Bank 2004):

1. Interventions must be evidence-based.
2. It is essential to select an appropriate target audience for each intervention.
3. The target audience must be large enough to permit a significant impact and to allow for evaluation of outcome.

4. Multiple interventions against a single risk factor are more likely to have an impact than single interventions.
5. Regulation and administrative orders are not likely to be enforceable unless the target population understands the value of compliance. Therefore, social mobilization is critical.

Fogarty International Center

From 2003 to 2007, with a grant from the FIC of the National Institutes of Health (NIH), the Johns Hopkins Bloomberg School of Public Health, in partnership with the Peking University Medical College (PUMC), conducted research on how to implement tobacco control in China. The program, "Towards a Smoke-Free China," focused on improving tobacco control capacity and supporting interventions in three provinces: Jiangxi, Henan, and Sichuan. The goals of the intervention sites were to increase awareness of the harm of passive smoking (or secondhand smoke), decrease passive smoking by women and children at home, create a model of passive smoking prevention based on Chinese norms and culture, and disseminate the experience throughout China (China CDC, PUMC, and JHUSPH n.d.). FIC provided additional support for a second phase of the project to expand the work to an additional seven provinces, and extended Phase II until 2012.

Outcomes from Phases I and II included the execution of a robust evaluation of the project, delivery of workshops to build capacity among the tobacco control program teams, development of the Global Tobacco Control Leadership Program (an annual two-week in-depth training held at JHSPH), and the creation of the Center of Excellence, designed to provide provincial and local-level CDC staff with the skills to conduct surveys and measure air nicotine. They worked with local officials to develop and implement smoke-free policies in public places and to educate the public on the harms of secondhand smoke, and developed community-based intervention models in rural schools, hospitals, homes, and communities to protect nonsmokers from secondhand smoke (Stillman et al. 2006).

American Cancer Society

The ACS established a representative office in Beijing in 2005 and fostered important relationships with organizations such as the China MoH, the China CDC Tobacco Control Office, Hong Kong University, the Chinese Anti-Cancer Association, and the John Tung Foundation of Taiwan. ACS focused their efforts on cessation, specifically on training counselors and establishing cessation clinics. Other activities included sponsoring the first Cross Strait Tobacco Control Conference in Taiwan, partnering with the China Tobacco Control Network to develop the *Cessation Clinic Operations Manual,* and cosponsoring a Smoke-Free Worksite campaign with the Chinese Preventive Medicine Association, the China Anti-Cancer Association, and the China Center for Disease Control. They also created a smoke-free workplace toolkit to provide instructions on creating smoke-free environments (ACS 2008).

The Bloomberg Initiative to Reduce Tobacco Use

The Bloomberg Initiative's objectives are:

1. To refine and optimize tobacco control programs to help smokers stop using tobacco and to prevent children from starting
2. To support public sector efforts to pass and enforce key laws and implement effective policies, including taxing cigarettes, preventing smuggling, altering the image of tobacco and protecting workers from exposure to second-hand smoke
3. To support advocates' efforts to educate communities about the harms of tobacco and to enhance tobacco control activities that work towards a tobacco-free world
4. To develop a rigorous system to monitor the status of global tobacco use (Bloomberg Initiative 2012c).

The Bloomberg Initiative partner organizations responsible for meeting the objectives of the initiative include the International Against Tuberculosis and Lung Disease, CTFK, the CDC Foundation, JHSPH, WHO, and the World Lung Foundation (Bloomberg Initiative 2012a). As of May 2012, the Bloomberg Initiative had issued 36 tobacco-related grants to China, totaling almost nine million dollars (Bloomberg Initiative 2012b). The following summaries provide details of the partner organizations' goals and projects:

International Union Against Tuberculosis and Lung Disease

The union's goals are to support public sector efforts to pass and enforce key laws and implement effective policies. It also supports and provides training to local organizations to build and manage tobacco control programs.[4] The union's key projects have included the following:

IMPROVING THE HEALTH OF TUBERCULOSIS (TB) PATIENTS AND THEIR FAMILIES BY ESTABLISHING SMOKE-FREE TB CENTERS AND PROMOTING SMOKE-FREE FAMILIES, HUNAN PROVINCE (2007–2009)

All of the 75 tobacco control centers adopted and enforced smoke-free policies, all patients (35,567) were included in the smoking survey, 14,547 homes were reached, and 41 percent declared their homes to be smoke-free. In addition, 119 of the TB clinic staff smokers quit smoking (27 percent), 11,639 village doctors were trained to give cessation support, 847 declared their homes smoke-free, and 2,762 patients had quit smoking by the end of their TB treatment. The government leadership committed to including tobacco control in its local health policy and a tobacco control and TB coalition was established for each city in the province.

ADVOCATING FOR THE REVISION AND STRENGTHENING OF
EXISTING SMOKE-FREE LEGISLATION AND REGULATIONS IN
PUBLIC PLACES' OLYMPIC CITY SITES (2007–2009)

The project aimed to make all taskforce agencies smoke-free, build capacity in Beijing and other Olympic sites (Qingdao, Shanghai, Shenyang, Tianjin, and Qinhuangdao), build public and government support for smoke-free legislation, revise and enforce smoke-free legislation, and raise public support for the smoke-free directive. As an outcome, the Beijing Regulations on Expanding the Scope of Banning Smoking in Public Places were adopted and implemented, and inspectors were trained to enforce the smoke-free policy. Two media campaigns were aired in Olympic site cities from May–December 2008, and evaluation results showed that, respectively, 74 percent and 66 percent of respondents who viewed the ads claimed the ads might make them stop smoking.

BUILDING ADVOCACY CAPACITY FOR TOBACCO CONTROL AMONG
THE PUBLIC HEALTH WORKFORCE IN CHINA (2007–2008)

The project aimed to develop a training program on tobacco control advocacy to be included in public health curricula in selected universities in an effort to build a tobacco control coalition among public health workers. Seven universities implemented the curriculum and created smoke-free campuses: Zhejiang University in Hangzhou, Beijing Medical University, Harbin Medical University, Ningxia Medical University, Nanjing Medical University, Guangdong Pharmaceutical University, and Shanxi Medical University.

DEVELOPING TOBACCO CONTROL COURSES IN SMOKE-FREE
UNIVERSITIES WITH PUBLIC HEALTH FACULTIES (2010–2011)

The project aimed to create smoke-free universities and to establish tobacco control courses in universities that included schools of public health. As an outcome, 22 universities offered the tobacco control courses and 16 of the selected universities adopted smoke-free policies. Eleven schools adopted policies that blanketed the entire campus and five universities adopted policies that applied to their public health schools.

ESTABLISHING 20 SMOKE-FREE TRADITIONAL
CHINESE MEDICINE HOSPITALS (2009–2011)

The project goal was to protect staff, patients, and visitors from exposure to secondhand smoke and increase cessation efforts among staff and patients. The outcome was that 16 of the 20 targeted hospitals adopted and enforced smoke-free policies.

ADVOCATING FOR THE ESTABLISHMENT OF EFFECTIVE SMOKE-FREE LEGISLATION IN WORKPLACES (INCLUDING BARS AND RESTAURANTS) AND PUBLIC PLACES IN SHANGHAI (2008–2011)

The project objectives included adoption of a smoke-free policy by 2008, and increased public support for smoke-free workplaces, including restaurants and bars.

CREATING SMOKE-FREE CITIES PROJECT (2009–2014)

The aims of the project are to strengthen the China CDC Tobacco Control office and to support its efforts to promote the creation of smoke-free environments in Shanghai (2008–2011), Chongqing (2009–2012), Lanzhou (2009–2012), Nanchang (2009–2012), Shenyang (2009–2012), Harbin (2010–2014), Shenzhen (2010–2014), and Tianjin (2010–2014).

FACILITATING TOBACCO CONTROL LEGISLATION FOR PUBLIC PLACES IN GUANGZHOU (2009–2013)

The aim of the project includes the facilitation of enactment of and compliance with legislation consistent with the policy banning smoking in public places in Guangzhou. Surveys, research, education, training, community interventions, and mass media campaigns were used to raise public awareness and support for smoke-free public places. Guangzhou passed the smoke-free legislation, with the ban going into effect on September 1, 2010. It was the first city in China to ban smoking in offices.

ACCELERATING INCORPORATION OF SPECIFIC SMOKE-FREE HOSPITAL REQUIREMENTS INTO TRADITIONAL CHINESE MEDICINE (TCM) HOSPITAL MANAGEMENT POLICY AND PROMOTING A 100 PERCENT SMOKE-FREE ENVIRONMENT IN ALL TCM HOSPITALS (2011–2013)

The goal of the project is to advocate for an amendment to the TCM hospital management policy to include a requirement for all TCM hospitals to comply with the WHO Framework Convention on Tobacco Control and adopt a smoke-free policy. The Chinese Association on Chinese Medicine (CACM) is currently lobbying the State Administration of Traditional Chinese Medicine to include the smoke-free TCM hospital criteria in its policy.

ADVOCATING FOR THE ESTABLISHMENT OF EFFECTIVE
SMOKE-FREE LEGISLATION IN WORKPLACES AND PUBLIC
PLACES, GUANGDONG PROVINCE, CHINA, (2011–2013)

This project aims to promote the overall adoption and enactment of smoke-free
legislation.

EXPANDING TOBACCO CONTROL COURSES IN SMOKE-FREE
UNIVERSITIES WITH PUBLIC HEALTH FACULTIES (2012–2014)

The project's aim is to increase the reach of the tobacco control course model,
expanding it to an additional 60 Chinese universities.

PROMOTING TOBACCO CONTROL LEGISLATION AND
CREATING A SMOKE-FREE CITY, JINAN (2012–2014)

The aim is to create smoke-free public places and workplaces by promoting effective legislation consistent with Article 8 of the Framework Convention on Tobacco Control.

Campaign for Tobacco-Free Kids

CTFK's China programs aim to foster a political and social environment conducive to policy change, catalyze a sustainable tobacco control movement, and
promote the adoption and implementation of effective tobacco control policies
(Bloomberg Initiative 2012c). Although CTFK does not formally evaluate its projects, a description of the outcomes resulting from its activities was provided by
the organization.[5]

FOSTERING A CONDUCIVE POLITICAL AND SOCIAL ENVIRONMENT

CTFK has worked to change China's public opinion concerning tobacco control.
As a result of the organization's strategic media outreach, the media has inten-
sively covered tobacco control issues, with coverage increasing by 27 percent between 2008 and 2010 (Redmon et al. 2013). Influential bloggers have begun writing about smoking harms and voicing their support for tobacco control. CTFK
has helped raise awareness through journalism workshops, sponsored journalists' attendance at international conferences, and worked with grantees to implement media advocacy strategies. Working with Tsinghua University, the Xinhua
News Agency, and *Caixin* magazine, it has trained Chinese journalists, helped
educate journalists about tobacco control issues, and increased the quantity and
quality of media coverage on tobacco control.[6]

In an effort to denormalize tobacco and the tobacco industry, CTFK grantees and other partner organizations successfully convinced the Shanghai World
Expo's organizing committee to return the donation of two hundred million

renminbi by a tobacco company in 2010, stopped a tobacco company–sponsored sports event, played an instrumental role in having a tobacco researcher removed from the list of potential recipients of the Ministry of Science and Technology's 2012 National Science and Technology Progress Award, and contentiously questioned the claims made on behalf of "light" and "low-tar" cigarettes. To raise public awareness of the health risks of smoking and mobilize public support for a policy that would require graphic warnings on cigarette packs, in 2011 a CTFK grantee (the ThinkTank Research Center for Health Development) carried out a multicity pack warning campaign, "I Want to Tell You Because I Love You." The campaign covered 40 cities across China over a three-month period (Redmon et al. 2013).

CATALYZING A SUSTAINABLE TOBACCO CONTROL MOVEMENT

CTFK conducted annual media advocacy training and legal training workshops for government law-drafters, public interest lawyers, administrative law experts, and environmental protection lawyers. In a bid to broaden alliances beyond traditional tobacco control circles, CTFK has worked with children's rights protection groups and environmental groups, including the Beijing Children's Legal Aid Center, the Green Beagle Environment Institute, and the All-China Environment Federation (ACEF).

In 2012, CTFK partnered with the Emory Global Health Institute–China Tobacco Control Partnership to work with the Luoyang city government to strengthen its existing but weak smoke-free public places policy. CTFK also collaborated with other international partners to work with the government of Beijing to adopt smoke-free laws.

China-based organizations funded by CTFK include the ThinkTank Research Center for Health Development, the Chinese Association on Tobacco Control, China University of Political Science and Law, the Chinese Center for Health Education, the Ministry of Health, Beijing Dongfang Public Interest and Legal Aid Law Firm, the Green Beagle Environment Institute, Pioneers for Health Consultancy Center, the Health Inspection and Supervision Center, China CDC, and the city of Luoyang.

Johns Hopkins Bloomberg School of Public Health

JHSPH's aim is to refine and optimize tobacco control programs to help smokers stop and to prevent children from starting.[7] In addition to the aforementioned Global Tobacco Control Leadership Program, one of its key projects in China has been the 2007–2008 program "Towards a Smoke-Free China." An extension of its initial Fogarty International Center grant, this project was designed to complement the Bloomberg Initiative in China's efforts to promote the adoption and implementation of policies banning smoking in public places; to improve tobacco control capacity in China; and to reduce exposure to secondhand smoke. Forty cities and counties in 20 provinces were targeted for the program. As a result of this project, the overall evaluation showed a significant decrease in male smoking rates and in exposure to secondhand smoke. Nineteen cities or counties revised their smoking ban regulations, various mass media and publicity campaigns were launched, and evaluation results showed that the campaigns significantly impacted awareness of the harms of tobacco use and secondhand smoke. Observation checks to evaluate enforcement of the smoke-free polices showed that 85 percent of the sites visited showed strong enforcement intensity. Finally, it was determined that funding for tobacco control at the project sites was five times greater than the national average, demonstrating a strong government commitment to tobacco control (Yang 2009).

World Health Organization (WHO)

In addition to its organizational contributions, since 2008 WHO has also received funding from the Bloomberg Initiative for specific projects.[8]

FACILITATING THE SMOKE-FREE HOSPITAL STANDARD IN CHINESE HOSPITALS (2008–2010)

This project aimed to make at least 40 hospitals in China smoke-free, and to create a smoke-free hospital model for China. A smoke-free hospital standard was developed and endorsed by the MoH and the National Patriotic Health Campaign Committee in March 2008. WHO also developed technical guidelines for implementation.

PROMOTING SMOKE-FREE HEALTH CARE AND SUPPORTING THE MOH DECISION ON SMOKE-FREE HEALTH CARE FACILITIES (2011–2012)

This project aimed to improve the health of health care staff by reducing their smoking and their exposure to secondhand smoke in health care facilities, and developing a national smoke-free health care strategy to support the MoH smoking ban in medical and health systems. It also aimed to increase the number of smoke-free hospitals, to raise awareness of smoke-free policies and smoking cessation among health care administrators and professionals, and to increase quitting among doctors. Project outcomes were not available at the time of publication.

The World Lung Foundation (WLF)

WLF's focus is on developing mass media campaigns with hard-hitting public health messages. They have produced eight campaigns for China, working primarily with government agencies such as the Beijing Municipal Health Bureau, the Beijing Patriotic Health Campaign Committee, the Ministry of Health, the

China CDC, the National Center for Tuberculosis Control and Prevention, the Guangzhou Association on Tobacco Control, the Guangdong Provincial Health Education Institute, the Yunnan Health Education Institute, the Jiangsu CDC, the Tianjin CDC, Zhejiang University, Fudan University, the Yunnan Provincial Health Bureau, and the Yunnan Health Education Institute. WLF also collaborated with other Bloomberg Initiative partners and the Emory Global Health Institute to provide media-specific technical support to China cities. It also launched a national-level evidence-based tobacco control public service announcement in 2012, and will evaluate the efficacy of the effort.[9]

The CDC Foundation

The role of the CDC Foundation is to develop a rigorous system to monitor the status of global tobacco use. It partnered with the U.S. CDC and the China CDC's Tobacco Control Office to implement the Global Adult Tobacco Survey (GATS) in China in 2010. The survey is used to collect data on adult tobacco use and key tobacco control measures (Bloomberg Initiative 2012c).

The 2010 China GATS results provided valuable information on the following topics: tobacco use prevalence, smoking and smokeless tobacco products, secondhand tobacco smoke exposure and policies, cessation, knowledge, attitudes and perceptions, exposure to media, and economics (CDC 2010).

The China Medical Board (CMB)

CMB has promoted anti-tobacco activities among its associated academic health science center grantees, who submitted proposals for smoke-free areas, curricula on smoking and its hazards, efforts to decrease smoking among physicians, and research projects on the economics and epidemiology of tobacco use. CMB's goal is to help establish tobacco control programs and research as legitimate and robust areas for academic inquiry, teaching, and service. The Bill & Melinda Gates Foundation funded the initial tobacco control efforts, but the continued funding to encourage the development of tobacco prevention and control as appropriate topics for health science academic careers has been from CMB. The board also cosponsored in 2011 the first academic conference on tobacco control in China, and funded a September 2013 *Tobacco Control* journal supplement to highlight research presented at the symposium ("China Tobacco Control Research Symposium—From Research to Action" 2013).

The Bill & Melinda Gates Foundation (BMGF)

BMGF has supported tobacco control activities in China since 2007. The foundation provided partial funding for the CMB tobacco control program, and currently supports the Emory GHI-CTP, the China Red Cross, and the Campaign for Tobacco-Free Kids (BMGF 2012).

The Emory Global Health Institute–China Tobacco Control Partnership (GHI-CTP)

The GHI-CTP's goal is to reduce the health, social, environmental, and economic burdens of tobacco use by increasing China's in-country capacity to develop and implement effective, accountable, and sustainable tobacco prevention and control initiatives. The two main initiatives are the Tobacco Free Cities (TFC) program and the Programs of Excellence (PoE). The objective of the TFC program is to build sustainable, comprehensive city-level tobacco control programs to prevent initiation among youth, young adults, and women; to promote quitting among adults and youth; and to eliminate exposure to environmental tobacco smoke. The objective of the PoE is to establish sustainable national tobacco control resource centers to conduct research and to provide expertise to support national and local tobacco control efforts (EGHI 2012).

The GHI-TFC initiative builds on the model of the World Bank Health VII project, with a goal of providing successful models of tobacco control at a city level that can be disseminated to other sites. The GHI partnered with the ThinkTank Research Center for Health Development, a health-focused NGO in Beijing, to develop and manage the initiative, which funds 17 cities throughout China. The pilot programs launched in 2009 were in cities including Luoyang, Tangshan, Changsha, Qingdao, Ningbo, Shanghai, and Wuxi. Ten additional cities were subsequently selected and began the program in 2010, including Anshan, Bayannaoer, Changchun, Dalian, Hangzhou, Kelamayi, Nanning, Nanjing, Suzhou, and Yinchuan. Each city developed a program aimed at changing the social norms of tobacco use based on its own unique situation, partnerships, and abilities.

While the TFC program evaluation is ongoing, preliminary assessments show that its grantees' progress in establishing tobacco control policies and in raising public awareness through targeted programs and education activities has varied from modest to substantial. Currently 17 of the cities have goals of creating smoke-free sectors including hospitals, schools, government buildings, businesses, religious sites, and homes, and 14 of them have made significant progress toward their goals while continuing to expand their efforts. Two cities, Anshan and Kelamayi, adopted smoke-free public places policies in late 2012, and Qingdao successfully adopted such a policy in 2013. Three additional cities—Changchun, Luoyang, and Tangshan—are now working with their legislative staffs to draft and adopt strong, citywide smoke-free public places policies. All of the TFC grantees have engaged local media outlets to promote their efforts, and a few have launched mass media campaigns to educate the public on the harms of tobacco use and secondhand smoke (Redmon et al. forthcoming).

The PoE initiative is designed to encourage tobacco control research, scholarship, and expertise among faculty and staff. Five universities were selected, and programs were launched in 2010. The programs and objectives include (EGHI 2012):

- Kunming University, School of Public Health, was funded to provide a comprehensive analysis of dangers associated with smoking and secondhand smoke and their associated economic costs in rural China. The program is also analyzing socioeconomic factors influencing tobacco use and exposure to secondhand smoke in this specific population.
- Yunnan Agricultural University, College of Economics and Management Pioneers for Health Consultancy Center, was funded to determine the feasibility of alternatives to growing tobacco in rural China. The program includes (1) community engagement to better understand the needs and concerns of tobacco-growing communities; (2) participatory research on the feasibility of alternative crops; and (3) message development for policymakers on the benefits of alternatives to tobacco crops, including for the health and income of the farmers and their families as well as for tax revenues.
- Tsinghua University Law School, Health Research Centre of Tsinghua University, was funded to conduct analysis on policy and legal issues related to tobacco control in China, and to establish a Legal Center on Tobacco Control to provide expertise and resources to the tobacco control workforce in China.
- Shanghai Jiao Tong University, School of Public Health, was funded to address gaps in behavioral and social science research in the area of tobacco control in China. The program implemented a study to determine behavioral, social, family, and community-level factors that influence smoking initiation in youth.
- Shandong University, Department of Epidemiology and Health Statistics, was funded to explore appropriate, effective, and sustainable tobacco control strategies and model practices in tobacco control in rural areas in China. The program aims to become a resource for comprehensive tobacco control program interventions and strategies for rural China.

In addition to these main initiatives, GHI-CTP also co-funded and served as the lead organizer for a tobacco control research conference, the aforementioned 2011 China Tobacco Control Research Symposium; published an electronic monthly tobacco control newsletter (TCAlliance 2012); and hosted a website providing up-to-date information on the program (EGHI 2012). It also provides funds to the ThinkTank Research Center for Health Development to develop and maintain a robust online resource center and to produce a monthly newsletter highlighting current tobacco control activities (TCRC 2012).

China Red Cross

The aim of the China Red Cross grant (2011–2014) is to increase support for tobacco control among China's leaders, and to help socially stigmatize smoking among the population in order to ensure long-term political and social change. This will entail providing support to universities and both government and non-government organizations (Redmon et al. 2013).

"Philanthropy" from China's Tobacco Industry

While the international philanthropic community has played a major role in accelerating tobacco control in China, China's tobacco industry has not been silent. Rather, they have actively worked to counteract these efforts. Tobacco companies worldwide use "corporate social responsibility" contributions as a means to counter tobacco control efforts and increase goodwill among policymakers and the general public (WHO 2009). The China National Tobacco Corporation (CNTC) is no exception. CNTC's "philanthropy" funding has been used to reduce poverty, invest in environmental sustainability, provide donations to education, and support disaster relief (STMA 2011).

CNTC and subsidiary companies have made significant contributions targeting youth in an effort to attract new smokers by providing funding support for schools and educational services as well as youth events and activities (Sunflower Cup Charity 2011; Moore and Adams 2011). A number of the funded schools even bear the name of the tobacco company. A slogan of one of the schools, Sichuan Tobacco Hope School, reads, "Talent comes from hard work—tobacco helps you become talented" (Moore and Adams 2011).

International tobacco control companies have also made philanthropic donations to China, including the British American Tobacco Company, which funded the Beijing Health Promotion Society (initially named the Beijing Liver Foundation) in 1997 to divert attention from secondhand smoke. They have also used the society to foster relationships with CNTC and the State Tobacco Monopoly Association, and to help them undermine China's smoke-free legislation (Muggli et al. 2008).

China's Government Response to Tobacco Control

The national and international public health communities' attention to the tobacco use epidemic, China's place at the epicenter of the epidemic, and the attention of international philanthropic organizations have prompted action by the central government. In 2006 China ratified the WHO Framework Convention on Tobacco Control, with a commitment to implement its obligations (WHO 2012b). The Ministry of Health issued a smoke-free hospital policy in 2009, with guidelines for health care facilities to be smoke-free by 2011,[10] and in 2010 the MoH and the Ministry of Education also issued a policy with guidelines for creating smoke-free schools.[11] The MoH authorized a policy prohibiting smoking in indoor public places starting on May 1, 2011,[12] and the National People's Congress included a statement of commitment to tobacco control in the 12th Five-Year Plan. While these actions are important, there is little evidence that the policies are being adequately implemented and enforced. Also, a significant financial commitment from the central and local governments to establish effective and sustainable programs and policy efforts has yet to be realized.

Discussion

Why did foreign foundations choose tobacco control as a health priority in China? The tobacco epidemic, or at least its recognition and subsequent attempts to actively control it, occurred many years earlier in the West. The dramatic effect of tobacco control measures has been researched and documented in North America, Western Europe, and Australia over the past 40 years. When observed at a distance by health leaders from these regions, China is seen as having the largest preventable cause of death in the world, and as being ripe for intervention and application of what has been learned in countries with successful control efforts. Foreign philanthropies have made a similar observation and have considered smoking as having two features that make infectious diseases so appealing to control—proven effective control measures and a large burden of illness. Thus, it seems to afford them an opportunity to play a catalytic role in effectively preventing the problem, and not just in controlling it. But as the authors of this chapter have noted elsewhere, the arrival of foreign foundations has not been without counterattack in China. Pro-tobacco interest groups in China have accused these foundations of meddling in Chinese priorities, of harboring ulterior motives. For example, it has been asked why American foundations invest in tobacco control in China when the United States remains one of the world's largest tobacco producers. The charge of foreign interference may also serve to weaken Chinese partner groups who can be accused of being aligned with foreign priorities. On the other hand, many Chinese public leaders have exercised public health leadership in advocating for tobacco control, and many Chinese admire foreign foundation work as valid and legitimate because of the foundations' genuine public health commitments (Redmon et al. 2013).

In Western nations with longstanding and effective tobacco control programs, philanthropy has not generally played a major supporting role, with the notable exception of the generous and forceful leading role played by the Robert Wood Johnson Foundation. Given the adversarial nature of tobacco control efforts, with the adversary being a legal corporate entity with deep pockets and little scruples, philanthropists—whose own assets have been generated by business success—may be reluctant to choose tobacco as a health issue when there are so many other important areas of health concern. Similarly, domestic Chinese philanthropy remains on the sideline of tobacco control. Even with the emergence of Chinese philanthropy in recent years, tobacco has not yet attracted Chinese foundation support. But there are a few very active anti-tobacco groups, including ThinkTank, an NGO headed by retired public health officials, and the China Tobacco Control Association, a GONGO organized by the Ministry of Health

(Redmon et al. 2013). Chinese philanthropists' reluctance to invest in tobacco control may reflect the current situation in China, and their reluctance may be compounded by the government's monopoly over the tobacco industry, the likelihood that these donors smoke themselves, and the very early stage of the maturation of China's philanthropic culture.

Many leaders in China's central government recognize the health impact of tobacco and the need to reduce its use despite its prominent economic role. Nevertheless, other powerful voices at all levels of governmental leadership are strongly supportive of tobacco as a crop, a manufactured product, a personal habit, a source of employment, and a source of government revenue. China's path from a tobacco-promoting culture to an anti-tobacco culture is dependent upon changes in social norms and government tobacco policies, and, depending on the speed of progress, those changes will translate into millions of lives saved or lost.

Summary

While philanthropic support for tobacco control in China is relatively recent, it has markedly changed the energy and enthusiasm for the topic in Chinese government, academia, and civil society. The value of the philanthropic support goes far beyond the dollars spent. An even greater contribution is the added attention and visibility to the issue given by foreign philanthropic interests. In addition, there has been a great need to elevate the level of technical capability in operating tobacco control programs, and the philanthropy-supported efforts have markedly increased this capacity as well as the sophistication of tobacco control staff.

Since international tobacco control efforts began in 1987, the Chinese government has issued a ban on smoking in public places, ratified the WHO Framework Convention on Tobacco Control (2006), and issued bans on smoking in hospitals (2009) and schools (2010). In 2011, the National People's Congress approved for the first time the inclusion of language, in the 12th Five-Year Plan, calling for China to "comprehensively promote a ban on smoking in public places." The hazards of tobacco are becoming more widely recognized and smoke-free spaces are increasingly common in cities.

Even though national and local support for tobacco control efforts has increased since the mid-1980s, China remains at the center of the global tobacco epidemic. It is important that the major global health philanthropies maintain their attention to China and its need to diminish its addiction to tobacco. It will also be vitally important for Chinese philanthropists to recognize the health threat of tobacco use and to invest their funds and influence in reducing this hazard. Any philanthropy whose goal is to have the biggest impact in reducing the global burden of disease must address the biggest preventable cause of deaths in the country with the biggest burden from tobacco.

Acknowledgments

We thank Jacob L. Wood for providing interview information and references on many of the philanthropies described in this paper. We also thank Shuyang Li for editing and providing references for this chapter.

Notes

1. Dan Xiao (director of the Epidemiological Department at the Beijing Institute of Respiratory Medicine and professor at the WHO Collaborating Center for Tobacco or Health), in discussion with Jacob Wood, June 21, 2012.

2. Ibid.

3. Ibid.

4. Yan Lin (head of Union China Center), in discussion with Jacob Wood, June 4, 2012; Honge Liu (project officer of the Union China Center), e-mail to Jacob Wood, June 5, 2012; Quan Gan (project officer of Union China Center), in discussion with Jacob Wood, June 4, 2012; Ning Dong (project officer of the Union China Center), e-mail to Jacob Wood, June 5, 2012.

5. Xi Yin (director of China programs, Campaign for Tobacco-Free Kids), e-mail to the authors, August 1, 2012.

6. Ibid.

7. Frances A. Stillman (co-director of the Institute for Global Tobacco Control, Johns Hopkins Bloomberg School of Public Health), e-mail to Jacob Wood, June 2, 2012; Stephen A. Tamplin (associate scientist at the Department of Epidemiology, Johns Hopkins Bloomberg School of Public Health), e-mail to Jacob Wood, June 2, 2012.

8. Xiao, discussion.

9. Yvvette Chang (associate director and marketing and communications country director for China and Indonesia at the World Lung Foundation), telephone interview with Jacob Wood, June 22, 2012; Winnie Chen (China communications manager at the World Lung Foundation), telephone interview with Jacob Wood, June 22, 2012.

10. Ministry of Health, "Decisions on Completely Prohibiting Smoking in the National Health Care System from 2011," 2009.

11. Ministry of Health and Ministry of Education, "Suggestion on Enhancing Tobacco Control Efforts in Schools," 2010.

12. Ministry of Health, "Rules for the Implementation of Sanitation Administration Ordinance in Public Places," 2011.

References

ACS (American Cancer Society). 2008. *Greater China Cancer Control Initiative—2007–2008 Project Overview*. Atlanta: American Cancer Society.

Beijing Institute of Respiratory Medicine. 2012. "About Us: WHO Collaborating Centre for Tobacco or Health." http://www.birm.cn/aboutjiey8.asp?ArticleID=148.

Benedict, Carol. 2011a. *Golden-Silk Smoke: A History of Tobacco in China, 1550–2010*. Berkeley: University of California Press.

Benedict, Carol. 2011b. "Between State Power and Popular Desire: Tobacco in Pre-Conquest Manchuria, 1600–1644." *Late Imperial China* 32 (1): 13–48.

Bloomberg Initiative. 2012a. "Bloomberg Initiative Partners—Tobacco Control Grants." http://www.tobaccocontrolgrants.org/Pages/45/BI-Partners.

Bloomberg Initiative. 2012b. "Bloomberg Initiative to Reduce Tobacco Use Grants Program." http://www.tobaccocontrolgrants.org/.

Bloomberg Initiative. 2012c. "About the Bloomberg Initiative." http://www.tobaccocontrol grants.org/Pages/44/About-the-Bloomberg-Initiative.

BMGF (Bill & Melinda Gates Foundation). 2012. "Bill & Melinda Gates Foundation—Tobacco Overview." http://www.gatesfoundation.org/topics/Pages/tobacco.aspx.

CDC (Centers for Disease Control and Prevention). 2010. "Statement Regarding First Release of Global Adult Tobacco Survey Result by China." http://www.cdc.gov/media /pressrel/2010/s100818.htm.

China CDC (China Center for Disease Control and Prevention), PUMC (Peking Union Medical College), and JHUSPH (Johns Hopkins Bloomberg School of Public Health). n.d. *Towards a Smoke-Free China Program Summary Report, January 2007–December 2008.* Beijing: China CDC.

"China Tobacco Control Research Symposium—From Research to Action." 2013. Supplement, *Tobacco Control* 22 (S2). http://tobaccocontrol.bmj.com/content/22/suppl_2.toc.

CRI English. 2011. "More Chinese Cities Committed to Anti-Smoking Campaign." http:// english.cri.cn/6909/2011/01/13/1461s615294.htm.

EGHI (Emory Global Health Institute). 2012. "Emory Global Health Institution–China Tobacco Control Partnership." http://www.ghi-ctp.emory.edu/.

Eriksen, Michael, Judith Mackay, and Hana Ross. 2012. *The Tobacco Atlas.* 4th ed. Atlanta: American Cancer Society; New York: World Lung Foundation.

External Evaluation Panel for Health VII Project of World Bank. 2004. *The Disease Prevention Project with the Loan of World Bank (Health VII Project) Sub-Project on Health Promotion External Evaluation Report.* http://lnweb90.worldbank.org/oed/oeddoclib .nsf/DocUNIDViewForJavaSearch/8525682E00686037852570450052D51E?open document.

Gan, Quan, Kirk R. Smith, S. Katharine Hammond, and Teh-wei Hu. 2007. "Disease Burden of Adult Lung Cancer and Ischaemic Heart Disease from Passive Tobacco Smoking in China." *Tobacco Control* 16:417–422.

Giovino, Gary A., Sara A. Mizra, Jonathan M. Samet, Prakash C. Gupta, Martin J. Jarvis, Neeraj Bhala, Richard Peto et al. 2012. "Tobacco Use in 3 Billion Individuals from 16 Countries: An Analysis of Nationally Representative Cross-Sectional Household Surveys." *Lancet* 380:668–679.

Ministry of Health. 2007. *WHO Collaborating Center in China Work Report.* http://www .whocc.org.cn/publish/index.html.

Moore, Malcolm, and Stephen Adams. 2011. "Chinese Primary Schools Sponsored by Tobacco Firms." *Telegraph* (London), September 21. http://www.telegraph.co.uk/news /worldnews/asia/china/8779180/Chinese-primary-schools-sponsored-by-tobacco-firms .html.

Muggli, Monique E., Kelley Lee, Quan Gan, Jon O. Ebbert, and Richard D. Hurt. 2008. "'Efforts to Reprioritise the Agenda in China': British American Tobacco's Efforts to Influence Public Policy on Secondhand Smoke in China." *PLoS Medicine* 12:251.

Redmon, Pamela, Lincoln C. Chen, Jacob L. Wood, Shuyang Li, and Jeffrey P. Koplan. 2013. "Challenges for Philanthropy and Tobacco Control in China (1986–2012)." In "China

Tobacco Control Research Symposium—From Research to Action," supplement, *Tobacco Control* 22 (S2). http://tobaccocontrol.bmj.com/content/22/suppl_2/ii4.full.

Redmon, Pamela, Michael Eriksen, Kean Wang, Shuyang Li, and Jeffrey Koplan. Forthcoming. "The Role of Cities in Reducing Smoking in China." *Global Health Promotion*.

Stillman, Frances A., Gonghuan Yang, V. Figueiredo, Mauricio Hernandez-Avila, and Jonathan Samet. 2006. "Building Capacity for Tobacco Control Research and Policy." *Tobacco Control* 15 (suppl. 1): i18–i23.

STMA (State Tobacco Monopoly Association). 2011. "Community Service." http://www.tobacco.gov.cn/html/19.html.

Sunflower Cup Charity. 2012. "Sunflower Cup." http://www.sfy.cn/.

Tang, Kwok-Cho, Don Nutbeam, Lingzhi Kong, Ruotao Wang, and Jun Yan. 2005. "Building Capacity for Health Promotion—A Case Study from China." *Health Promotion International* 20:285–295.

TCAlliance. 2012. "Newsletter for Tobacco Control in China." http://www.tcalliance.org.cn/home/?action-forumdisplay-fid-39.

TCRC (China Tobacco Control Resource Center). 2012. "China Tobacco Control Resource Center—Publications." http://www.tcrc.org.cn/Item/list.asp?ID=1228&page=1.

WHO (World Health Organization). 2009. "Tobacco Industry Interference with Tobacco Control. Geneva: WHO." http://www.who.int/tobacco/resources/publications/tob_ind_int_cover_150/en/index.html.

——. 2012a. "GATS (Global Adult Tobacco Survey)." http://www.who.int/tobacco/surveillance/gats/en/index.html.

——. 2012b. "Parties to the WHO Framework Convention on Tobacco Control." http://www.who.int/fctc/signatories_parties/en/index.html.

World Bank. 2005. *World Bank Implementation Completion Report*. Report No. 30613. http://documents.worldbank.org/curated/en/2005/04/5855192/china-disease-prevention-project.

Yang, Gonghuan. 2009. *Fogarty Project Book Series: Building Epidemiology, Surveillance and Intervention Capacity of Tobacco Control in China*. Beijing: Peking Union Medical College Publishing.

PART III
TRANSITIONS AND PROSPECTS

10 GONGOs in the Development of Health Philanthropy in China

Deng Guosheng and Zhao Xiaoping

Introduction

In China, the philanthropic and nonprofit sector is unique and distinctive. The nongovernmental organizational (NGO) landscape in China is largely divided into two groups—government-linked and independent NGOs—the latter of which ranges from grassroots to international organizations. The distinction between the two is based on whether government or civil society has started the organization and, thus, controls its governance and operations (Wang and Liu 2004). Government-organized nongovernmental organizations, or GONGOs, dominate China's NGO and philanthropic landscape.

GONGOs are not unique to China and are found around the world, although they may be more prevalent in socialist countries transitioning to a market economy, like the former Soviet satellite states (Young 2004). Often, they are seen as "extended arms of the government" (Wu 2002) or considered in opposition to "legitimate civil society." Among some groups, GONGOs may be viewed with suspicion as "nothing but agents of governments that created and funded them" (Moisés 2007). Yet nonsocialist countries also have government-linked bodies that are widely considered to be part of the nonprofit sector, such as the Japan Foundation, the British Council, the International Center for Human Rights and Democratic Development in Canada, and the National Endowment for Democracy (NED) in the United States. These organizations were founded or encouraged by the government, receive government funding, and are usually legally registered as charitable organizations in their home countries.

However, China's GONGOs are distinctive as legacies of China's socialist history. They are far more numerous in China than in Western countries, and they continue to fulfill a wide array of social welfare and other functions.[1] The role of GONGOs is important to China's future, for the development of both health and the nonprofit sector.

GONGOs Defined

GONGOs evolved as function of China's transition from a socialist to a market-based economy in the late 1970s.[2] Before China's reentry into the global market economy, the government controlled and managed all social welfare activities in China. Therefore, organizations working in this sphere were entirely sponsored and supported by the government. The state established GONGOs primarily to mobilize citizens for social work, receive assistance from multilateral, bilateral or international nongovernmental organizations, strengthen technology and information support, or solve new problems (Wu 2002). GONGOs were created to fulfill a specific need (i.e., foreign interaction and domestic function) that a social organization, industry association, or private NGO would satisfy in a more developed country (Deng 2004).

Economic reforms beginning in the late 1970s led to a relaxation in the management and control of these organizations, which was further accelerated after China's entry into the World Trade Organization in 1995. Although such an opening created, at least in concept, new opportunities for private NGOs to emerge, the development of independent NGOs has been hampered by various impediments. Instead, GONGOs continue to dominate the NGO landscape.

GONGOs may be defined as nonprofit organizations initiated or funded by the government, but GONGOs are not government departments or units. Technically, GONGOs may have legal status as nonprofit organizations equivalent to formal registration in the civil affairs sector, but GONGOs are not, by their nature, completely autonomous. Usually, the government controls their governance structure and leadership. In theory, GONGOs may seek independence with their own boards, as the board chooses the executive leadership of the organization, but in reality, the board chairman or secretary-general is appointed by the government. Other aspects and major decisions, including personnel, finances, and administrative procedures, can also be heavily influenced or even controlled by the government. This contrasts with GONGOs or NGOs in Western countries, which may receive government funding but without a similar degree of government intrusion. In China, official legitimacy enables GONGOs to operate from a preferential position relative to other NGOs, especially unregistered NGOs. Registered NGOs face lower barriers to obtaining resources than unregistered NGOs, and GONGOs have even more privileges in this regard. For instance, only after successful registration are GONGOs and other registered NGOs allowed to seek approval for an official seal and open a bank account. GONGOs also benefit from special regulations that allow them more room to maneuver with regard to financing and administration. GONGO foundations, for instance, are able to conduct public fundraising, collect tax-exempt donations, and mobilize resources through the domestic media.

GONGOs in China may overlap with other organizational forms in other countries, including grant-making or direct operating foundations. Especially relevant to the public health field are GONGOs that assume the role of professional societies or associations, organizations that customarily belong to the professional group. GONGOs are not unique due to their source of financing, since many NGOs receive government funds and also secure private or corporate donations. But since GONGOs are mandated to perform as an "extra arm" of the government, they therefore rarely criticize or oppose government policies. While the daily operations of most GONGOs are fairly autonomous, the extent of government penetration into organizational affairs varies. NGOs that are fully independent or autonomous stand in the greatest contrast to GONGOs. Yet, in China, many of these NGOs lack legal legitimacy because they cannot officially register as nonprofit entities. They may be international or domestic organizations, the latter of which are sometimes called grassroots NGOs.

An Overview of the Place of GONGOs in China's Nonprofit Landscape

Understanding the place of GONGOs is critical to understanding China's nonprofit landscape. Although few in number compared with the total number of

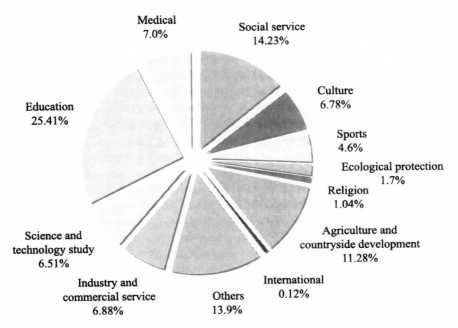

Figure 10.1. Landscaping China's GONGOs and NGOs by Field of Work (%). *Source: China Ministry of Civil Affairs (2012).*

organizations within the NGO landscape, GONGOs occupy a leading and dominant role largely due to their favored status, whereby their governmental linkages
grant them legal legitimacy, easier access to national-level operations, and more
favorable financing. According to statistics from the Ministry of Civil Affairs
(MoCA), China has 462,000 officially registered NGOs with an annual growth
rate of 8 percent in the five years leading up to the end of 2010, indicating a stable
but positively increasing trend (Ministry of Civil Affairs 2011). Although many
registered NGOs are GONGOs, this figure also includes registered grassroots
NGOs.

The range of work that GONGOs and NGOs do is wide. Figure 10.1 summarizes China's GONGOs and NGOs by various fields of social work—including
agriculture, sports, culture, science and technology, and industrial and commercial services. Noteworthy is the large share (26 percent) devoted to education.
Health receives a modest share of GONGO-NGO attention at 7 percent, or
32,000 NGOs.

These data do not present a complete picture of China's NGO landscape.
Truly independent unregistered NGOs have been estimated at more than three
million, or six times the number of officially registered organizations (Gao 2008).
Many of these informal or grassroots NGOs register under company law as for-
profit corporations subject to taxation, or they simply operate informally under
the radar of the government. The government does not officially recognize these
grassroots NGOs, but as long as they do not threaten state security or social stability, the government has mostly not impeded their work (Deng 2010). The government's policy toward unregistered organizations, known as the "Three 'No'"
policy, is: "No recognition, no banning, no intervention." In other words, as long
as they do not harm state security or social stability, the government will not ban
them or interfere with their internal affairs. Therefore, grassroots NGOs lacking official registration operate on a large scale, despite not having official legal
status.

GONGO and NGO Registration

Because unregistered NGOs constitute the overwhelming majority in China,
the defining characteristic of GONGOs, conversely, is their registration status.
All legitimate NGOs, including GONGOs, must register with MoCA or, like the
Chinese Red Cross Society, have special status that exempts them from registration. Registration sets GONGOs apart from the many independent grassroots
NGOs, which under the rules of the current Chinese system of governance have
not been able to achieve registration. The registration process is complex, shut-
ting out most grassroots NGOs and thus conferring legitimacy only on GON-
GOs and a handful of other registered NGOs.

Successful registration brings government supervision, confers official legitimacy, and enables access to standard banking, auditing, personnel, and other

policies essential for smooth operations in China. Registration usually requires "dual registration"—legal status secured from MoCA (called the "registration administration") and another governmental department related to the field of work for supervision (known as the "competent business unit" or "supervisory unit").[3] The practice of dual registration may persist, although there is local experimentation in relaxing requirements in cities like Shenzhen and Beijing, as well as in regulation reform more generally across Guangdong, Hunan, Jiangsu, and Yunnan Provinces.

For instance, in 2009, MoCA announced a Cooperative Agreement on Advancing Integrated Reforms in Civil Affairs with the municipal government of Shenzhen, under which Shenzhen has become an "experimental site" for registration and management of social organizations. In 2008, Shenzhen allowed social organizations in the spheres of business, social welfare, and charity to register directly with the civil affairs department, effectively dropping the dual registration system (ICNL 2013).

Beijing has also experimented with regulation reform. It tested a "free-of-supervision-unit model" in Zhongguancun Industrial Park in 2010, and Dongcheng district established a service center to ease the registration process of small and mid-sized charitable associations (Zhang 2011).

Beyond city-level experimentation, some provinces are experimenting with changes to regulations and management of NGOs more generally. Guangdong is working on reforms to do away with the professional supervising agency requirements and decentralize the authority to register social organizations at the township and subdistrict government levels. Jiangsu and Hunan have been working on more general reforms to NGO regulation, including local-level regulations governing foundations and fundraising (ICNL 2013).

Registration distinguishes NGOs by type and assigns each NGO a sphere of operations. China classifies NGOs into three categories: (1) social associations (*shehui tuanti*), including societies, professional and industry associations, etc.; (2) private non-enterprise units (*minban feiqiye danwei*), including private hospitals, private schools, etc.; and (3) foundations (*jijinhui*), of both the public and private variety.[4] Public foundations can receive donations from the public, but private foundations cannot receive donations or conduct public fundraising.

Registration may also take place at different governmental levels, including national, provincial, and municipal. NGOs that register in a specific local area are limited in their operations and activities to that particular area. Most of the currently successfully registered grassroots NGOs are locally registered. For example, the Jiangxi Medical Association, which is registered only in Jiangxi Province, has activities confined to the province and only allows membership in Jiangxi. In contrast, nationally registered NGOs register with MoCA and can conduct activities throughout the country. As national-level registration is extremely difficult to achieve, successful national registration is almost exclusively enjoyed by GONGOs. In 2011, China had only 2,300 national NGOs, less than 0.5 percent of the total registered NGOs.

It is noteworthy that the focus of this chapter is on national GONGOs because most organizational modes in China are top-down and national GONGOs usually shape regional ones, which ensures the relative uniformity of organizations across different levels. The difficulty of categorizing NGOs and the plethora of information available at various levels makes analyzing data for regional and municipal GONGOs cumbersome. Data on national GONGOs, on the other hand, are relatively accessible because of the limited number of organizations.

China's Health-Related GONGOs

National health GONGOs evolved in China mostly after the market economic reforms in the early 1980s, and they were brought about to address emerging health challenges. There are two types of national health GONGOs. Some are founded by the Ministry of Health (MoH),[5] while some are founded by other government units or People's organizations (*renmin tuanti*). Except for the China Medical Association, which was founded in 1915,[6] all 74 national health GONGOs were established after market reforms. Altogether, there are 53 GONGOs under the MoH. Such associations, societies, and foundations include the China's Women Medical Association, the China Rural Health Association, and the China Sexology Association. Twenty-two health-related GONGOs are under other supervising departments, including the Chinese Medical Association, the China Charity Federation, the Chinese Red Cross Foundation, the China Foundation for Poverty Alleviation, and the China Children and Teenagers' Fund. In 1978, the China Healthy Birth Science Association was founded, and since 2009, three new organizations have been registered: the China Health Inspection Association, the China Association for Plastics and Aesthetics, and the China Association for Disaster and Emergency Rescue Medicine.

Financing of China's Health GONGOs

China's health-related national GONGOs are nonprofits, most of which are financed by government funding, donations, and supplementary sources like fees and funds raised through commercial activities. Financial size can vary greatly in terms of annual revenue. The smallest is the China Transplantation Development Foundation with 31,000 RMB annually. The largest is the China Charity Federation, which received 8.6 billion RMB in 2010, consisting of 4.4 billion RMB of donated materials (of which 4 billion RMB was in medicines and medical equipment) and 4.2 billion RMB in cash donations.

Table 10.1 shows the high variability in government financing and sources of revenue, using the China Medical Association (CMA) and Cancer Foundation of China as examples. The Cancer Foundation of China has total revenue of 310 million RMB, the third largest in size. A full 99 percent of this revenue consists

Table 10.1. Funding Sources (%) of the Cancer Foundation of China and the Chinese Medical Association

	Cancer Foundation of China	Chinese Medical Association
Donation	99.2	N/A
Membership fee	N/A	0.1
Service fee	00.4	76.7
Commercial sales	0	18.1
Government assistance	00.2	3.9
Miscellaneous	00.2	1.2
Total	100.0	100.00

Source: Cancer Foundation of China *Annual Report 2010*; China Medical Association *Annual Report 2010*.

of donations, while the remaining 1 percent is made up of small fees for services charged and government support. CMA's annual income of 434 million RMB is second in size, but is mostly dependent upon service fees and commercial income, at 77 percent and 18 percent, respectively; government support constitutes only 4 percent.

But even if GONGOs do not receive direct government funding, they still enjoy something of a monopoly on donations because of their favored legal status.[7] Unlike grassroots NGOs, which cannot legally fundraise in public and whose support can only come from donations from enterprises or individuals, GONGOs can mobilize resources more easily, both because they can seek public support through media and because donations to them are subject to tax reductions or tax exemptions (MoCA Legislative Affairs Office of the State Council 2004).

GONGOs' Roles in the Health Field

National health-related GONGOs play different roles in advancing health. These roles are largely dictated by their organizational type, which determines major constituencies and funding sources. Table 10.2 shows an analysis of the scope of activities of 75 national health-related GONGOs. The data in the table also demonstrate that foundations and social associations have different financial and social orientations, which lead them to do different types of work. Many of these organizations carry out more than one type of activity, and the definitions of the types of work or activity in table 10.2 are as follows: (1) academic exchanges, which include academic meetings and conferences, research collaboration and funding, and the production of journals that disseminate academic work; (2) consultation services, which involve experts from organizations advising other organizations, for instance providing expertise to hospitals, schools, local governments, etc.; (3) training, which involves the training of health professionals and includes free

Table 10.2. The Main Activities of National Health-Related GONGOs

Activities	Foundations		Social Associations	
	Quantity	Ratio (%)	Quantity	Ratio (%)
Academic Exchanges	11	39.3	25	53.2
Consultation Services	7	25.0	46	97.9
Training	12	42.9	42	89.4
Medical Assistance	22	78.6	0	0.0
Fundraising	28	100.0	0	0.0

Source: Data were compiled from the articles of association and information on the activities of 75 national GONGOs in the field of health philanthropy. If a type of activity was mentioned in the GONGO's articles of association or described in information about its activities, it was counted; activities not mentioned in the articles of association or described in supporting information were not counted in the above figures.

and tuition-based programs, as well as continuing education programs; (4) medical assistance, which consists of the provision of medical services to vulnerable populations, including the poor, people in rural areas, women and children, and those who have been affected by disastrous events; and (5) fundraising, which involves the mobilization of social resources and fundraising campaigns via media outlets.

Foundations were created to mobilize resources from society and apply those resources to the provision of social services. In China, public foundations are the only social organizations allowed to conduct public fundraising, and because GONGOs are the only national-level foundations,[8] they get the lion's share of funding. About 9.3 percent of total annual charitable giving, or 9.6 billion RMB, was allocated for health-related philanthropy in 2010. Grassroots NGOs received less than 5 percent of this total (Meng, Peng, and Liu 2012).

All foundations engage in fundraising, collecting, and redistributing capital and services. In order to provide direct medical assistance, both cash and in-kind donations of medicines and medical equipment are provided for those who cannot afford medical treatment, particularly for poor patients in poverty-stricken areas (Pan 2012). Although the government provides medical assistance to poor patients through medical insurance and direct medical care programs, including government allocations of 5 billion RMB for urban areas and 8.3 billion RMB for rural medical assistance in 2010 (Ministry of Civil Affairs 2013), health-focused GONGOs essentially supplement government provisions of health services, including public health services (Ji, Chu, and Tian 2012). Medical assistance, including the provision of equipment and medicines, treatment of special diseases, and public health education and services, is targeted at vulnerable groups such as those in poverty, children, women, and ethnic minorities.

The capacity to provide medical assistance through the mobilization of social resources gives foundations a special role in disaster relief, which can be considered a specific form of medical assistance. After the 2008 Wenchuan earthquake, 13.8 billion RMB was donated to relief efforts (He 2013), most of which went through GONGOs, which often work in collaboration with official government relief efforts. Disaster relief galvanizes the mobilization of more charitable giving. According to figures provided by the China Charity Alliance Donation Data Center, since the Wenchuan earthquake more than 100 billion RMB has been donated each year to GONGOs, grassroots NGOs, and government relief efforts (China Charity Net 2013).

As an example, the China Charity Federation (CCF), China's largest national health-related GONGO in terms of size of donations received, works primarily in the areas of medical assistance and fundraising. CCF, founded in 1994, is governed by a council, a standing council, and a president. Its current president is Baojun Fan, who is a member of the 9th and 10th Standing Committee CPPCC, former deputy secretary of the Party Leadership Group, and deputy minister of civil affairs. As one of China's largest charity organizations, CCF conducts programs in disaster relief; care for the disabled, orphaned, elderly, and poor; medical aid; and education aid. The federation also provides medical care, equipment, and medicines to support medical treatment for poor and neglected populations. From 2010 to 2011, CCF provided over twenty thousand patients with free medicine, donated ultrasound and mammography machines, and provided operations for children with cleft lips and palates and senior citizens with cataracts in poverty-stricken areas (China Charity Federation 2013). CCF has also helped in disaster relief, raising nearly 1.75 billion RMB for disaster relief efforts, including the reconstruction of disaster-affected areas. After the Lushan earthquake in 2013, CCF raised over 40 million RMB and worked in cooperation with the local government to provide purified drinking water to earthquake victims (Yu 2013). As with all GONGO foundations, a major component of CCF's activities involves fundraising. According to the federation's statistics, between January 1, 2007, and December 31, 2012, CCF raised 30.4 billion RMB in donations of money and goods, allowing it to carry out more than 60 charity projects affecting over one million people (China Daily 2013).

Some GONGO foundations, like the Chinese Foundation for Prevention of STD and AIDS, work across the full range of activities. That foundation's organizational structure, which includes a Publicity and Education Department; an Academic Exchange Department; a Medicine, Science and Technology Department; an Expert Consulting Services Department; and a Fundraising Department, reflects this wide range of activities. In terms of fundraising, the Fundraising Department, together with assistance from the International Liaison Department, works to collect donations from Chinese society and from international donors (Chinese Foundation for Prevention of STD and AIDS 2009).

In the area of academic exchange, the foundation hosts and attends conferences and symposia on HIV and AIDS, including the World AIDS Conference and the Asia-Pacific AIDS Conference. It also reinforces academic exchange through publications, such as the *International Newsletter of STDs and AIDS*. It conducts education and training targeted both at the public, via public education campaigns and exhibitions, and at health professionals, through programs such as STD and AIDS testing technique workshops. The foundation also engages in consultation activities, including the establishment of clinics used for demonstrations. Often, these activities involve interaction with grassroots NGOs, local health departments, and the general public. For instance, the foundation provides public AIDS prevention and treatment consultation services through the AIDS Online website, which has been operational since November 2001. Finally, in terms of medical assistance and care, the foundation provides support to individuals with AIDS, especially orphans and women. Since 2005, the foundation has worked on projects in Yunnan, Henan, Sichuan, and Xinjiang to provide children with medical care, mental support, and educational training. The foundation also provides health services in the form of screening programs for early detection and management of STDs and AIDS.

In contrast to foundations, social associations provide services directly to their members. These associations cannot legally engage in fundraising, and therefore they must depend on other sources of financing. Due to their obligation to their members, financing constraints narrow the scope of their work (i.e., they do not engage in medical assistance). Most associations, therefore, work on professionally oriented, technical areas of knowledge generation, academic exchange, and training. Nevertheless, they still provide social services and offer social value, but more indirectly, by improving the quality of health professionals, which helps produce better health outcomes.

The Chinese Medical Association (CMA) is China's oldest GONGO and arguably its most prominent health-related social association. Since its founding in 1915, it has grown into an academic and professional association covering 85 specialties with over five hundred thousand members in China. As a social association, it cannot conduct public fundraising activities, but instead generates revenue primarily through service fees, commercial sales, government assistance, and membership fees.

CMA's activities are focused on academic and professional programs such as conferences, training activities, consulting, research collaboration, and the publication of academic work, and it convenes national conferences across a number of medical disciplines. In 2011, CMA held conferences on pediatrics, pathology, trauma medicine, and endemic diseases, bringing together leading scholars and practitioners of medicine for the exchange of ideas and professional development. Additionally, it conducts training activities, which include, among other things, courses on how to use the latest medical technologies, such as practical training on ultrasound technologies. CMA also allocates funding in support of medical research projects. For instance, it has funded studies on the treatment of ovarian cysts at Peking University Third Hospital, surgical weight loss treatments for Type 2 diabetes patients at the First Affiliated Hospital of Xi'an Jiaotong University Medical College, and on the effectiveness of selenium in treating Graves' disease at the First Affiliated Hospital of China Medical University. The association also disseminates research results through the publication of over 125 medical and popular science journals, including high-level medical journals like the *Chinese Medical Journal.*

Overall, GONGOs like the Chinese Medical Association, as membership-based social associations, focus primarily on academic and professional activities that service their members. These CMA activities, by strengthening the professional abilities and academic quality of China's medical practitioners, also contribute to improving the quality of China's health system.

It is important to note that professional training is one area of convergence between government-organized foundations and social associations. Almost 90 percent of social associations engage in training programs, while 43 percent of foundations do so as well. For instance, the Chinese Red Cross Foundation (CRCF) cooperates with academic partners like the Peking Union Medical College and Capital Medical University as well as the Ministry of Health to coordinate free training programs for rural doctors. A CRCF 2006 program in conjunction with Capital Medical University trained over ten thousand rural doctors.

Implications of GONGOs for Health Philanthropy

China's GONGOs have a special role in China's health philanthropy sector because they "straddle and sometimes bridge the worlds of governmental agencies and NGOs" (Wu 2002). The two worlds delineate some of the strengths and weaknesses of GONGOs. On the one hand, linkages with the government allow GONGOs to innovate in the areas of health and social policy, making them the "innovation arm" of the government. Whereas government departments reward civil servants for not making mistakes, encouraging risk-aversion and discouraging innovation, most GONGO staff are not civil servants, so GONGOs do not face the same procedural and cultural pressures as departments directly under government administration.[9] Their relative degree of separation from government means that they are more likely to generate innovations than government bodies are. At least in theory, the relatively independent financing of GONGOs allows the freedom to experiment. Additionally, close relationships with the government, high levels of political trust among leadership, and top-down administrative systems allow GONGOs to enter and implement programs in communities quickly. These factors give GONGOs an efficiency advantage over other NGOs in conducting pilot projects, disaster relief, and awareness campaigns. Their degree of separation from government allows for experimentation, while their government affiliation allows successful pilots to expand in government programs backed by government policy.

On the other hand, while close government linkages allow GONGOs (such as the China Social Welfare Foundation and the China Foundation for Poverty Alleviation, discussed below) higher relational and implementation power, closeness to government also limits GONGOs. The appointment of major leaders and tight guidelines on operations and financial controls compromise their independence (Xu 2008). Similarly, GONGOs with government connections may suffer from bureaucratization. GONGOs are designed to serve the government and be responsible to the government, so there is also the question of loyalty. In contrast to GONGOs' being somewhat beholden to the government, grassroots organizations believe that they are accountable to vulnerable groups and the general public. Ultimately, grassroots NGOs might be more innovative and more capable of working with fewer resources. While GONGOs have also shown they can innovate, they may have more opportunities than NGOs simply because of their favored position vis-à-vis the government.

The China Social Welfare Foundation's linkages with government, for example, have allowed it to influence policymaking. In 2011, the foundation launched the Free Lunch Project, together with Deng Fei, a journalist from *Phoenix Weekly*, and five hundred other journalists. The project sought to mitigate the problem of child malnutrition by calling on the public to donate 3 RMB every day to provide free lunches to students at impoverished rural schools. Within three months, the Free Lunch project mobilized over ten thousand donors via microblogs, collecting over 16.9 million RMB. On average during 2011, the China Social Welfare Foundation bank account received 65,000 RMB each day (China Daily 2012). By the end of June 2012, the project had collected over 35 million RMB and provided free lunches for over 34,000 children across 163 schools.

The Free Lunch Project not only drew attention to the problem of child malnutrition, but also demonstrated an innovative method for solving public health issues that the government has adopted in other cases. Adopting a standard of 3 RMB per day per student for a nutritious lunch, the central government encouraged local governments to implement programs like the Free Lunch Project. In October 2011, the State Council implemented a program to improve the nutrition of students' diets. The Chinese central government began allocating 16 billion RMB annually for a new compulsory nutrition improvement scheme for rural students. Government programs now cover 26 million students across 680 counties and cities in China (Xinhua News 2012).

In another case, the rural maternal and infant health programs of the China Foundation for Poverty Alleviation (CFPA) stimulated policy changes by local governments. Sparked by reports that maternal mortality rates in poor areas of China were about 10 times higher than those in urban regions, CFPA launched the Action 120: Maternal and Infant Health Project in Yunnan Province in 2000 (China.org.cn 2006). The project aimed to strengthen maternal and infant health by reducing or exempting medical treatment fees for poor mothers, especially by providing financing for in-hospital or attended births. The project also established an integrated system of county-level maternal and child health rescue centers working in coordination with village-level health workers to identify, track, and follow up with high-risk mothers and infants. During the project's duration from 2000 to 2009, the project raised over 52 million RMB in financial and material donations. By 2010, it had covered 12 counties in six provinces and municipalities, helping 127,000 women and infants and saving 287 women from critical health problems (National Working Committee on Children and Women under the State Council 2010). Recognizing the success of these interventions, local governments of project sites in Yunnan and Anhui Provinces began providing allowances for births in hospitals (Zhou 2008).

Opportunities and Challenges for GONGOs

GONGOs also have a unique relationship with truly nongovernmentally organized groups such as domestic grassroots NGOs. Although GONGOs can compete with independent NGOs, they may also complement them by working together toward mutually shared goals. But as NGOs are given more opportunities to flourish in China, competition between GONGOs and grassroots NGOs may increase in the future. Meanwhile, GONGOs have developed complementary partnerships with international and domestic NGOs and funding sources. Most domestic grassroots NGOs are unregistered, and without fundraising qualifications, bank accounts, invoices, or tax-exempt status, they cannot collaborate with international donors. GONGOs can play an intermediary role by supporting and creating a platform for grassroots NGO development as pass-through organizations or sources of funding.

For example, the Global Fund sought to involve grassroots NGOs in AIDS prevention and control in China. Instead of working directly with grassroots NGOs, the Global Fund supports grassroots NGOs through the Chinese Association of STD and AIDS Prevention and Control, a GONGO serving as an intermediary. The Chinese Association in this case not only channels funding from the Global Fund to the grassroots NGOs, but also, in working with grassroots NGOs, can provide training and enhance their capacity. In addition, a small number of GONGOs in China provide direct financial support to domestic grassroots NGOs. For example, after the Wenchuan earthquake, the China Foundation for Poverty Alleviation collected donations that were then used, through a tender and bidding process, to support projects by grassroots NGOs, including those providing medical assistance and psychological counseling.

At the same time, GONGOs also compete with grassroots NGOs and private foundations, especially for resource acquisition in the forms of donations and government funding. The tax status of donations to GONGOs in relation to NGOs is an important factor. GONGOs can both obtain funds for their own operations and distribute funds to support other groups, in effect "managing" grassroots NGOs by choosing to whom they channel funds. GONGOs and NGOs compete for both government contracts and funding from the government. Increasingly, more grassroots NGOs have received government funding, yet they are often in direct competition with GONGOs.

Starting in 2011, the government of Beijing's Dongcheng district began funding community and social service projects. The government funded some projects of grassroots NGOs but not some GONGO projects, indicating that GONGOs may face stronger competition from grassroots NGOs for resources in the future. As grassroots NGO numbers increase and their capacities improve, GONGOs may face increasing pressure from the competition. Yet even without pressure from newly emerging NGOs, GONGOs themselves face increasing pressure from Chinese society at large in terms of efficiency, transparency, and client responsiveness. Previously, with strong government linkages and little pressure to be transparent or demonstrate efficiency, many GONGOs did not have an incentive to be transparent about the sources of their funding. Increasingly, though, GONGOs with a continued lack of transparency are coming under scrutiny and facing problems in terms of social credibility (Tao 2008). Recent scandals have demonstrated the importance of public trust to a public fundraising organization's ability to collect donations.

The Red Cross Society of China—a GONGO set apart from the rest with its own law granting it special status—is a prime example of how scandal and lack of public trust can handicap fundraising power. In 2008, the society received roughly 90 percent of the 13.8 billion RMB donated after the Wenchuan earthquake. But after a young woman known as Guo Meimei posted pictures of herself with luxury vehicles and designer handbags and claimed she worked for the "Red Cross Chamber of Commerce," the Red Cross was harshly criticized for being corrupt. Even though Guo Meimei's claims turned out to be false, the scandal had a striking impact on donations to the Red Cross Society. According to the *Beijing News,* in April 2013, after an earthquake in Lushan, the Red Cross Society received only 570 million RMB of the over 1 billion RMB donated. The remainder of donations went to another 115 other charity groups, who have agreed to disclose information about their earthquake fundraising on a website established by Jet Li's One Foundation.

Conclusion

With their many advantages over other NGOs in terms of human and capital resources and organizational networks, GONGOs play important roles in health-related philanthropy in China, including academic exchanges, training, medical assistance, and fundraising. The continued strengthening of cooperative partnerships between GONGOs and other NGOs in China will help the development of both GONGOs and health-related philanthropy in China. Yet GONGOs face serious limitations in terms of autonomy, credibility, and vitality, and they must also strive for more efficiency. Administrative policy reforms aimed at increasing autonomy could potentially enhance the impact of GONGOs. Currently, revisions are being made to the Regulations on the Registration and Management of Social Organizations (1998) and the Regulations on the Management of Foundations (2004). Registration reform may reduce the involvement of government departments in the personnel, finances, and major activities of GONGOs. Such administrative reform may increase independent decision-making and autonomy, but at the same time could reduce government financial support.

GONGOs will continue to be important in China for the foreseeable future because they are likely to maintain a monopoly on, or at least a considerable advantage in, serving as a conduit for public donations and mobilizing resources for charity. As much as netizens and others complain about the lack of transparency of these organizations, the truth of the matter remains: Chinese society does not yet have the capacity to engage in substantial philanthropic activities in the health sector without GONGOs, but it remains to be seen if they will be needed in the future.

Notes

1. It is impossible to develop accurate statistics on the number of GONGOs and the ratio of GONGOs to NGOs in China, for no organization will expressly label itself as a GONGO or an NGO. In this study, organizations were categorized based on information about their organization type, registration status, and whether they label themselves a "competent business unit" or not.

2. For a description of health-related NGOs in China, including government relations, see chapter 1.

3. For a more complete description of the regulatory landscape of NGOs in China, see chapter 2.

4. See Regulations on the Registration and Management of Social Organizations (1998), Interim Regulations on the Registration Management of Civil Non-Enterprise Units (1998), and Regulations on the Management of Foundations (2004).

5. Now the National Health and Family Planning Commission (NHFPC), *Guojia weisheng he jihua shengyu weiyuan hui.*

6. The Red Cross Society of China has been operating in China since 1904. However, this article does not include the Red Cross Society as a GONGO because the society is not registered with the Ministry of Civil Affairs; its operations are instead based in the 1993 Red Cross Law. It is therefore not considered an NGO under current law; however, the Chinese Red Cross Foundation, Chinese Medical Association, and Children and Teenagers' Fund are are all legally registered NGOs under the current law. For more on the Red Cross Society of China, see

Caroline Reeves's chapter, "The Red Cross Society of China: Past, Present, and Future," in this volume.

7. In Guangdong, new regulations may potentially help break the monopoly that GON-GOs enjoy on public fundraising. The regulations are experimenting with allowing social organizations (*shehui tuanti*), civil non-enterprise units (*minban feiqiye danwei*), and nonprofit public institutions (*shiye danwei*) to fundraise publicly, especially in priority areas of disaster relief and caring for the elderly, disabled, solitary, and poor.

8. By the end of 2011, only a few NGOs were registered and recorded as local public foundations, allowing them the ability to collect donations from the public. One example is the One Foundation in Shenzhen, founded by film star Jet Li. All national-level public foundations are GONGOs.

9. Owing to historical reasons, there are still some Chinese GONGOs whose key staff are civil servants.

References

China Charity Federation. 2013. "China Charity Federation." http://cszh.mca.gov.cn/article/english/.

China Charity Net. 2013. "China Charity Alliance." http://www.charity.gov.cn/fsm/sites/newmain/index2.jsp.

China Daily. 2012. "Free Lunch Project Feeds 15,000 Kids in 2011." http://www.chinadaily.com.cn/china/2012-04/09/content_15005593.htm.

China Daily. 2013. "China Charity Federation Raises 30b Yuan in 6 Yrs." http://usa.chinadaily.com.cn/business/2013-04/03/content_16374996.htm.

China.org.cn. 2006. "Action 120: Maternal and Infant Project." http://www.china.org.cn/english/features/cw/168334.htm.

Chinese Foundation for Prevention of STD and AIDS. 2009. "Jijinhui jigou shezhi" [Foundation's Organizational Structure]. http://www.cfpsa.org.cn/html/guanyujijinhui/2009/1102/175.html.

Deng Guosheng. 2004. "Yetan GONGO" [On GONGOs]. *China Development Brief*, no. 18: 18.

Deng Guosheng. 2010. "The Hidden Rules Governing China's Unregistered NGOs: Management and Consequences." *China Review* 10 (1): 183–206.

Gao Bingzhong. 2008. *Zhongguo gongmin zhehui gazhan lanpishu* [Bluebook on Civil Society Development in China]. Beijing: Peking University Press.

He Huifeng. 2013. "Red Cross Society of China Sees Smaller Share of Donations after Quake." *South China Morning Post*, April 13. http://www.scmp.com/news/china/article/1225522/red-cross-society-china-sees-smaller-share-donations-after-quake.

ICNL (International Center for Not-for-Profit Law). 2013. "NGO Law Monitor: China." http://www.icnl.org/research/monitor/china.html.

Ji Ying, Chu Hong, and Tian Zhen. 2012. "NGO zai gonggong weisheng fuwuzhong de juese fenxi" [The Role of NGOs in Public Health Services]. *Zhongguo xingzheng guanli* [Chinese Public Administration], no. 5: 54–57.

Meng Zhiqiang, Peng Jianmei, and Liu Youping. 2012. *2011 Zhongguo cishan juanzhu baogao* [Annual Report on Charitable Donations in China 2011]. Beijing: Chinese Society Press.

Ministry of Civil Affairs. 2011. *Minzhengbu fabu 2010 nian shehuifuwu fazhan tongji baogao* [Ministry of Civil Affairs 2010 Report of Statistics on Social Services Development]. http://www.mca.gov.cn/article/zwgk/mzyw/201106/20110600161364.shtml?2.

Ministry of Civil Affairs. 2013. "Tongji shuju" [Statistical Data]. http://www.mca.gov.cn /article/zwgk/tjsj/.

Ministry of Civil Affairs, Legislative Affairs Office of the State Council, eds. 2004. *Jijinhui zhinan* [Commentary on the Regulation and Administration of Foundations]. Beijing: China Society Press.

Moisés, Naím. 2007. "What is a GONGO? How Government-Sponsored Groups Masquerade as Civil Society." *Foreign Policy.* http://www.foreignpolicy.com/articles/2007/04/18 /what_is_a_gongo.

National Working Committee on Children and Women under the State Council. 2010. "127,000 Benefit from Maternal and Infant Health Project." http://www.nwccw.gov .cn/?action-viewnews-itemid-154737.

Pan Jintang. 2012. *Shehui baozhang tonglun* [Introduction to Social Security]. Jinan: Shandong People's Press.

Tao Chuanjin. 2008. "Shehui xuanze: mujuan zuzhi de weilai zouxiang" [Social Choice: The Future of Fundraising Organizations]. *Zhonggao caifu* [China Fortune], no. 8: 24–25.

Wang Ming, and Liu Peifeng. 2004. *Minjian zuzhi tonglun* [A General Survey of Nongovernmental Organizations]. Beijing: Current Affairs Press.

Wu Fengshi. 2002. "New Partners or Old Brothers? GONGOs in Transnational Environmental Advocacy in China." *Wilson Center China Environment Series*, no. 5: 45–47. http:// www.wilsoncenter.org/publication/china-environment-series-5-2002.

Xinhua News. 2012. "Free Lunch Project Improves Diets of Rural Students." http://news .xinhuanet.com/english/culture/2012-11/01/c_131944569.htm.

Xu Yushan. 2008. "Fei duichenxing yilai: Zhongguo jijinhui yu zhengfu guanxi yanjiu" [Asymmetric Dependence: Research on the Relationship between Foundations and Government in China]. *Gonggong guanli xuebao* [Journal of Public Management] 5 (1): 33–40.

Young, Nick. 2004. "GONGO, Not Made in China." *China Development Brief*, no. 18: 19.

Yu Qingfan. 2013. "Zhonghua cishan zonghui wei Lushan dizhen huoqu chouji kuanwu chao 4000 wanyuan" [China Charity Federation Raises over 40 Million Yuan for Lushan Earthquake Relief]. Zhongguo zaixian xiaoxi [China Online News]. http://gb.cri.cn/42 071/2013/04/26/5892s4098135.htm.

Zhang Dongya. 2011. "NGO Registration May Ease in 2011." *Beijing Today.* Accessed May 24, 2013. http://www.beijingtoday.com.cn/news/ngo-registration-may-ease-in-2011.

Zhou Mingzhu. 2008. "Muying pingan xingdong dao Jixi" [Maternal and Infant Safety Project Comes to Jixi]. *Jianghuai chenbao* [Jianghuai Morning Post], January 2. http:// www.hf365.com/html/01/02/20081128/187193.htm.

11 The Red Cross Society of China

Past, Present, and Future

Caroline Reeves

THE RED CROSS Society of China has operated uninterrupted since 1904, out-lasting diverse governments and helping millions of Chinese over a more than one-hundred-year history. The organization began as a civic-run Chinese group building on the Chinese tradition of local charity and expanded into a national-level philanthropic organization with international ties. It provides an historic example of a successful Chinese federated charitable organization of autonomous societies with their own fundraising, decision-making, and personnel capabilities.

Philanthropy in Early Twentieth-Century China

At the start of the twentieth century, China's natural and political landscapes were rocked by disaster and civil violence as China's last dynasty crumbled and China was pushed into the modern world. Internationally, imperialism and geo-politics encroached on China's sovereign integrity, worsening the domestic situation. Poverty, increased mortality, political instability, and social conflict became the norm for many Chinese, of whom more than 90 percent were rural peas-ants. China's elite—and, increasingly, China's general populace—wanted better for China domestically and in the world comity. Working together, they drew on China's past and innovated for China's future to improve the social welfare environment for their nascent nation.

By 1900 China's tradition of philanthropy had been well established. China boasted mutual-aid societies from the Han dynasty on (206 BCE–220 CE), and charitable activity was encouraged by all major religious and philosophical sys-tems in the empire. Beginning in the Ming dynasty (1368–1644), social welfare institutions caught the attention of the imperial government, which encour-aged them, and whose prestige, in turn, was reinforced by their work. In fact, these groups acted as an arm of the government, providing what Max Weber has termed informal "liturgical governance," where "local elites were called upon to perform important public services on the state's behalf, at their own expense" (Mann 1987, 12–13). Medical philanthropy was an important part of this charitable endeavor, and the distribution of medicines and the establishment of clinics often targeted at specific seasonal diseases were staples of Chinese outreach to the disadvantaged.

The understanding of state responsibility for social relief provision was well articulated and popularly entrenched by the late imperial period (1368–1911). Public officials, including the emperor himself, were seen as parental figures by the ethnically Han people. These "Father-Mother Officials" (*fu-mu guan*) acted, in a sort of cosmological way, *in loco parentis*, mitigating between a judgmental Heaven and a vulnerable populace. This fundamental equation between social welfare provision and the state has proven to be one of the most enduring facets of China's philanthropic *habitus*, prevailing through periods of weak states (the Republican period, 1911–1927), strong states (arguably the Nationalist era, 1927–1937; and the People's Republic of China, 1949–present), and even states fundamentally opposed to traditional cosmologies (the Maoist state, 1949–1976). Despite this equation, the Chinese state often had to rely on its unofficial representatives to provide the services it was too poor or too fragmented to provide itself, as it did in 1904 when the Chinese Red Cross Society was founded.

Founding of the Chinese Red Cross

In 1904, the Russo-Japanese War spilled onto Chinese territory. Foreign nationals were quickly evacuated from the war area (Central Committee of the Red Cross Society 1924). Russia, however, refused Chinese entry into the Manchurian ports to help distressed Chinese refugees. Afraid of being drawn into hostilities, the imperial government, too weak to hold its own if forced into war, would not challenge the blockade, even to rescue Chinese citizens (*Zhongguo Hongshizihui zazhi* 1913). Responding to the crisis, Chinese community leaders in Shanghai met to pledge their financial support if some way could be found to help "repatriate" the Chinese sufferers (*Beijing zazhi* 1904a).

The civic rescue initiative and the eventual establishment of a Chinese Red Cross society was led by Shen Dunhe, a prominent Shanghai tea merchant, modernizer, and government official who had studied international law at Cambridge University (Tiao 1911). Shen's exposure to Western organizations and his knowledge of international law alerted him to the existence of an organizational vehicle that could cross closed "borders": the Red Cross Society. The Red Cross organization had recently become well known internationally after Henri Dunant, founder of the group, won the Nobel Peace Prize in 1901 (Moorehead 1998, 168). As Shen knew, the Red Cross organization offered well-publicized political neutrality, accepted by the world community (Reeves 1998, chap. 1). Red Cross neutrality would allow Chinese workers unchallenged access to sensitive war zones.[1]

The International Committee of the Red Cross (ICRC) had been conceived in Switzerland in 1863 by a group of Europeans intent on changing the nature of war (Boissier 1963, 201). The formation of the group was inspired by the 1862 book *A Memory of Solferino*, written by Genevan Henri Dunant (1828–1910). Overwhelmed by the sight of scores of wounded men left to die on the battlefield of Solferino, Dunant proposed a remedy for the horrors he witnessed: the creation of internationally recognized, permanent, national volunteer relief societies to care for the war-wounded. Gustave Moynier, a prominent Genevan lawyer and later first president of the Red Cross, contacted Dunant after reading the book to suggest the formation of a committee to turn Dunant's ideas into reality (Checkland 1994, 4). Thus was born the International Committee to Aid the Military Wounded, which by 1884 became known as the International Committee of the Red Cross (Hutchinson 1996, 6).

The ICRC, which deals only with international disasters at the invitation of the involved national societies, was created to encourage the formation of nationally based, voluntary aid societies around the world to work under a flag of neutrality on the battlefield. This neutrality became guaranteed by the international Geneva Conventions, first instituted in 1864, promoted by the ICRC, and signed by member states. The formation of national societies was and still is left to individual nations. In the ICRC's early years, the primary thrust of the national societies was the formation of medical auxiliaries for a nation's army, intended to serve impartially as medical charities during wartime. A secondary mission evolved over time, which was service as peacetime providers of relief, particularly medical relief, in natural disasters and for disease prevention.

In 1904, armed with this knowledge, Shen moved quickly to contact Shanghai's Chinese and foreign community leaders to form a Red Cross group. Anticipating a negative reaction from the Japanese and Russians to a Chinese organization, Shen crafted an *international* Red Cross group to represent China, composed of prominent men from neutral Western countries (Great Britain, France, Germany, the Netherlands, and the United States) living in Shanghai, as well as Chinese elites. He named this group "the International Red Cross of Shanghai," which began operations in April 1904 (Wong and Wu 1985, 571; Richard 1916, 322; *Shenbao* 1904). Thanks to donations from the Chinese Railway authorities and the Telegraph Administration, elites from Shanghai were able to travel by train to the northeast and communicate by telegraph free of charge, facilitating relief efforts and drumming up local Chinese patronage (*Beijing zazhi* 1904b; Red Cross Society 1912). These new technologies helped spread the word about the new Red Cross organization and improved its effectiveness across the country.

By the close of the Russo-Japanese War, the new Red Cross group had evacuated over 130,000 refugees from Manchuria and coordinated more than 20 relief centers and hospitals across the area, aiding more than a quarter of a million people. They had raised well over half a million Shanghai taels of silver through public subscription drives in 1904–1905, 120,000 taels more than they actually spent. Building on its initial successes, the Red Cross organization in China continued to grow after the war, and was increasingly staffed by the Chinese themselves, displacing earlier Western missionary organizers and medical men. The Red Cross's medical focus dovetailed with China's long-term enthusiasm for medicine and more recent engagement with biomedicine, creating a potent synergy. After the war, the balance of the initial fund drive was applied to starting a Red Cross medical school and building Red Cross hospitals in Shanghai (Zhang 2004, 108–115).

Institutional Organization

Although the Red Cross Society was initially funded by impressive donations from Chinese across the social spectrum, by 1911 the board of directors decided to offer membership in the society, which would become its major revenue source. Three classes of membership with graduated dues were designed, allowing members voting rights in the society as well as a mention in the annually published membership directory (its actual publication record is unclear). Within ten days of opening the membership rolls in 1911, the society enrolled one thousand members. In 1920 the organization added two more membership categories, Ordinary and Student. By 1924 membership had soared to over forty thousand. The public support for this organization confirms current scholarship on the salience of civic action in the constitution of national citizenship during the pre-Sino-Japanese War period (Culp 2007; Mitter 2011, 243–275).

Like most national Red Cross Societies, the Chinese group incorporated a national headquarters—in China's case, in Shanghai—which coordinated widely dispersed local branch societies (*fenhui*) commanding their own administrative and financial operations. On the national level, the Shanghai headquarters was initially set up within the Silk Merchants' guild hall, and later moved to its own headquarters on Jiujiang Road (Central Committee of the Red Cross Society 1924). Local branches, formed in county seats as well as in larger cities, operated nationally as well as locally. Drawing personnel from the surrounding areas, the chapters initiated relief and medical activities for their own communities as well as participated in the larger organization, functioning with remarkable autonomy in terms of the activities they participated in, how they financed their operations, and even how they conceptualized the Red Cross mission. These branch societies were often run by the same men who had previously served in traditional philanthropic activities in their locality, sometimes even in the same buildings. The new local Red Cross activities allowed the creation of social networks and capital for the donors and organizers of Red Cross efforts, building local reputations, leadership capacities, and a sense of participatory community involvement.

The centralized national Red Cross organizational structure facilitated coordinated responses to disaster relief and an ordered movement of resources and personnel across large distances. The innovation of local branch societies feeding into a national network fit well with China's preexisting local philanthropic structures (*shantang*)—and also played a critical role in expanding China's philanthropic organization to the national level. The national reach of this model meant that the association had its own network that could operate independently of a national government, and that the society could penetrate deep into the hinterlands to mobilize social actors to participate in its activities. Within 20 years of the Red Cross's founding, the connection between the Red Cross symbol and medical aid was well known across China.[2] Shen Dunhe's innovation was a resounding success.

The Chinese Red Cross in the International Arena

As the newly institutionalized international Red Cross movement spread around the world at the beginning of the twentieth century, it quickly established itself and the laws and principles it espoused as international norms (Reeves 2005, 64–93). The formation of national societies affiliated with the international parent became a hallmark of an increasingly internationalized global landscape. Recognition as a Red Cross member was important for all modern states, and acknowledgment of a national Red Cross Society by the International Committee of the Red Cross was and still remains "a standard early sign of Statehood," conferring powerful international legitimacy on the sponsoring government (Best 1980, 345). Emerging and embattled powers alike looked to membership in the Red Cross organization to bolster their reputations domestically and internationally. Across Asia, the clout of this new organization was widely recognized, and its imprimatur highly sought.

In China, the international cachet of having a national Red Cross Society was clear to the governments of the early twentieth century. The Qing dynasty had seen the formation of a national Red Cross Society primarily as a diplomatic initiative, designed to boost China's image in the international community and improve its army (Reeves 2005). Individuals such as Shen Dunhe, who actually created a working, effective society, saw the Red Cross mission as a mandate both to enhance China's international stature and to improve domestic social welfare along traditional lines. This confluence of goals meant that while the society operated during its first decades as an autonomous organization, it did so with the explicit blessing of the government.

China, through its new society, became a full international participant in the Red Cross movement. Its gradual movement toward official recognition was fully consonant with the trajectory of other emerging national Red Cross Societies.[3] In 1904 the Qing adhered to the international Geneva Convention, paving the way for international recognition of China's Red Cross group ("Accession de la Chine à la Convention de Genève" 1904).[4] In 1912 China's Red Cross was officially recognized by the ICRC in Switzerland and became a full-fledged member ("Reconnaissance de la Societe Chinoise de la Croix-Rouge" 1912). The new Chinese Red Cross Society engaged actively overseas, in many ways representing China abroad. Much like the society's activities in the national arena, these international dealings were neither dictated nor directed by China's national government. But the confluence between China's diverse governments' desires to be recognized as world players and the prestige afforded by being part of the international Red Cross movement meant that these governments would and did continue to back China's new Red Cross organization. Similarly, in these early years, the Swiss-based ICRC, nominally interested in the national societies, did not become actively involved in the direction of its national affiliates. Stipulating a few fundamental rules, such as the sanctity and exclusivity of the Red Cross symbol, the ICRC mostly left the national societies to their own devices.

The Chinese Society reached out to the international Red Cross organization and contributed to other national societies' relief activities, particularly in areas where there were large Chinese communities. The Chinese Red Cross donated significant funds to international Red Cross disaster relief, such as after earthquakes in San Francisco in 1906, in Kagoshima in 1914, and in Tokyo and Yokohama in 1923. It also worked to help overseas Chinese outside the Red Cross network. For example, in 1919, the Society put forward twenty thousand American dollars to repatriate Chinese workers who were stranded in Germany and Austria-Hungary after World War I. In turn, China's Red Cross was a recipient of internationally coordinated Red Cross aid (Central Committee of the Red Cross Society 1924, 25–26). In 1917, for example, during record-breaking floods in Zhili, Japan's Red Cross sent the Chinese Society a donation of five thousand Japanese yen (Central Committee of the Red Cross Society 1924, 20).

The success of China's Red Cross association could be measured not only by the international recognition it commanded, but also by its national growth: by 1924, it boasted over 40,000 members and 286 chapters, and by 1934, almost 120,000 members and 500 chapters (Central Committee of the Red Cross Society 1924, 55; Zhang 2004, 269–279). It also had a profound influence on other philanthropic groups within China, inspiring the formation of other internationally oriented charities, such as the Red Swastika Society. This initial growth and establishment of the society in the early Republican period made statements about the growth of China's national philanthropic network, China's increasingly optimistic international position, and the success of a citizen-run social welfare organization.

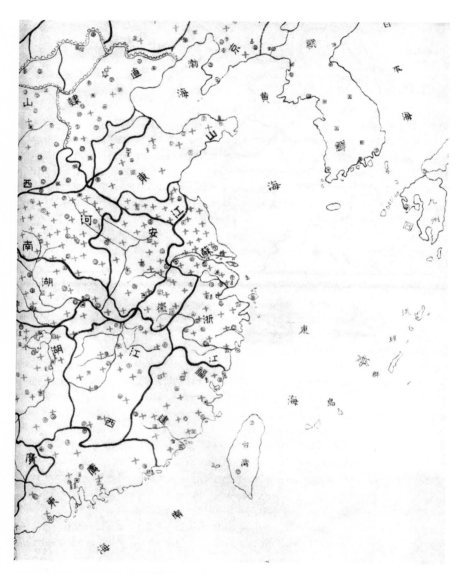

Map 11.1. Map showing the locations of Red Cross chapters across China, included in the society's 20th anniversary celebration volume. *Source: Central Committee of the Red Cross Society (1924).*

By the early twentieth century, the Red Cross movement was "flourishing mightily, and the meaning of the Red Cross was well understood throughout the European-American dominated world. The National Societies . . . had become natural features of the landscape of modern civilization" (Best 1980, 151). China, by being an active participant in the international Red Cross movement, established a degree of credibility as a functional, international state that countries without these trappings of civilization could not hope to claim.[5] Despite clearly articulated reservations about discontinuities between the Western-dominated ideology of the Red Cross movement and China's own ideological and logistical positions, Chinese citizens and government officials wholeheartedly joined the movement, fully cognizant of the international political clout the organization commanded. Finding resonance where they could, such as between the (fifth-century BCE) ancient philosopher Mozi's conception of *jian'ai* and Dunant's contemporary idea of humanity, and ignoring dissonance where they had to, China's initial embrace of the Red Cross movement was both instrumentalist and idealist (Reeves 2005).

The ICRC Comes to China

The duality of the state/society relationship, always blurred in the case of China, became further complicated in the late 1920s as the independence of peripheral elites rubbed up against the centralizing impetus of the Nationalist Guomindang (GMD) state. Increased visibility and assertiveness of local power, which had grown since the Taiping period, posed both a threat and an opportunity for the relationship between centralized and centralizing power structures and society (a conflict still extremely powerful in the PRC today). Setting the ball in motion for one of the most complete state-societal takeovers in modern history by the Chinese Communists, the GMD state began trying to assert control over local civic organizations soon after its formal assumption of power in 1927. Ironically, the ICRC encouraged this takeover.

In the early 1930s, the ICRC twice sent its secretary, Sidney Brown, to China. In this pre–World War II period, a statist paradigm of governance had become increasingly popular around the world. The ICRC was not immune from this trend and began actively promoting an understanding of national Red Cross societies as quasi-state military organizations. During his second visit to China in 1934, Brown made his opinion about the proper way for a national Red Cross Society to operate clear to the Chinese Red Cross personnel and the government ministers with whom he met. In his confidential report back to Switzerland, Brown wrote, "I insisted—perhaps too strongly?—on the traditional role of national Red Cross Societies as voluntary aid organizations to Military Medical Services."[6] He notes that he gave former Chinese Red Cross Society managing director B. Y. Wong, MD, explicit instructions to press this agenda with the Nationalist government.

Brown also included similar exhortations in his written report to the Chinese Committee.[7]

These instructions from the ICRC were in agreement with the GMD's own inclinations. The Nationalist government tightened control over the Society, particularly its autonomy in choosing its personnel. Brown applauded this shift in staffing, despite what seems to be the glaring unsuitability of many of the new principals, including known gangster and druglord Du Yuesheng.[8] With Brown's blessing, by 1935, a government takeover of the appointment of Red Cross Society officials—functional as well as honorary—was all but complete.

In September 1937, as the war with Japan escalated, the Chinese Red Cross Society gave up its mandate as the sole Red Cross Society in China and offered a "charter" to a new group of philanthropists: the Shanghai International Committee of the Red Cross Society, or, in Chinese, the Shanghai International Committee of the Chinese Red Cross Society. In its new incarnation, the society lost touch with many of its branches and became, in essence, an international association, relying on aid contingents and donations sent to China from national societies around the world, including those in the United States, England, and Belgium, as well as donations from societies in Germany and the Soviet Union (*Hongshizihui yuekan* 1946). The Chinese Red Cross was assimilated into the international atmosphere of the world war being fought in China and ceded control of the organization to the government. It would never again regain the autonomy it had before the war.

The Sino-Japanese War

The war years provided new challenges to the Red Cross organization. With the disruption of the national network, the central office no longer had control over—or often even a connection with—local branches. Routine activities were subsumed into the war with Japan. A new kind of Red Cross unit was created to deal with the emerging situation: the Red Cross Medical Relief Corps (MRC). These units initially operated independently of the Central Committee of the Red Cross Society, arising spontaneously as the need for them became all too obvious. China's Red Cross had worked with refugees and victims of civil war in the past, but now the scale of the disruption and the number of refugees and wounded, as well as the acuity of the need for surgical care, changed the nature of Red Cross work for the period 1937–1942.

Funding for this war work came primarily from outside China—from overseas Chinese groups in Southeast Asia and North America and from other charitable agencies in North America, Britain, the Dutch East Indies, Australia, and New Zealand. Fundraising led by just one doctor from Batavia (Jakarta today), Kwa Tjwan Sioe (Ke Quanshou), between July 1937 and December 1941 raised 50 million Hong Kong dollars (the 1945 equivalent of $27 million), a sum split between the Red Cross and Song Qingling's China Defense League (Watt 2014, 18). Much of this funding was inspired and brokered by the head of these new Red Cross units, Robert K. S. Lim (Lin Kesheng), MD.

Trained as a British officer in the Royal Army Medical Corps and having served in World War I, Lin became head of one of the first Red Cross mobile units in Shanghai during the January 28 (1932) Shanghai bombing relief effort. Subsequently, Lin was appointed head of the personnel division of the Red Cross North China Medical Relief Commission, organizing 12 mobile medical teams to provide care for soldiers fighting the Japanese in North China. These teams treated around 20,000 casualties. Under Lin's supervision and guidance, standardized first aid kits were developed for these teams, and Peking Union Medical College students, sponsored by the Beiping Red Cross branch, produced a Red Cross field service manual.

When war broke out in Shanghai in August 1937, provisional Red Cross Medical Relief Corps teams were formed yet again. Twenty-two rescue and first aid teams, 24 emergency hospitals, and 98 ambulances were employed, as well as 16 public and private hospitals requisitioned to serve Chinese troops fighting around Shanghai. The provisional MRC supplemented woefully inadequate Army medical teams. By October 1937, the Red Cross also set up a hospital in Nanjing with three hundred doctors and nurses and four hundred orderlies. Although short-lived due to the Japanese advance, it was the largest of its kind at the time. In the spring of 1938, the Medical Relief Corps was formally inaugurated, and Lin was appointed general director.

From 1938 to 1940, the Red Cross Medical Relief Corps "grew into a substantial healthcare agency supplying field armies with on-the-spot training, surgical, medical and sanitary services" (Watt 2014, 129). As the war wore on, battle conditions changed, and the understanding of logistics deepened. The MRC developed as well. Initially attached to army base hospitals, the corps then moved closer to the front to serve army field hospitals. Finally, in its longest and most effective phase, the MRC was reorganized into small mobile units consisting of one physician, one nurse, four staff, and up to ten stretcher bearers/sanitary assistants (Watt 2014, 131). Between 1938 and 1941, the number of these units grew from 75 to 172, and the corps performed over 67,000 operations. They treated millions of patients, from delousing and malaria prevention to control of cholera epidemics. Under Lin's supervision, the MRC was more than an emergency relief operation: it also spread the basic tenets of preventive health care and sanitary services through China's vast countryside.

Meanwhile, on the organizational front, in May 1943 the International Committee of the Red Cross in Geneva received a letter from the National Red Cross Society of China: "Dear Sirs: This is to inform you that as a war measure, the national government has taken over the direction of all the activities of the National

Red Cross Society of China. . . . Very sincerely yours, Chengting T. Wang."[9] Thus the government takeover of the organization was complete.

The Civil War Years

After World War II ended in 1945, the Chinese Red Cross tried valiantly to recover its pre-war organization and mission. The internationalized groups and emergency medical corps were disbanded, and the Central Committee reasserted control under a board of directors. In 1946 Wang Zhengting was replaced as the head of the Red Cross, but many other Nationalist operatives, including former gangster Du Yuesheng, stayed on. One priority for the newly reorganized society was to reestablish control over Red Cross branches in the northeast and on Taiwan that had been taken over by the Japanese Red Cross during the war. A revitalization of the national network of branch societies and active membership was also in the works. By 1947, however, due to the escalating civil war, these prerogatives had to be put aside and the organizational recovery mission scrapped to focus on reactivating Red Cross emergency medical relief corps. Some non-war-related activities were still performed by the Chinese Red Cross, such as flood relief in Guangdong, Guangxi, and Sichuan in the summer of 1947 and the launch of a campaign in 1948 to develop a Red Cross Youth Corps. The repatriation of prisoners of war and displaced persons was also on the agenda, and the Chinese Society began communicating with other Red Cross groups around the world to help bring soldiers back to their homes. On the whole, however, the majority of these peacetime projects came to a standstill as civil war overwhelmed China yet again.

"The Right Arm of the State": 1949–1966

As the Communists swept across China in 1949, the Chinese Red Cross remained active. With the capture of Nanjing in April 1949 came a crucial question: where would the loyalties of Red Cross actors fall? In fact, a minority of Red Cross leaders chose to go to Taiwan, with the majority of Red Cross management staying in China (Chi 2005, 116).[10] Many administrators moved back to Shanghai, home of the Red Cross headquarters before the war. The International Committee of the Red Cross sent word from Geneva that the Chinese Red Cross should and would act with strict neutrality as the civil war ended, and this principle was upheld. The continuing need for relief work that had initially inspired so many Chinese to join the Red Cross gave them a cause in mainland China that kept them there for the long haul.

The transition to a "new" Red Cross in the new Red China was a relatively smooth one. The convergence of the CCP's prerogatives and the historical mission of the group eased the process. Zhou Enlai was personally involved in overseeing much of the Red Cross's new administration, amending the Red Cross constitution himself and dictating the line of command between the Society and the Ministry of the Interior, the Foreign Ministry, and the Ministry of Health. In 1950, Zhou mandated that the Red Cross headquarters move from Shanghai to Beijing's Ganmian Hutong in the heart of the city (now the site of the Red Cross Hotel). The Red Cross became subordinate to the Ministry of Health and the Emergency Relief Committee (Chi 2005, 119).

As in the earliest years of the organization's existence, the importance of the Red Cross organization to China's international relations became paramount. This potential was immediately obvious to the new government. In April 1950, Zhou Enlai sent a telegram to the International Committee of the Red Cross to proclaim the Chinese Red Cross of the PRC as the only legitimate Red Cross Society of China. Zhou also demanded that the ICRC expel any Guomindang Red Cross representatives from the international organization. This gambit paid off, and in 1952, after the new PRC government signed onto the Geneva Conventions (including the most recent 1949 convention), the ICRC granted full recognition to the PRC's Red Cross Society as "China's sole lawful, nationwide Red Cross" (Wang and Chen 2008, 87). This diplomatic coup guaranteed the preservation of the organization under the new regime.[11]

After 1949, the Chinese Red Cross became highly politicized both in and outside China. As Chinese scholars have pointed out, "Although the post-[1949] Red Cross continued to emphasize its independence, under the circumstances of that era, in reality it was a work unit under central government leadership" (Wang and Chen 2008, 87). On the international stage, the group often served as a mouthpiece for the PRC. At the 19th Plenary Session of the International Red Cross, Red Cross President Li Dequan (widow of General Feng Yuxiang and the PRC's first minister of health) gave a speech denouncing Taiwan and the "two-China plot manufactured by the United States." In the late 1960s, China publicly refused to come to an ICRC board meeting because the Saigon chapter of the Red Cross was in attendance. Despite its often-antagonistic stance, however, China's Red Cross chose not to drop out of the international arena, instead maintaining a high international profile and often using that profile as a bully pulpit for government proclamations. In 1957 Mao Zedong himself welcomed Red Cross officials from Romania in Tiananmen Square.

Domestically, the Red Cross also became increasingly political, serving as a propaganda machine for CCP initiatives. The state arrogation of control begun under the Nationalists was complete, with Communist penetration from the highest to the lowest levels of society. With the outbreak of the Korean Conflict, Chinese Red Cross teams denounced American aggression in Korea and took part in anti-American demonstrations. Similarly, the Red Cross participated in and held demonstrations against British colonialism in Malaya. Meanwhile, Red Cross domestic disaster relief, the Chinese Red Cross military medical corps in Korea, and routine Red Cross public health work were able to continue. Throughout the early 1950s, the Chinese Red Cross was one of three groups to sponsor efforts to repatriate Japanese stranded in China, assisting significantly in normalizing postwar Sino-Japanese relations (Chi 2005, 138). Throughout the 1950s and early 1960s, branch societies were reorganized and reactivated, despite (or as part of) the politically charged atmosphere. By 1964, there were more than three hundred branches and five million members of the Chinese Red Cross Society (Gu 1994, 131).

The Cultural Revolution and the Red Cross: Feudal, Capitalist, and Revisionist, but Good to Posture with

Not surprisingly, the Red Cross group was not viewed well during the Great Proletarian Cultural Revolution (1966–1976). Branded "Feudal, Revisionist, and Capitalist," the Chinese Red Cross Society all but shut down domestic operations during this time (Qu 1999, 57). Internationally, however, the Chinese Red Cross entered one of its most active periods of the Mao years, reaching out globally to potential "friends" to offer both moral and material disaster relief support. Telegrams from this period document Chinese Red Cross support to 138 countries, including Somalia, Tanzania, Zambia, Senegal, Madagascar, Algeria, Albania, North Vietnam, Cyprus, Romania, Bolivia, Peru, and Myanmar. This aid totaled over one billion renminbi (Chi 2005, 187–213). Although many other organizations were shuttered during this period of revolutionary activity, the Red Cross Society was allowed to remain open.

Reopening: 1977–1990

As did so many other parts of Chinese life, the Chinese Red Cross Society experienced a revival after the conclusion of the Cultural Revolution and the death of Chairman Mao. Reprising the post–Sino-Japanese War period, the organization decided to focus on the domestic arena and prioritize the rebuilding of the national network of Red Cross branches. As China's reopening progressed, so, too, did the loosening of government control over the Red Cross organization. Although the Chinese Red Cross would never again regain the autonomy or grassroots credentials of its earliest years of operation, this period began to see a repositioning of the organization vis-à-vis the government and an opportunity for genuine civic input and involvement in the society. Growth in this early period of liberalization was slow, perhaps reflecting popular exhaustion with "joining," or perhaps due to a lingering distrust of the organization, severely discredited during the Cultural Revolution. By 1984, membership had reached only 1,870,000 (including 410,000 youth members), a far cry from 1964's figures (Gu 1994, 193).

In 1980, the deputy chairman of the Standing Committee of the People's Congress welcomed Alexandre Hay, then president of the ICRC (1976–1987), on a state visit to the PRC. This welcome of Hay, praising the ICRC's "outstanding accomplishments for world peace" signaled a sea change in the PRC's stance toward the international organization. No longer decrying the ICRC as a lackey of

Western imperialists, now China welcomed the opportunity to become involved in multilateral international organizations. As Chinese political scientists Wang Ronghua and Chen Hanxi have commented, "The activities of the Chinese Red Cross within the International Red Cross Movement thus evolved from 'using the Red Cross Movement as a platform for government propaganda' to 'positively becoming a member of the International Red Cross Movement'" (Wang and Chen 2008, 91). In 1983, the PRC signed onto the most recent Geneva Convention, the *sine qua non* of participation in the International Red Cross Movement. In 1990, China publicly affirmed its new attitude by hosting a regional Red Cross meeting in Beijing.

The Chinese Red Cross also began to recognize a need for domestic legislation defining the organization's status under state law. In 1988, the society proposed legislation to the National People's Congress to clarify "the character, status, and international and domestic function of the Red Cross" (Wang and Chen 2008, 92). In the early 1990s, the imminent return of Hong Kong and Macau exacerbated the need for clarification, pushing this legal process forward. The Hong Kong Red Cross's legal statutes were based on British Red Cross Law. This discrepancy would not stand after 1997, because, as articulated by the Chinese Red Cross, "if at the appointed time the Chinese Red Cross appears to rely on Hong Kong's or Taiwan's law, this will obviously be inappropriate. This requires that we see the importance and urgency of [creating] China's [own] Red Cross Law" (Wang and Chen 2008, 103). This line of argument brought the case to the forefront of legislative attention, and in 1993, "the Standing Committee of National People's Congress officially promulgated the Red Cross Law of the People's Republic of China, which provides legal protection to the Chinese Red Cross and its work." Today, the Hong Kong and Macao Red Cross chapters enjoy "highly autonomous status" in China, but are governed by the PRC's own 1993 Red Cross Law, providing a template for the Red Cross as a marker of sovereignty if or when Taiwan "returns" (Red Cross Society of China n.d.).[12]

According to the Chinese Red Cross, the period from 1987 to 1999 was one of considerable growth. The organization raised more than two billion renminbi in contributions. By 1993, 99.5 percent of China's provinces and regions and 90 percent of its counties had Red Cross branches, with a total of 140,000 branches and 19,000,000 members (Gu 1994, 225). During this period, the Red Cross echoed its post-WWII work building bridges with former enemies by serving as a conduit for people-to-people exchanges with Taiwan, and continuing its traditional work with medical philanthropy (Gu 1994, 264–274).

A Second Century of Work: 2004–2104

The national Red Cross Society of China has begun its resurgence as a quasi-private charity, a GONGO (government-operated nongovernmental organization) through which Chinese individuals can show their concern for fellow citizens.[13] The society's name and mandate are well-recognized across China, and this "brand name recognition" is important within China, as it has been since the early twentieth century. As in many countries, the Red Cross symbol, although protected fiercely by the ICRC, has become synonymous with health care provision. The Red Cross runs over two thousand hospitals across China (Evans 2012). On the emergency relief front, the 2008 Sichuan earthquake showcased the organization on both a national and an international stage, and the Red Cross provided the main venue through which private funds were collected for relief (Teets 2009, 338, 340, 342). The domestic Red Cross organization is trusted by the Chinese government, and thus the government relies on the society to carry out many of its social welfare duties.

The Red Cross Society of China is also active in domestic public health work, such as a national campaign involving blood donation (since 1982) and tobacco control. Although the Red Cross's recent public health campaigns have met with varied success—organ donation being a particularly hard sell in a Confucian country where the body is seen as a sacred gift from one's parents (Chao and Sommer 2011)—the prominent role the Red Cross plays and is asked to play demonstrates how uniquely positioned and irreplaceable this quasi-governmental organization is in the context of China. Despite what many saw as negative publicity in a series of scandals in 2011—elaborate banquets funded by donations (Xinhua 2011), glamorous Red Cross "associates" boasting Maseratis and fancy handbags (Hong and FlorCruz 2011), and mysterious "Red Cross training fees" collected along with driver's license payments—when seen from a distance, the overall domestic picture for the Society looks positive.

The public's obvious interest and pride in the organization and its much-used internet watchdog capabilities show an organization that is subject to a civic-minded national community which demands that it be worthy of its public support. In fact, this unofficial oversight has already brought significant change to the Red Cross Society of China. In August 2012, in direct response to the scandals of the previous year, Executive Vice President of the Red Cross Zhao Baige announced a "top-down reform in the organization to address existing problems and gradually meet public expectations" (*China Daily* 2012). The speed of the Society's response to the scandals and its subsequent crackdown on corruption has not gone unnoticed by China's citizens. While the overall feeling toward the Chinese Red Cross as of this writing is still negative, time will heal some of the distrust as the Society continues to try to eradicate corruption, improve transparency in its operations, and continue its good work.

This kind of financial scandal in the context of philanthropic work is neither new nor in any way specific to China or any other country. Other national Red Cross Societies have been similarly marred by unscrupulous principals. For example, the American Red Cross has been plagued by constant scandals in the last decade: fundraisers donating charitable contributions to their own bank accounts, chapter managers embezzling donations to support drug habits, and a CEO of a major chapter stealing more than a million dollars from the American Red Cross to fund his and his lover's gambling habit (Holguin 2009). These figures may seem small in the Chinese context, but the response to these scandals bears analysis. These embarrassments—crimes!—go all but unnoticed in the American context, as do similar scandals in the international community (or they pass quickly from public attention, as did rock star Bono's One Foundation scandal), whereas in China, the national audience expects more, demands more, and is already getting a more responsible, responsive charitable organization because of its watchdog stance and its optimistic belief in the potential of the Red Cross organization (Blucher 2012).

On the international front, the ICRC and the Federation of National Red Cross and Crescent Societies are cognizant of and work with the Chinese national society and government. Programs sponsored by the ICRC are run in China to educate the Chinese army and the larger public on the tenets of international humanitarian law, a mandate of the Red Cross movement. The international humanitarian community needs to continue this trend, to embrace China's potential role as a major Red Cross participant, and to bring China back into the fold of its supporters. The national society could play an important role in working with the government to encourage this facet of soft-power creation, and the Chinese Red Cross could emerge as a major powerhouse in the public health philanthropy community.

In the twenty-first century, as China's potential to participate in global humanitarianism grows, China's current "state-centric" approach to the humanitarian enterprise is considered suspect, and this suspicion often revolves around the relationship between the Chinese Red Cross and the Chinese government. Yet most Red Cross Societies are linked to their sponsoring government—even the American Red Cross, often considered a "private charity," is deeply linked to the American state (Allen 2005).[14] The Chinese Red Cross's position vis-à-vis its government is neither outstanding, surprising, nor cause for undue concern: the relationship between the two is simply more transparent than in many other nations.

The Red Cross in China is built on a philanthropic tradition that goes back more than one thousand years, and it has organized international humanitarian activities for over one hundred years. These traditions have emerged in cooperation with the state, rather than in opposition to it. Their legitimacy and efficacy are no less valuable than Western traditions or conceptions of compassion, philanthropy, and humanitarianism. Historically and culturally contingent, suspicion of the state's role in the humanitarian enterprise is not an immutable, insurmountable tenet of humanitarianism. As Pichamon Yeophantong has observed, "Humanitarianism is not static, nor monolithic. It *has* evolved and it *is* influenced by a variety of historical and political factors" (cited in Hirono and O'Hagan 2012, 8). China's pre-Maoist history plays an important role in China's future—and indeed, in the future of the rest of the world. To develop a truly global notion of humanitarianism, then, we need first to understand and then to embrace this Asian tradition of philanthropy, to appreciate how even Western notions of humanitarianism can vary through time and space, and to try to incorporate these ideas into our "universalist" principles.

Notes

1. Articles in the *Shenbao* written by Shen prominently proclaim the Red Cross's intrinsic neutrality; for example, he provides a translation of the Red Cross Treaty (the Geneva Convention), which immediately discusses neutrality, in *Shenbao*, March 30, 1904, 3.

2. The map showing the locations of Red Cross chapters across China, included in the society's 20th anniversary celebration volume (Central Committee of the Red Cross Society 1924), is a stunning visual that reveals the depth of Red Cross penetration across China's hinterlands (see map 11.1).

3. Unfortunately, few of these stories have been documented except in Red Cross–sponsored hagiographies. The history of the Japanese Red Cross is an exception; see Olive Checkland's work.

4. There is much confusion over the actual date of China's adherence to this convention and to the Geneva Convention of 1906. For documents on China's participation in the early Geneva Conventions, see the Academia Sinica's Waiwubu Archives, section 02-21, Baohehui, Hongshizihui (the Hague Conventions and Red Cross Society), Academia Sinica, Nangang, Taiwan.

5. The lack of an internationally recognized national Red Cross Society is still considered a telltale sign of a certain international precariousness; consider, for example, the cases of Israel and Taiwan. Similarly, groups and states that do not recognize the sanctity of the Red Cross symbol are dismissed as "barbaric" or "rogue states"; see, for example, Ignatieff (1997, 109–163).

6. Sidney Brown, "Report [to the ICRC] from Mr. Sidney H. Brown on his Stay in China from 17 December 1934 to 15 January 1935," January 18, 1935, 4–5, ICRC Archives CR00/14, Geneva (translated from the French). This report is quite different than the one presented to the Chinese Red Cross. This assessment is echoed in much more disparaging tones in the new managing director Y. S. Tsao's 1936 *China Quarterly* article.

7. Ibid.

8. Sidney Brown, "Memorandum Submitted to the Red Cross Society of China," January 14, 1935, ICRC Archives CR00/14.

9. Chinese Red Cross, "Letter, February 12, CRC to ICRC," 1943, ICRC Archives CR00/14.

10. The Taiwanese account concurs with this assessment, although the word it uses for those who stayed, "xian" (defected), is different (Zhang 2004, 343).

11. This decision would eventually so divide the ICRC that from 1957 to 1965, the International Conference of the Red Cross and Crescent would suspend meetings (Buignon 2009, 677).

12. Red Cross Societies have frequently served as markers of sovereignty in the past. For an earlier instance in China, see Reeves (2011).

13. This public involvement was amply demonstrated by the online outpouring of support after the 2008 Sichuan earthquake (Nicholas 2012, 68).

14. Despite the biased source of this article (the *Socialist Worker*), the information included is actually quite accurate. "People who think of the [American] Red Cross as a 'private charity,'" its author writes, "would be shocked to discover its actual legal status. Congress incorporated the Red Cross to act under 'government supervision.' Eight of the fifty members of its board of governors are appointed by the president of the United States, who also serves as honorary chairperson. Currently [in 2005, when this article was written], the Secretaries of State and Homeland Security are members of the board of governors. This unique, quasi-governmental status allows the Red Cross to purchase supplies from the military and use government facilities—military personnel can actually be assigned to duty with the Red Cross. Last year, the organization received $60 million in grants from federal and state governments. However, as one federal court noted, 'A perception that the organization is independent and neutral is equally vital.'"

References

"Accession de la Chine à la Convention de Genève" [China's Adherence to the Geneva Convention]. 1904. *Bulletin International des Sociétés de la Croix-Rouge* 35 (139): 190.

Allen, Joe. 2005. "The Truth about the Red Cross." *Socialist Worker,* October 21. http://socialistworker.org/2005-2/562/562_04_RedCross.shtml.

Baudendistel, Rainer. 2006. *Between Bombs and Good Intentions: The Red Cross and the Italo-Ethiopian War.* New York: Berghahn Books.

Beijing zazhi [*Beijing* magazine]. 1904a. "Yanshuo Hongshizihui jinggao quanguo" [Addressing the Nation about the Red Cross Society Imperial Decree]. No. 2 (Guangxu 30.5.30): 22–23.

Beijing zazhi [*Beijing* magazine]. 1904b. "Wanguohongshizihui zhangcheng" [Constitution of the International Red Cross Society]. No. 3 (Guangxu 30.8.30): 32–36.

Best, Geoffrey. 1980. *Humanity in Warfare.* New York: Columbia University Press.

Blucher, Alexandra. 2012. "Red Cross Society of China Reforms." November 6. http://english.cri.cn/7146/2012/11/06/2702s731280.htm.

Boissier, Pierre. 1963. *Histoire du Comite International de la Croix-Rouge de Solferino a Tsoushima* [The History of the International Committee of the Red Cross from Solferino to Tsoushima]. Paris: Plon.

Buignon, Francois. 2009. "The International Conference of the Red Cross and Red Crescent: Challenges, Key Issues and Achievements." *International Review of the Red Cross* 91 (876): 675–712.

Central Committee of the Red Cross Society. 1924. *Zhongguo Hongshizihui ershi zhounian jiniance* [The 20th Anniversary Celebration of the Red Cross Society of China]. Shanghai: Central Committee of the Red Cross Society.

Chao, Sunny, and Gisela Sommer. 2011. "China's New Organ Donation Registry Unlikely to Take Off." *Epoch Times,* May 1. http://www.theepochtimes.com/n2/china-news/chinas-new-organ-donation-registry-unlikely-to-take-off-55639.html.

Checkland, Olive. 1994. *Humanitarianism and the Emperor's Japan.* New York: St. Martin's.

Chi Zihua, ed. 2005. *Zhongguohongshizihui lishibiannian 1904–2004* [A Chronological History of the Red Cross Society of China, 1904–2004]. Hefei: Anhui People's Publishing.

China Daily. 2012. "Red Cross Society Promises Reforms." August 3. http://www.china.org.cn/china/2012-08/03/content_26111618.htm.

Culp, Robert. 2007. "Synthesizing Citizenship in Modern China." *History Compass* 5 (6): 1833–1861.

Evans, Michael. 2012. "China's Red Cross Fights Online Rumors as Hospital Investigation Continues." *Asian Correspondent Online*, November 8. http://asiancorrespondent .com/91650/chinas-red-cross-fights-online-rumors-as-hospital-investigation -continues/.

Gu Yingji, ed. 1994. *Zhongguohongshizihuide jiushinian* [Ninety Years of the Red Cross Society of China]. Beijing: China Friendship Press.

Hirono, Miwa, and Jacinta O'Hagan, eds. 2012. *Cultures of Humanitarianism: Perspectives from the Asia-Pacific*. Canberra: ANU College of Asia & the Pacific Department of International Relations.

Holguin, Jaime. 2009. "Disaster Strikes in Red Cross Backyard." CBS News, February 11. http://www.cbsnews.com/stories/2002/07/29/eveningnews/main516700.shtml.

Hong Haolan, and Jaime FlorCruz. 2011. "Red Cross China in Credibility Crisis." CNN World, July 6. http://www.cnn.com/2011/WORLD/asiapcf/07/06/china.redcross/index .html.

Hongshizihui yuekan [Red Cross Monthly]. 1946. "Huixun" [Society News] Section. December 31, 2.

Hutchinson, John. 1996. *Champions of Charity: War and the Rise of the Red Cross*. Boulder, CO: Westview.

Ignatieff, Michael. 1997. *The Warrior's Honor: Ethnic War and the Modern Conscience*. New York: Metropolitan Books.

Mann, Susan. 1987. *Local Merchants and the Chinese Bureaucracy, 1750–1950*. Stanford, CA: Stanford University Press.

Mitter, Rana. 2011. "Classifying Citizens in Nationalist China during WWII, 1937–1941." *Modern Asian Studies* 45 (2): 243–275.

Moorehead, Caroline. 1998. *Dunant's Dream: War, Switzerland, and the History of the Red Cross*. New York: Carroll & Graf.

Nanjing Daxue Chubanshe. 1993. *Hongshizihui lishiziliao xuanbian, 1904–1949* [Selected Historical Documents of the Red Cross Society, 1904–1949]. Nanjing: Nanjing Daxue Chubanshe.

Nedostup, Rebecca. 2009. *Superstitious Regimes: Religion and the Politics of Chinese Modernity*. Cambridge, MA: Harvard University Press.

Nicholas, Jenna. 2012. "21st Century China: Does Civil Society Play a Role in Promoting Reform in China?" Unpublished thesis, Stanford University Center for Democracy, Development and the Rule of Law. http://iis-db.stanford.edu/docs/642/JENNA _NICHOLAS.pdf.

Qu Zhe, ed. 1999. *Zhongguohongshizi shiye* [The Accomplishments of the Red Cross Society of China]. Guangzhou: Guangdong Economics Press.

Red Cross Society. *Red Cross Society Articles of Association*. 1912. Shanghai: Red Cross Society.

Red Cross Society of China. n.d. Accessed December 11, 2013. http://www.china.org.cn /english/MATERIAL/132108.htm.

Reeves, Caroline. 1998. "The Power of Mercy." PhD diss., Harvard University.

——. 2005. "From Red Crosses to Golden Arches? China, the Red Cross, and the Hague Peace Conference, 1899–1900." In *Interactions: Regional Studies, Global Processes, and Historical Analysis*, edited by Jerry Bentley, 64–93. Honolulu: University of Hawaii Press.

———. 2011. "Sovereignty and the Chinese Red Cross Society: The Differentiated Practice of International Law in Shandong, 1914–1916." *Journal of the History of International Law* 13 (1): 155–177.

"Reconnaissance de la Societe Chinoise de la Croix-Rouge" [Recognition of the Chinese Red Cross Society]. 1912. *Bulletin International des Sociétés de las Croix-Rouge* 43 (169): 8–9.

Richard, Timothy. 1916. *Forty-Five Years in China.* New York: Frederick A. Stokes.

Shenbao. 1904. "Shijun Zhaoji biyi Shanghai chuangshe Wanguohongshizizhihui huiyi dazhi" [Mr. Shi Zhaoji Translates an Account of the Meeting Creating the Shanghai International Red Cross Society]. March 14.

Teets, Jessica C. 2009. "Post-Earthquake Relief and Reconstruction Efforts: The Emergence of Civil Society in China?" *China Quarterly* 198 (June): 330–347.

Tiao Shui Waishi [pseud.]. 1911. *Shen Dunhe.* Shanghai: Jicheng Tushugongsi.

Tsao, Y. S. 1936. "The Red Cross Society in China." *China Quarterly* 1 (4): 55–63.

Xinhua and Staff Reporter. 2011. "China's Red Cross Banquet Scandal." *China Times*, April 20. http://www.wantchinatimes.com/news-subclass-cnt.aspx?id=20110420000103&cid=1103.

Wang Ronghua, and Chen Hanxi. 2008. "International Institutions and the Chinese Red Cross Legislation." *Chinese Journal of International Politics* 2:73–108.

Watt, John. 2014. *Saving Lives in Wartime China: How Medical Reformers Built Modern Healthcare Systems Amid War and Epidemics, 1928–1945.* Boston: Brill.

Wong, K. Chimin, and Wu Lien-Teh. 1985. *History of Chinese Medicine.* 2nd ed. Taipei: Southern Materials Center.

Zhang Yufa, ed. 2004. *Zhonghua Minguo Hongshizihui bainian huishi, 1904–2003* [An Organizational History of One Hundred Years of the Red Cross Society of the Republic of China 1904–2003]. Taibei: Red Cross Society of the Republic of China.

Zhongguo Hongshizihui zazhi [Chinese Red Cross Society magazine]. 1913. "Zhongguo Hongshizihui guoquji jianglai" [The Chinese Red Cross Society, Past and Future]. May: 1–4.

12 More than Mercy Money

*Private Philanthropy for
Special Health Needs*

Li Fan

Background and Introduction

This chapter examines Chinese innovation in philanthropy for people with disabilities and other special health needs. According to the Second China National Sample Survey on Disability, conducted in 2006, approximately 83 million people in China—around 6 percent of the population—are considered to be disabled. The Chinese term used itself reflects how much has changed for those with special health needs: now called *canji*, a compound with a literal meaning close to "incomplete and ill," disabled persons had previously been pejoratively called *canfei,* or "incomplete and useless." The change in their standing goes beyond mere semantics, however. Economic development and the rapid growth of private wealth in China over the past five years, and the attendant boom in philanthropy, have made more resources available to support this population than ever before. Newly wealthy families with firsthand experience of the challenges faced by people living with disabilities have started foundations to tackle neglected and marginalized health problems, and, in pursuing such philanthropy, have developed many innovations particularly suited to the Chinese context. This chapter characterizes these developments through six case studies and concludes with a call for continuing public education and advocacy for people with special health needs in China, as well as new approaches to help nonprofit organizations become sustainable and self-sufficient, and thus capable of better serving the special health needs community in the future.

The overall living conditions and social status of people with disabilities in China have greatly improved in the past 30 years due to a series of administrative and legislative actions, as well as the tireless work of organizations dedicated to helping those with special health needs. The most powerful and widely influential organization in this area has been the China Disabled Persons' Federation (CDPF), or *Zhongguo canji ren lianhe hui*, founded in 1988. CDPF is a ministerial-level governmental disability advocacy organization founded by Deng Pufang, the son of Deng Xiaoping. Paralyzed due to a broken back suffered during the Cultural Revolution, Deng was the prime mover behind a national survey of people with disabilities in 1987, which resulted in the establishment of the Law on the Protection of Persons with Disabilities (*Zhonghua renmin gongheguo canji ren baozhang fa*) in 1991. The law is the most important legal decree that protects the rights of people with special health needs in China, containing 54 articles that address rehabilitation, education, employment, cultural life, welfare, physical accessibility, and legal liability. As the official state representative body for disabled communities in China, CDPF participated in the amendment of the law, as well as in investigations, inspections, and visits by members of the National People's Congress and the National People's Political Consultative Committee to both monitor enforcement of the law and evaluate its efficacy.

In the Law on the Protection of Persons with Disabilities, the term "disabled persons" (*canji ren*) is used in reference to people with visual, aural, linguistic, bodily, intellectual, psychological, multiple, and other disabilities.[1] In China, the definitions of disabilities and the criteria for classifying them have been strongly influenced by a medical model of disability, and in particular by the International Classification of Impairments, Disabilities, and Handicaps (ICIDH) developed by the World Health Organization in 1980. Used internationally as a tool for social policy, the ICIDH has been amended many times since its original formulation. Today it is known as the International Classification of Functioning, Disability, and Health (ICF), and stresses the social aspects of disability, including contextual and environmental factors.

With medically focused solutions moving toward a conceptual framework that recognizes that people are disabled by environmental factors as well as by their bodies, international initiatives such as the United Nations Standard Rules on the Equalization of Opportunities of Persons with Disabilities have incorporated a concern for the human rights of people with disabilities, culminating in 2006 with the adoption of the United Nations Convention on the Rights of Persons with Disabilities (CRPD). In April 2008, China amended the law and introduced for the first time content regarding the "prohibition of discrimination on the grounds of disability." In line with international standards, the Chinese government has moreover formulated and implemented several hundred sets of national standards relating to barrier-free construction practices and the provision of devices to assist people with disabilities.

In March 2010, China's State Council issued its Guiding Opinions on Accelerating the Promotion of the Social Security System and Services System for

Persons with Disabilities (*Guanyu jiakuai tuijin canjiren shehui baozhang tixi he fuwu tixi jianshe de zhidao yijian*). The guiding opinion requires that a social security system and a social service system for people with disabilities be established by 2020 to ensure that people with disabilities are guaranteed a basic livelihood, including essential medical care and rehabilitation services.

This will not be easy to achieve. According to the report *Implementation of the Convention on the Rights of Persons with Disabilities* submitted to the United Nations by the Chinese government in August 2010, the per capita income of urban families of people with disabilities in 2009 was 8,578 RMB, as compared with the national per capita income of urban families of 17,175 RMB. The per capita income of rural families of persons with disabilities was only 4,066 RMB. Until December 2009, 2.4 million disabled people in urban areas and 6.2 million in rural areas—around 10 percent of the entire disabled population—were receiving the minimum subsistence allowance.[2] The monthly allowance is only available to people who applied for and were certified as "disabled," with the amount varying by city and region. For example, autism was officially recognized as a "mental disability" in 2006. According to a national survey conducted by the Shenzhen Autism Research Network, 50 percent of the interviewed families spent over 50 percent of their monthly expenses on rehabilitation treatment; government support only accounts for around 8 percent of the costs (Shenzhen Autism Society 2012, 78–79). Families that live in big cities can receive up to 200 RMB per month; one family from a small town said that they received "a bag of rice" as an allowance from the local authorities.

The report also stated that 6.2 million people with disabilities—about 8 percent of the entire disabled population—received varying types of rehabilitation services in 2009. In recent years, the Chinese government has invested 711 million RMB to implement its Salvage Therapy and Rehabilitation Project for Poor Children with Disabilities (*Pinkun canji ertong qiangjiuxing kangfu xiangmu*). However, as the Enable Disability Studies Institute (*Yi neng yi xing shenxin zhang'ai yanjiusuo*) pointed out in its *Observation on the Implementation of CRPD in China*, Chinese law's great emphasis on the importance of rehabilitation as a medical treatment to "fix the physical problems" of people with disabilities means that less attention is paid to rehabilitation as a long-term process aimed at facilitating the inclusion of disabled people in society (Enable Disability Studies Institute 2010, 9). This is particularly important for people with mental disabilities and autism.

With regard to education, the report stated that by the end of 2009, 1,672 special schools had been established nationwide, serving some 428,000 blind, deaf, or mentally disabled children and teenagers. Although these numbers seem to indicate progress in this area, they do not reveal anything about the quality of education. China has a mixed system of "inclusive education" by mainstream schools and "special education" by special schools for children and teenagers with disabilities. In theory, children or their parents choose a mainstream or special school, with most children who have a modest level of physical or mental disability preferring to be enrolled in the mainstream school system. The Law on the Protection of People with Disabilities stipulates in Section 25 that "ordinary primary and junior high schools must accept children with disabilities who are able to adapt themselves to life and study there." The schools are not obliged to improve accessibility on campus to include these children, and as such the duty of "being adaptable" is placed on the disabled children. As a result, the majority of children with disabilities cannot go to normal schools. According to a 2009 survey conducted by CDPF, 42 percent of disabled people aged 18 years or older have never been to school in their entire life (China Disabled Persons' Federation 2010, 12).

Educational barriers also result in employment difficulties for people with special health needs. For decades, China employed many disabled people in subsidized "welfare factories," where they performed simple tasks for modest salaries. Economic reform resulted in the closing of money-losing state industries and closed many of these so-called welfare factories. Currently, the Chinese government has a proportional employment allocation system for people with disabilities. Employers who fail to meet the quota have to pay a fine, but most companies are reluctant to hire people with disabilities or to offer them a fair wage. The Enable Disability Studies Institute pointed out in its report *Observation on the Implementation of CRPD in China* that many companies purchase the ID of a disabled person instead of actually hiring them, or simply falsify their numbers of disabled employees (Enable Disability Studies Institute 2010, 5).

Despite the unique political power of CDPF and its efforts to support China's disabled population, there are still huge gaps. Private philanthropy has the opportunity to play a key role in developing new sources of funding and social services for China's large disabled population. Supporting the disabled community has long been considered the government's responsibility, but since over 40 percent of the disabled population have literacy problems and 70 percent are unemployed, their livelihood largely depends on family members. Poverty is thus a common characteristic of households with disabled family members. Furthermore, the barriers to involving disabled communities in social life and in public matters are still very high, a reflection of low public awareness of their difficult living conditions.

Among people with disabilities, there are a growing number of people with impairments that have yet to be recognized by the law or the government as "disabilities," including children and teenagers with cerebral palsy and brittle bone disease. Since no social or medical benefits are available to them, familial financial difficulties mean that many of these children do not receive timely medical treatment and rehabilitation. Facing enormous economic and psychological pressure, parents of these children often find themselves isolated and hopeless, leading to extreme behavior. In November 2010, for instance, a mother in Dongguan city killed her thirteen-year-old twin boys and committed suicide. Both children were born with cerebral palsy, and the mother could no longer afford to take care of them at home (Sun 2011).

The economic development and rapid growth of private wealth in the past five years has generated a boom in philanthropy, with a range of philanthropists and foundations eager to put their money to good use. More resources from private wealth and public giving are available to support people with special health needs, and grassroots initiatives have been established to put those resources to work serving those in need. The founders of these nonprofit initiatives, often hailing from the disabled community or having disabled family members, work tirelessly to learn from the best practices of other countries, to use their social networks to raise awareness among the general public, and—most importantly—to improve the living conditions of disabled communities. At the same time, innovative approaches, such as social enterprises, have been adopted to support people with special health needs in a sustainable way.

Private Philanthropy's Outreach to the Special Health Needs Community: From Financial Aid to Social Inclusion

The growing force of philanthropists, foundations, and nonprofit organizations in China supports the disabled community through three main types of initiatives: financial support to people with special health needs and their families, to help them receive timely medical treatment and escape poverty; education and rehabilitation courses for disabled people, especially children and teenagers with rare diseases and with mental and physical disabilities; and activation of the special talents of disabled communities, providing skill training and facilitating job creation so that disabled people are able to secure working opportunities, support themselves financially, and better integrate into society.

The Smile Angel Foundation

The Smile Angel Foundation was founded in 2006 by celebrity couple pop star Faye Wong and actor Li Yapeng to help children born with cleft palates. The foundation is named after the couple's daughter, who was born in the same year with a severe cleft palate. The Smile Angel Foundation was the first family foundation registered under the umbrella of the Chinese Red Cross Society. Although the Regulations on the Management of Foundations were enacted in June 2004 to encourage giving by a growing wealthy class in China, the rapid growth of private foundations did not really start until 2007.[3] Before that time, truly private foundations were virtually impossible, meaning that collaborating with large GONGOs such as the Chinese Red Cross Society was the only option for those organizations wishing to receive public donations.

According to research conducted by the Smile Angel Foundation in November 2007, there are around 2.4 million Chinese children with cleft lips and palates, with over 30,000 babies born with them in China every year (Smile Angel Foundation n.d.). A large number of these children go untreated, and some are even abandoned by their parents due to the expensive cost of surgical repair. In rural areas and in western China, very few local doctors and facilities are capable of performing the surgery. Furthermore, continuous physical and psychological support is needed after the surgery so these children can attend school instead of facing difficult lives filled with shame and isolation.

The Smile Angel Foundation provides free surgery to children under 14 years old who cannot afford the surgical procedure. The foundation partners with nine hospitals throughout China, in Beijing, Tibet, and Xinjiang, among other places. Smile Angel also organizes routine medical trips to remote areas for patients without access to hospitals and clinics. As of February 2011, the foundation had provided over eight thousand free surgeries for poor families nationwide.

After five years of work, Li Yapeng realized the limitation of partnering with large state hospitals that treat millions of patients in total every day, and decided that a specialized hospital was needed to provide long-term, systematic support to children born with cleft palates. In May 2012, Smile Angel launched the first children's charity hospital in Beijing's Wangjing district, its investment totaling 30 million RMB. The hospital provides surgery to children with cleft palates as well as post-surgical rehabilitation, including speech-language therapy and psychological treatment. The hospital aims to provide free service to six hundred underprivileged children each year; children from high-income families will be charged for medical treatment and the resulting profits will be used to subsidize the charitable gifts.

Although the Smile Angel Foundation is well known in China and benefits from the fame of Faye Wong, 90 percent of its donations have come from the couple's celebrity friends and their social connections. The foundation raised over 70 million RMB at its annual fundraising dinner in 2009, for example. Publicly, Li Yapeng has announced that attracting small donations from the general public will be the foundation's main goal in the future, and on its website the foundation has promised to spend less than 10 percent of all donations on administrative costs. Smile Angel was selected as one of the 10 most influential charities in 2009 by the minister of civil affairs.

The Beijing Stars and Rain Autism Education Institute

According to research published in April 2012 by Beijing Normal University's China Philanthropy Research Institute, there are an estimated 1.6 million children with autism in China (Beijing Normal University 2012). The Beijing Stars and Rain Autism Education Institute is China's first and perhaps best-known nongovernmental education agency for children with autism. Until the 1990s, there was an overall lack of knowledge about autism in China, and families were unable to find education and treatment for their children. When Stars and Rain was founded in 1993 by Tian Huiping, whose son Yang Tao had been diagnosed as autistic in 1989, no such educational institutes or medical services were available. Tian and her colleagues started the Applied Behavior Analysis (ABA) program with just six children in a small space inside a kindergarten. Widely recognized as a safe and effective treatment for autism, the program applies the techniques and principles of behavior analysis—which focuses on explaining how learning takes place—to bring about meaningful and positive behavioral change. In particular, ABA principles and techniques can foster basic skills such as looking, listening, and imitating, as well as complex skills such as reading, conversing, and interacting and communicating. After failing to pay rent to the kindergarten for two months, Tian was forced to leave and ended up paying home visits to the children and staying overnight with their parents so as to continue the program. Like many grassroots nongovernmental organizations (NGOs) in China in the 1990s, and still for millions of grassroots groups today, there are huge hurdles to achieving official NGO status due to China's underdeveloped legal and regulatory environment. Until recently, Stars and Rain encountered many crises, relying on donations and grants from international organizations.

Since its establishment, Stars and Rain has helped more than seven thousand children with autism and trained 210 teachers from all over China. Currently the institute has 27 employees, including 10 ABA teachers and 3 teachers in the training department. Stars and Rain's pre-school education program, which is based on ABA, helps children aged 3 to 12 as well as their parents. Since it is impossible to serve all the autistic children in China, Stars and Rain focuses on educating parents in the skills and techniques required to aid children in their daily lives. In order to spread its impact, it has fostered an outreach community among the families who have benefited from the training program, with parents who received training at Stars and Rain starting programs of their own upon returning to their home communities (Beijing Stars and Rain Autism Education Institute).

In 2005, Stars and Rain established a national alliance, the Heart Alliance Autism Network, which has grown to include 145 member organizations throughout China. Initially supported by Miserior (the German Catholic Bishops' Organization for Development Cooperation), the Heart Alliance Autism Network provides capacity-building courses and technical support to grassroots organizations that serve children with autism and their families. The network functions as a platform for information and resource sharing, and also aims to establish a coalition for advocacy to improve the living conditions of the autistic community.

In November 2006, Stars and Rain opened a group home to provide residential care and education for teenagers with autism aged 12 to 16 who cannot enroll in the regular education system. The teenagers live in the home from Monday to Friday and are taught practical skills using the TEACCH (Treatment and Education of Autism and Related Communication-Handicapped Children) methodology,[4] developed by German-American psychologist Eric Schopler at the University of North Carolina at Chapel Hill in the 1960s and still commonly used in U.S. public schools today. The group home aims to establish a model that can be replicated nationally so as to maximize the provision of care for autistic teenagers in China.

The One Foundation and Ocean Heaven Project

The rapid development in recent years of Stars and Rain and the Heart Alliance has been intimately connected with the work of the One Foundation. Formerly known as the Red Cross Society of China Jet Li One Foundation Project, it was founded by movie star Jet Li in strategic partnership with the Chinese Red Cross Society. In December 2010, the One Foundation successfully registered as a public foundation in Shenzhen, with registered capital of 50 million RMB.

In 2008 the One Foundation launched the One Foundation NGO Role Model Award to encourage and promote outstanding grassroots nonprofit organizations. Each award winner receives one million renminbi, the largest amount ever given in a single instance in the history of China's philanthropy sector. In 2009, Stars and Rain was selected as a million-renminbi award winner along with six other NGOs, among them the Shenzhen Autism Research Network, the most well-known autism-focused organization in southern China (One Foundation n.d.).

Through its role model award, the One Foundation became aware of the needs of autistic children and their families. In July 2011, Jet Li announced the launch of the Ocean Heaven Project, which aims to help autistic children with urgent needs for financial support, medical treatment, and education. The project reaches out to these children and their families through core support organizations—i.e., Stars and Rain, and members of the Heart Alliance Network—and its own network. The One Foundation invested ten million renminbi in the Ocean Heaven Project in 2011, supporting a total of 103 grassroots organizations nationwide aimed at helping children with autism and rare diseases. An estimated ten thousand children have benefited from the project (One Foundation 2011). In order to provide high-quality professional care and education to children with special health needs, the Ocean Heaven Project also aims to enhance the capacity-building of NGOs and educational institutes through training courses, regular seminars, and lectures.

Public Education and Advocacy to Raise Awareness of People with Special Health Needs

As a growing number of Chinese domestic NGOs and foundations take actions to support the disabled community, many of them have started to realize the limited number of people they can help relative to the huge number with need, the complex situation of the disabled in China, and the importance of advocacy in raising the government's and the public's awareness of the problems they face.

When Stars and Rain was established 20 years ago, there were only three doctors in China who had made the diagnosis of autism (Beijing Stars and Rain Autism Education Institute n.d.): in remote rural areas, many autistic children were simply considered to be mentally ill. The Heart Alliance Network helped spread awareness, linking organizations and parents' groups that support autistic children, but it was the One Foundation Ocean Heaven Project, with the network of the Heart Alliance as its foundation, that helped connect the autistic community and its families to the outside world. Key to its efforts was the nationwide broadcast in June 2010 of the film *Ocean Heaven*, which told the story of a father terminally ill with liver cancer, and his struggle to ensure the future safety and happiness of his 22-year-old autistic son. For many Chinese, this film marked the first time they realized that autistic children cannot be cured and become "normal children." A Stars and Rain volunteer wrote the script; a large part of the story was based on the life of the son of the founder of Stars and Rain. Jet Li not only discovered the script and played the father in the film, but through his personal connections helped enlist some of the most popular movie stars in China, as well as Oscar-winning musicians and photography crews, to work on it. *Ocean Heaven* was a success both financially and socially.

Named after the movie, the Ocean Heaven Project is now expanding its support to other children with rare diseases such as cerebral palsy and brittle bone syndrome. The China-Dolls Care and Support Association, an advocacy group that provides popular education on rare diseases in China, is another important participant in the project.

The China-Dolls Care and Support Association

Twenty-nine-year-old Wang Yi'ou, a brittle bone sufferer who endured frequent bone fractures throughout her childhood, founded China-Dolls in May 2008. Officially known as osteogenesis imperfecta (OI), brittle bone disease is a genetic disorder that often results in bone fragility and deformities. The name of the organization, a play on the common Western term for dolls made of glazed porcelain, signifies that OI patients are fragile and require gentle care.

Despite the fact that—according to research conducted by China-Dolls—there are around one hundred thousand people in China who suffer from OI, Wang did not meet anyone else with OI until she was in her twenties. "For a very long time my parents thought that I was the only person in China who had this horrible disease, and the feeling of isolation was almost unbearable," Wang recalled in a CCTV interview in 2010 (Wang 2010). The mission of the China-Dolls Care and Support Association is to increase social awareness and understanding of OI and other rare diseases; to reduce social discrimination against patients afflicted with these conditions; to ensure their equal rights to treatment, education, and employment; and to advocate for the development of policies to increase social benefits for people with rare disorders (China-Dolls Center for Rare Disorders n.d.).

The first project of China-Dolls was an informational website that provided medical advice and consultations to OI patients. Additionally, a bimonthly newsletter was distributed for free to readers who registered online, enabling China-Dolls to quickly gain access to over three hundred patients with OI around the country. In December 2008, China-Dolls conducted and published its *Livelihoods of People with Osteogenesis Imperfecta Research Report,* the first report of its kind in China. According to the report, OI patients in China face serious problems in medical treatment, education, and employment. Between 2007 and 2008, 37 percent of respondents had dropped out of school; more alarming still, 29 percent had never attended school. Since China's social welfare system does not cover medical treatment for rare diseases like OI, most patients have to rely on help from family members. Medication for each treatment costs between 1,500 RMB and 3,000 RMB, a monthly salary for many Chinese living in small and mid-sized cities.

According to the World Health Organization, rare diseases have a prevalence of between 0.65 and 1 percent of the total population (China Charity Federation Rare Diseases Relief Public Fund n.d.). But medications for rare diseases are in short supply because the pharmaceutical industry has little interest in developing "orphan drugs"—i.e., medications treating conditions so rare as to offer little potential for profit. Many countries, including the United States, Japan, Australia, and the members of the European Union, have laws that provide financial incentives for companies to develop such treatments. No such policies exist in China, and the cost of imported orphan drugs is prohibitively high.

Because the pool of OI patients is not large enough to attract attention from the general public and from policymakers, in 2009 China-Dolls collaborated with six rare-disease advocacy groups, including ones supporting patients afflicted with hemophilia and Duchenne muscular dystrophy, and submitted a proposal to the National People's Congress calling for new legislation to improve medical and social welfare support for the over ten million people with rare diseases in

China. The proposal also urged the government to support new drug research and development by the Chinese pharmaceutical industry so as to ease access to orphan drugs. In May 2011, Minister of Civil Affairs Li Liguo commented at a conference that children with rare diseases would soon be included in the social welfare system (*Jinghua Times* 2011).

In August 2009, China-Dolls set up a fund under the umbrella of the government-linked China Social Welfare Education Foundation. Open to public donations and dedicated to patients with rare diseases who need medical aid and other social services, the fund currently supports a medical aid project for OI patients under 18 years old; grants for young people with rare diseases who want to start their own businesses; and the publication of *Rare Disease in China* magazine to disseminate information on rare-disease issues. In 2009, China-Dolls became the only Chinese participant in International Rare Disease Day,[5] and in the 2011 Rare Disease Day campaign, China-Dolls launched an advocacy program that was widely reported on by national television, print media, and social media.

New Endeavors to Generate Resources to Support People with Special Health Needs

Today, the primary source of support for people with special health needs in China is their government stipend. Other financial support comes from foundations that collect public donations on their behalf and make private grants. In recent years, some organizations have started to adopt the social enterprise model, which generates income through the provision of services so as to make them sustainable and self-sufficient and thereby empower them to better serve the special health needs community in the long term. The CanYou Group is a good example of how a profit-making company can generate resources capable of providing lifetime support to the disabled.

The CanYou Group and the Zheng Weining Charity Foundation

The CanYou Group is a high-tech firm founded by Zheng Weining in 1999 and based in Shenzhen. Originally a small internet café, CanYao is now a group company with roughly 1,200 employees, many of whom are disabled young graduates who could not otherwise find employment. The name of the company, CanYou, means "friends of the disabled." Many disabled people in China see themselves as a burden on their family and society, but Zheng was an exception. Born with hemophilia and later diagnosed with diabetes and hepatitis, his conditions confined him to a wheelchair. In 1999, Zheng's mother died and left him three hundred thousand renminbi, which he used to launch a website called Disabled People 101, aimed at providing useful information for people like himself, such as tips on rehabilitation, dating, and job opportunities. In 2001, Zheng and his friends opened an internet café with five computers. That business having proved profitable, in 2002 Zheng started a software business with Li Hong, a physics graduate from Tsinghua University who had been diagnosed with progressive muscular dystrophy. With Li's help the company quickly developed from a website operator into a software and animation production company.

Today, CanYou is a multimillion-renminbi corporate group with 28 branches in Shenzhen, Zhuhai, and Hainan, and a client list that includes Microsoft, Intel, Bank of China, and other well-known national and international companies. CanYou chose to focus on information technology not only because of its high demand, but also because it has proven to be a sector in which disabled people have shown to be capable of matching and even exceeding the job performance of nondisabled people. Once the basic needs of daily life are met, disabled individuals—having developed significant mental discipline and fortitude in the process of coping with their condition—can sit patiently in front of a computer for a whole day, whereas some non-disabled people can more easily succumb to distraction.[6] Given the often tedious nature of software coding, this is a considerable virtue, and at CanYou, less-expert employees are often assigned such repetitive tasks as a first step toward mastering more complex ones.

Compared with other companies in the IT industry, CanYou has an extremely low employee turnover rate. One possible reason for this is that other companies do not offer similar benefits. As part of its compensation package, CanYou not only provides accommodation, laundry, and cooking services for its employees but also pays for medical insurance and offers lifelong employment with the promise of a pension. If health problems force workers to retire, the company will still pay their salary and house them in the company living facilities regardless of the length of their tenure with the company.

When social enterprises and social entrepreneurs became hot topics throughout China in 2008, CanYou started to gain recognition as a model social enterprise due to its success in providing both financial and social support to the disabled community. In 2009, Zheng established the private Zheng Weining Charity Foundation in Shenzhen and donated 90 percent of his personal stake in the company to it. As a result of the transfer of his shares, the foundation obtained ownership of the CanYou corporate group. The foundation decides the overall mission, strategy, and profit management policy of CanYou, while the company is responsible for providing jobs and making profits. In addition to establishing the foundation, CanYou also launched four nonprofit organizations under its umbrella, including the CanYou Social Service Agency for the Disabled and the China Volunteer Association for People with Special Needs. The CanYou Social Service Agency takes care of all the employees of CanYou after work, including meal delivery, on-site housing, and medical consultation services. The Volunteer Association, meanwhile, organizes events for users of the Disabled People 101 website. Every year the company donates one-third of its profits to the foundation.

The Shanghai Puki Coordination Agency for Deaf People

Another recent example of a successful social enterprise is the Shanghai Puki Coordination Agency, which aims to help young people with hearing problems find promising employment opportunities. Puki has an easy-to-remember and meaningful Chinese name for nondeaf people: it is referred to as *"xiaolong bao"* for short, which plays on the term for steamed Shanghai-style dumplings in a bamboo basket—both "basket" and "deaf" are pronounced *"long."* The organization's founder, Xiao Liang, believes that deaf people have certain affinities with these dumplings: although they look calm and unremarkable on the outside, they are quite hot, fiery, and passionate on the inside (Shanghai Puki Coordination Agency for Deaf People n.d.).

Xiao Liang is a healthy and happy young man whose philanthropic efforts are motivated not so much by his own experiences as by his empathy for others. While working in the aftermath of the 2008 Sichuan earthquake as a volunteer for an NGO that provides palliative care, he met a deaf designer who proceeded to introduce him to the deaf community in Shanghai. Discovering that most of the jobs available to Shanghai's 175,000 hearing-impaired residents entailed low-paid manual labor such as that of masseurs and cleaners, Xiao Liang concluded that their biggest obstacle in finding solid employment was communication. Companies willing to hire deaf people often have to spend extra money, time, and effort on training, while students from special schools for the deaf have little opportunity to learn how to communicate with the outside world before graduation.

In 2010, Xiao Liang—who then had six years' experience in the design and advertising industry—decided to quit his job and set up his own business, establishing a design company and coordination agency that provides internships and job opportunities to young people with hearing impairments. Puki provides a variety of design services—including logos and brochures, exhibition displays, event planning, and website design—for businesses, government agencies, and NGOs. Puki is now a team of six young people, four of whom are hearing impaired. Puki also established a "one-plus-one" internship program for students majoring in design and graphics at schools for the deaf in Shanghai. During the month-long internship, one deaf student is paired with one nondeaf student from the same major who knows sign language, and both are given the opportunity to participate in design work at Puki. At the end of the internship, excellent students are recommended to other design and advertising companies for an additional month-long internship. This two-month internship has proven to be a great opportunity for students to gain an advantage in securing jobs after graduation.

Puki is also actively working with writers and publishing houses to popularize sign language through picture books, which Xiao Liang hopes can help more people to communicate with the deaf. Puki generates its income mainly from its design services: Xiao Liang does not like to emphasize the charitable aspects of Puki, preferring to compete with other companies under the same rules. Even so, Puki benefits from the support of the Nonprofit Incubator (NPI), a nonprofit organization with offices in Shanghai, Beijing, Chengdu, and Shenzhen that incubates and supports grassroots NGOs and social enterprises. NPI provides free office space to Puki and introduces Puki to big companies, NGOs, and government agencies. With the help of NPI, Puki successfully registered as a nonprofit organization in Shanghai in August 2011.

Conclusion

Through financial assistance, education, and other support to the disabled population, these NGOs, foundations, and social enterprises are not only serving the community directly, but are also striving to educate the general public and address government policies that affect these populations. Through collaboration with the media and active use of social networks, they raise the general public's awareness of the living conditions and needs of people with disabilities. Through their advocacy roles, they also urge the government to provide a larger safety net to the disabled population.

As can be gleaned from the above cases, there are three key characteristics of how the young and growing Chinese philanthropic organizations working today to assist the special health needs community generate resources and raise awareness.

First, they are "insider-oriented." With very few exceptions, people with special health needs or their family members establish the majority of organizations that support them. Without their passion and devotion, and sometimes their self-sacrifice, most of these groups would not survive. Although an increasing number of people are starting to get involved as volunteers or donors, it is still quite rare for a complete "outsider" to take the initiative to fight for the rights of the disabled. Second, the celebrity effect has been a powerful force in attracting attention to special health needs populations. From Faye Wong and her Smile Angel Foundation to Jet Li and the One Foundation and the film *Ocean Heaven,* promotion by and engagement with well-known celebrities is the quickest way to raise public awareness, which is particularly important in a country as large and diverse as China. Finally, media and social media have increasingly played an important role, with successful organizations actively engaged with a variety of media ranging from CCTV and major newspapers to online media, blogs, and *weibo* (the Chinese version of Twitter). Another unique medium in China is so-called "touch media," interactive videos playing on screens installed in millions of taxis in major cities. In March 2011, as part of the campaign for International Rare Disease Day, NGOs participating in the Ocean Heaven Project released advertisements on touch media in Beijing, Shanghai, Shenzhen, and Guangzhou, generating an estimated 7.7 million plays.

While more private resources are becoming available to support people with special health needs in China, this philanthropic community remains relatively closed, consisting of stakeholders, related nonprofits, and a few foundations. Philanthropists, foundations, NGOs, and social enterprises are beginning to make a powerful impact on the disabled population through financial assistance, education, and other support. But sustained efforts are required to influence both the general public's awareness and policymaking. "Mercy money" is not enough. More innovative and comprehensive approaches are needed to truly help the 6 percent of the Chinese population with special health needs.

Notes

1. Law on the Protection of Persons with Disabilities (2008), http://www.gov.cn/jrzg/2008-04/24/content_953439.htm.

2. As part of the social protection system, China established a Minimum Livelihood Guarantee Scheme in 2003 for urban and rural residents whose per capita income is lower than the local minimum living standard.

3. Before 2004, very few foundations operated in China. The 2004 Regulations on the Management of Foundations defined the work scope of private foundations, differentiated between public and "non-publicly funded" (or private) foundations for the first time, and enhanced tax incentives for personal and corporate donations to foundations.

4. The organization's acronym represents its "core values": Teaching, Expanding, Appreciating, Collaborating and Cooperating, and Holistic (UNC School of Medicine).

5. Rare Disease Day was established in 2008 by the European Organization for Rare Diseases (EURORDIS). It is an observance held on the last day of February to raise awareness of rare diseases and to improve access to treatment and medical representation for individuals with rare diseases and their families.

6. Interviews with CanYou representatives were conducted by the author informally between 2008 and 2013 at conferences focusing on philanthropic issues. Since permission could not be obtained from the interviewees, their names have been withheld.

References

Beijing Normal University. 2012. "Baogao gu Zhongguo zibizheng huan er yu 160 wan, qi-cheng jiating nankan jingji zhongze" [Over 1.6 Million Children with Autism in China, 70% of Families Face Financial Crisis]. *Beijing Normal University News*, April 4. http://news.bnu.edu.cn/mtsd/44158.htm.

Beijing Stars and Rain Autism Education Institute [Beijing xingxing yu jiaoyu yanjiusuo]. n.d. Accessed December 12, 2011. http://www.guduzh.org.cn.

China Association of Disabled People Rehabilitation Department [Zhongguo can lian kang fu bu]. 2009. "Guduzheng ertong kangfu gongzuo xianzhuang, wenti ji duice" [The Present Situation, Challenges, and Responses in Rehabilitation Work for Autistic Children]. December 9. http://www.cnautism.com/Article/cnnews/200912/291.html.

China Charity Federation Rare Diseases Relief Public Fund [Zhonghua cishan zonghui hanjianbing jiuzhu gongyi jijin]. n.d. Accessed August 12, 2013. http://www.chinararedisease.cn/1-5-dingyi.html.

China Disabled Persons' Federation. 2010. *Monitoring Report on Status and Progress towards a Comfortable Life for Persons with Disabilities 2009.* http://www.cdpf.org.cn/ . . . /0026b978bfceof90d7b007.doc.

China-Dolls Center for Rare Disorders [*Ci wawa guanhuai xiehui*]. n.d. Accessed January 12, 2012. http://www.chinadolls.org.cn.

Committee on the Rights of Persons with Disabilities. 2010. *Implementation of the Convention on the Rights of Persons with Disabilities (China).* Report of the People's Republic of China State Party for the United Nations Committee on the Rights of Persons with Disabilities, August 30. http://www2.ohchr.org/SPdocs/CRPD/6thsession/CRPD-C-CHN-1_en.doc.

Enable Disability Studies Institute. 2010. *Observation on the Implementation of CRPD in China.* http://www2.ohchr.org/SPdocs/CRPD/6thsession/EDSIO_China_en.doc.

Hui Wang. "CanYou: High-Tech Firm for Disabled People." Zheng Weining Charity Foundation. Accessed December 3, 2013. http://www.zwncf.org/html/xinwenzhongxin/detail_2011_12/16/675.shtml.

Jinghua Times. 2011. "Aizi huan er jiang naru fuli baozhang fanwei" [AIDS-Infected Children Will Be Brought into the Purview of Welfare]. May 31. http://epaper.jinghua.cn/html/2011-05/31/content_665767.htm.

One Foundation [*Yi jijin*]. 2011. "Yi jijinhui Haiyang tiantang jihua quanmian qidong, wan ming teshu ertong shouyi" [One Foundation Ocean Heaven Project Benefits Ten Thousand Special Children]. November 11. http://onefoundationbj.blog.163.com/blog/static/12253685520111127311132538/

———. n.d. Accessed February 10, 2012. http://www.onefoundation.cn/html/en/introduction.htm.

Shanghai Puki Coordination Agency for Deaf People [Shanghai Xiaolong bao longren xieli shiwu suo]. n.d. Accessed February 10, 2012. http://www.pukidesign.org.

Shenzhen Autism Society [Shenzhen shi zibizheng yanjiu hui]. 2012. *Zibizheng renshi xianzhuang diaoyan fenxi baogao* [Investigative and Analytical Report on the Current Status of People with Autism]. The One Foundation. http://mat1.gtimg.com/gongyi/2012/zibizhengreport.pdf.

Smile Angel Foundation [Yanran tianshi jijin]. n.d. Accessed December 12, 2011. http://www.smileangelfoundation.org.

Sun Xuzhao. 2011. "Muqin nisi shuangbao tainaotan er an yishen xuanpan, Han Qunfeng huo xing 5 nian" [First Trial Verdict in a Case of a Mother Drowning Twin Children with Cerebral Palsy, Han Qunfeng Receives a Punishment of 5 Years]. Xinhua Net, June 28. http://news.xinhuanet.com/legal/2011-06/28/c_121595119.htm.

UNC School of Medicine. n.d. "About University of North Carolina TEACCH Autism Program." Acccessed December 3, 2013. http://teacch.com/about-us.

Wang Jing-Bo, Jeff J. Guo, Li Yang, Yan-De Zhang, Zhao-Qi Sun, and Yan-Jun Zhang. 2010. "Rare Diseases and Legislation in China." *Lancet* 375:708–709, doi:10.1016/S0140-6736(10)60240-1.

Wang Yiou. 2010. Interview. *Economy 30 Minutes.* CCTV Channel 2, July 27.

Zhang, Eric Guozhong. 2006. "Inclusion of Persons with Disabilities in China." *Asia Pacific Disability Rehabilitation Journal* 17 (2). http://www.aifo.it/english/resources/online/apdrj/apdrj206/inclusion-china.pdf.

13 Charitable Donations for Health and Medical Services from Hong Kong to Mainland China

David Faure

MEDICAL CHARITIES HAVE historically formed a key component of Chinese philanthropic organizations. Indeed, the linkage between philanthropy and physical well-being predates the advent of modern, scientific medicine; frequently this linkage had a religious cast. Traditional Chinese popular religion posits a spirit world closely integrated with that of the living, with spirits amenable to intercession in the affairs of the living if properly appeased through funeral rites and sacrifices. The exorcism ceremonies that have been held by Buddhist monasteries and village temples for centuries may be interpreted as philanthropy for both living and dead insofar as they ultimately serve the living: when the dead are appeased, the living are sheltered from disease, and appeasing the dead entails charitably satisfying their needs for food, clothing, and money. It is not far-fetched to say that beneficence, and especially medical charity, has always been a part of Chinese culture, and recognized as an essential part of social well-being.

The emergence of the hospital, along with the professionalization of medicine, may have reshaped philanthropic activity, but religious orientation and attachment to one's native place has continued to motivate modern health care philanthropy in China. One cannot however ignore the obvious Western origin of much of modern medicine, and the close association of medical service with missionary activity. On a cultural register, the turn toward modern medical charities has required Chinese institutions to take on two particular challenges: first, they have had to learn to accommodate modern medicine in its many forms, and, second, they have had to combine an informal attachment to their native place with formal practices concerning the control of funds, so as to make fundraising responsive and transparent to both donors and recipients. Philanthropic organizations in Hong Kong came to grips with such challenges over years of changes under the British colonial regime, and the continuation of this history is at the core of the philanthropic practices surrounding donations to mainland China today. This legacy empowers Hong Kong to play a unique and constructive role in the future of philanthropy for health in China by mediating between traditional prerogatives such as affinity for one's native place and international norms concerning organizational transparency and structure.

Medical Philanthropy as a Tradition in Hong Kong

The subtle shift in the history of Chinese philanthropic organizations in Hong Kong that took place toward the end of the 1860s was part and parcel of a much wider phenomenon embedded within Qing dynasty China's contact with the West. A similar process took place in many other cities with Chinese populations, including Chinese cities such as Shanghai and colonial cities with large overseas Chinese populations, such as Singapore and Batavia. The experience, as exemplified in Hong Kong, can be summarized as the application of Western ideas onto long-established Chinese practices for taking care of the ill and the deceased. In Hong Kong, that became the beginning of a major program in public hygiene, which, over time, led to government regulation of housing conditions and drainage, and the provision of clinics and hospitals for containing and treating contagious disease (Rogaski 2004).

In the late 1860s, the Hong Kong colonial government was shocked to find that the Chinese dead and dying were placed together in a communal temple that handled burial and sacrifice, and in 1870 it introduced the Tung Wah Hospital, a philanthropic institution run by local Chinese community leaders. In many ways, the Tung Wah Hospital retained strongly traditional Chinese characteristics. Its board of directors, for example, dressed in official robes for formal occasions, and paid annual homage to the gods of literary and martial skills housed in what was arguably the Hong Kong Chinese community's central temple. The hospital maintained a fierce dedication to the practice of Chinese traditional medicine, and, through its "coffin home," was engaged in the practice of shipping human remains from Chinese communities the world over back to the deceased's native place in China. Despite being very Chinese in sentiment, however, the hospital was closely supervised by the colonial government, and legislation enabled British officials to impose on it such un-Chinese administrative practices as the election of directors by members. Tung Wah was nonetheless a successful institution from its inception, and the colonial government recognized the dedication of its directors by consistently appointing one of its Chinese affiliates to the colonial legislative council from 1880 onward. This combination of recognition, contribution, and responsibility grounded in a strong communal consciousness proved key to Tung Wah's success (Sinn 1989; Ding 2010).

Still going strong today, the Tung Wah Hospital not only runs five hospitals but is moreover engaged in a wide variety of community services and educational initiatives. While it still champions the use of Chinese medicine—specifically, an integrated Chinese and Western medical approach to treatment—many of its doctors are trained in the Western medical tradition, and its hospitals are equipped with state-of-the-art Western-style medical facilities. Tung Wah is furthermore extremely successful in fundraising: in the 2011–2012 fiscal year (FY) alone, its income consisted of 293 million HKD (roughly $38 million) raised through donation and 353 million HKD (roughly $46 million) in rental income, the latter of which can be regarded as return on the investment of past donations. In addition, the Tung Wah is so well-established that it receives an annual subvention from the Hong Kong Special Administrative Region government on the order of 1.9 billion HKD (Tung Wah Group of Hospitals 2012, 183). Tung Wah is closely involved with the wider Hong Kong community as well: its annual fundraising extravaganza is a television hit, and it publishes information concerning its accounts and its governance structure annually.

In fast-moving Hong Kong, Tung Wah can in many senses be described as a traditional charity, though it has evolved considerably from the traditional charity that was built on folk religion. Still, it is important to recall the two extremes because much of Hong Kong charitable activity falls somewhere in between. The Buddhist charity Sik Sik Yuen—which runs the most popular temple in Hong Kong, the Wong Tai Sin Temple, which at Chinese New Year is thronged by believers seeking to have their fortune foretold by the resident deity—collects a donation income of 87 million HKD ($11 million) and an investment and rental income of 16 million HKD ($2 million), on top of a government subvention of 108 million HKD (roughly $13 million). It spends about 12 million HKD on medical services ranging from clinical care to dental services and from herbal medicines to acupuncture, but its temple still conducts communal exorcism ceremonies, and the god Wong Tai Sin answers prayers for medical cures by prescribing herbal medicines which the temple then distributes for free. As with Tung Wah, the tradition carried on by the religious side of the temple contrasts with the legalistic and modern aspects embodied by its financial and administrative structures. The temple, privately founded by a group of Daoists in the 1920s, is registered as a limited company engaged in charity, is governed by a member-elected board, is exempt from taxes, and publishes its certified accounts along with its annual report. Sik Sik Yuen even hires a CEO, who manages a staff of 600 people including 240 health care workers and 60 social workers (Sik Sik Yuen 2012, 86, 95).

Many other examples may be enumerated. The Chinese Temples Committee, a statutory body created in 1928 under chapter 153 of the Chinese Temples Ordinance, looks after some 40 temples as well as the General Chinese Charities Fund. Buddhist, Daoist, and Christian establishments run charities, including some well-supported hospitals. The institutions of the Tung Wah, in particular, have been replicated within the regional context of Hong Kong: the Pok Oi Hospital (with expenditures of 447 million HKD in FY 2011–2012, of which 32 million was raised via donation), was founded in 1919 and offers medical, educational, and social services to the northern parts of the New Territories; meanwhile, the Yan Chai Hospital (with expenditures of 767 million HKD in FY 2011–2012, of which 63 million was raised via donation) was founded in 1962 to serve Tsuen Wan district but has since extended its work to other parts of Hong Kong (Pok Oi Hospital 2012, 115; Yan Chai Hospital 2012, 210). As with Tung Wah and the Wong Tai Sin Temple, a substantial portion of the large discrepancies between donations and annual expenditures represents government subventions. The Hong Kong SAR has significantly maintained the legal framework of colonial days and requires strict financial accountability for philanthropic organizations. The Hong Kong SAR Inland Revenue Department (IRD) publishes on its website an 873-page list (with approximately 10 to 20 institutions per page) of charities operating in Hong Kong that have been granted tax-exempt status, many of which have religious or local connections (IRD 2013). The exceptions to this general rule tend to be specialist charities, some of which are affiliated with international organizations, such as Oxfam and Save the Children Fund. Hong Kong newspapers tend not to report on scandals connected with charity donations and expenditures in Hong Kong—a testament to the charities' integrity, the efficacy of rules concerning their transparency and accountability, their stature in the community, or some combination thereof. Tung Wah and the Wong Tai Sin temples are only two illustrations of a vibrant philanthropic scene characterized by extensive community involvement, and philanthropic donations to the Chinese mainland by Hong Kong residents must be seen in this context.

The Overseas Chinese Connection

Like other nineteenth-century colonial cities in Southeast Asia, British Hong Kong provided a haven for Chinese people. The Chinese diaspora and its related economic opportunities were closely tied to port cities such as Hong Kong, where steamships picked up passengers and banks handled the remittances they subsequently sent home. Some emigrants left for decades before returning, and many never did, but their bond with their native places was never broken. Temple steles recording donations for repairs in rural Hong Kong note that donations were collected not only from local people but also from former residents then living in Australia and the United States. The same donation pattern surfaced in contributions made to the revolutionary movement that in 1912 put Sun Yat-sen in power. It proved similarly effective on the local scale: villages with strong overseas-Chinese connections could afford more modern schools. Hospitals similar to Tung Wah could be found in Macau, Singapore, Bangkok, Cholon (today's Ho Chi Minh City), and San Francisco, and their directors were in constant communication concerning philanthropy.

Overall remittance was phenomenal, possibly accounting for 15 percent of all payments into China in 1930 (Remer 1968, 222). Nevertheless, until the beginning of the Sino-Japanese War in 1937, there were no systematic philanthropic donations from overseas Chinese to China—only sporadic donations in response to natural disasters (Deng 1910; Su and Wang 2010; Wu 2012). Most remittances were, moreover, sent to family members, though it would be reasonable to assume that some were subsequently directed toward more general local welfare—typically schools, policing, utilities, and transport, rather than medical service (Chen 1940). Explicit acts of philanthropy directed through institutional channels would typically involve Hong Kong, insofar as it served as the social hub of merchants within the huge overseas Chinese network. The directors of Tung Wah were closely involved with Guangzhou philanthropic associations, for instance, and Tung Wah's records show that they received donations from overseas that were subsequently directed to mainland China, especially for disaster relief.

Patriotism during the war years accounted for some donations from overseas Chinese, but seemingly not in very substantial amounts (Zeng 1988, 126–167). After 1949, Taiwan maintained strong connections with overseas Chinese associations, but in the People's Republic, the relationships of overseas Chinese with their hometowns were sundered by major policy shifts. With the advent of socialism in the 1950s and the total disruption of private trade and investment, no philanthropic donations as such were possible. By the time of the Great Proletarian Cultural Revolution, roughly 1966–1976, overseas Chinese connections were anathema to many in the mainland. When the economy opened up in the late 1970s, such connections resumed and provided sources of investment capital in both business and philanthropic senses (Young and Shih 2004). Initially, Hong Kong might have continued to serve as an intermediary for some donation efforts, but the pre-1949 philanthropic network no longer served as the nexus of philanthropic provisions. Before 1980, overseas Chinese channeled remittances home via Hong Kong, but since then, many would have likely sent donations directly to China. It is likely, therefore, that donations from Hong Kong to China prior to 1980 might well have originated outside of Hong Kong. Now that it is so easy to remit directly to China, donations from Hong Kong to China most likely come from donors in Hong Kong.

Donations to the Chinese Mainland

Hong Kong residents have a long tradition of sending gifts to families and friends back home, though this has, with the mainland's increasing prosperity, rapidly faded into the background. During the worst of times in the 1950s and 1960s, gifts took the form of food parcels, whereas by the 1980s, they were mostly daily necessities such as bicycles and refrigerators which could be purchased more readily in Hong Kong and then delivered to the mainland. By the 1990s, reform policies had

Table 13.1. Donations Earmarked for Health Care from Overseas Chinese and from Hong Kong, Macau, and Taiwan

Year	Donations (RMB)
1989	23,030,000
1990	104,530,000
1991	170,240,000
1992	391,540,000
1993	215,870,000
1994	320,070,000
1995	464,050,000
1996	18,600,000
1997	17,180,000
1998	88,360,000
1999	9,540,000
2000	4,940,000
2001	9,750,000
2002	4,520,000

Source: Guangdong Statistics Bureau, ed. 2004. *Guangdong Statistical Yearbook.* Beijing: Chinese Statistics Press, 489.

freed up the mainland's internal market—all that was needed was cash. Requests for donations were frequent, and any tour of villages in south China would reveal the vast amounts of overseas and Hong Kong investment in local reconstruction. It proved practically impossible to put numbers on those donations: in one instance where an educated attempt was made to do so, Zhang Guotao, on the basis of 29 major donors' activity in Xiamen, reckoned that through the 1990s Hong Kong donors donated 88 million HKD to that city. Donations to medical facilities did not constitute a major portion of the donations, which went toward education first and foremost—Xiamen University having attracted a substantial portion of the donations—and then toward other public services such as road and temple building (Zhuang 2001, 123–138; Guldin 1995 89–118).

The trend of making donations to one's native place has continued. Anecdotes aside, figures published by Guangdong Province show the sort of ebb and flow of donations from overseas Chinese and from residents of Hong Kong, Macau, and Taiwan. This might be expected based on China's soaring economic development. The data indicate that 23 million RMB was donated in 1989 toward health care, increasing steadily to 464 million in 1995 and declining very rapidly thereafter (see table 13.1). Donations from private individuals seem to have gone completely unrecorded.

Despite China's increasing prosperity, recent philanthropy has resembled that of the pre-1937 period insofar as it has focused on disaster relief. In response to the Wenchuan earthquake of 2008 alone, the Hong Kong public donated 18.7 million HKD, roughly matched by the pledges of 16 NGOs (for 17 million HKD); the total of these contributions was however a mere fraction of the 10.35 billion HKD pledged by the Hong Kong SAR government and by the Hong Kong Jockey Club, a nonprofit organization with a government-granted monopoly over horse racing and gambling which contributed roughly 1 billion HKD to that total.

Popular support was essential, certainly, for the donation of public funds to mainland China in emergency situations. Popular support also undoubtedly contributed in undetected ways, when individuals acting of their own accord donated to friends and relatives on the mainland, or through a volunteer service participated directly in relief work. Nevertheless, it seems probable that the business community would have been responsible for most such donations, with many—like those donations from small donors—going to their native places. Prominent among such major donors giving to their native places have been Sir Run Run Shaw, whose donation helped found the Sir Run Run Shaw Hospital in Hangzhou; Li Jiacheng (i.e., Li Ka-shing), whose donations have significantly if not exclusively been to Shantou; Huo Yingdong, who has given extensively to Guangzhou and specifically its Nansha district; Ho Shanheng, who has given to Guangzhou; and Tian Jiabing, who has given to Dabu in Guangdong. In terms of scope and magnitude, the Li Ka Shing Foundation has been the leader in the medical and health field, working closely with the China Disabled Persons' Federation (CDPF) to provide artificial limbs and training for disabled persons and with the Ministry of Civil Affairs to provide free operations for children suffering from hernias. (For linkages between the CDPF and Chinese mainland philanthropic organizations, see chapter 12.) Reflecting the donor's native-place connection, the foundation—together with the Hong Kong Chiu Chow Chamber of Commerce, the Federation of Hong Kong Chiu Chow Community Organizations, and other former Chaozhou resident associations in Hong Kong and elsewhere—runs rural clinics in Chaozhou and Shantou; moreover, Shantou University, to which the foundation contributes generously, operates numerous teaching hospitals in the region. Table 13.2, which builds on information culled from the internet, sets out those donations made from Hong Kong to the mainland by major philanthropists where place of origin might have been a motivating factor. Most of these donations have been made toward the provision of medical and health services, but even so, there is a preference, especially with the largest donations, for supporting universities. There is also a marked preference for supporting medical infrastructure, specifically the construction of buildings and the purchase of equipment. In terms of medical needs, donations tend to be channeled toward ophthalmology and the treatment of disability. Donors evince

Table 13.2. Major Medically Focused Donations to Native Place

Donor	Native Place	Donation Recipient(s)	Estimated Donation Amount
Sir Run Run Shaw Charitable Trust	Ningbo	Many, including Sir Run Run Shaw Hospital in Hangzhou, attached to the Zhejiang University School of Medicine	10 billion HKD (?)
Xing Liyuan	Wenchang, Hainan	The Yan Ai Foundation Ltd.; ultimate recipients include three medical facilities in Hainan	420 million HKD (100 million HKD to medical facilities)
Li Jiacheng (Li Ka-shing)	Chaozhou	The Shantou University Medical School and hospitals in Shantou	5.3 billion HKD (plus in-kind donations to hospitals)
He Shanheng	Panyu (Guangzhou)	Guangzhou Medical University; the Sun Yat-sen University Faculty of Medicine, a hospital in Zhuhai	50 million HKD
Huo Yingdong	Panyu	Hospitals throughout Guangdong Province and Guangzhou city, including Guangzhou Nansha Hospital	160 million HKD
Tian Jiabing	Hospitals in Meizhou and nearby counties		> 20 million HKD
Yang Hong and Brothers	Huizhou, Guangdong	The Gracious Glory (Buddhism) Foundation; ultimate recipients include several Huizhou towns and villages	2 million HKD worth of medical equipment
Liu Luanxiong	Chaozhou	The Sun Yat-sen University Faculty of Medicine	30 million HKD (in 2009)

Table 13.2. *continued*

Donor	Native Place	Donation Recipient(s)	Estimated Donation Amount
Chen Shouren	Quanzhou, Fujian	The Quanzhou Charity Association (since 2001); various local medical facilities providing cataract surgery, artificial limb fitting, and wheelchairs for the disabled (from 1980s until 2001)	> 10 million HKD
Zeng Xianzi	Meixian, Guangdong	Sun Yat-sen University No. 1 Hospital, Renmin University (for research on disability), Guangdong Province police medical services, and county hospitals	600 million HKD (total since 1978; includes 2 million HKD to Sun Yat-sen University No. 1 Hospital, 5 million HKD to Renmin University, 2 million HKD to Guangdong police medical services, and smaller donations to county hospitals)
Su Donglin	Zhaoqing, Guangdong	Hospital and medical facilities in Zhaoqing city and Sihui county.	67 million HKD/RMB[1] (inclusive of support for education and other nonmedical or health purposes)

Sources: This table was compiled using a number of websites, including but not limited to the following: http://charities.hkjc.com/charities/charities-overview/english/key-contributions.aspx; http://goldlion.com/tc/donation_tsang.php; http://www.sclf.org/mtjj/20101/t201011_1876g.htm; http://info.wenweipo.com/index.php?action-viewnews-itemid-47067; http://paper.wenweipo.com/2008/10/20/zt0810200018.htm; http://www.gdoverseaschn.com.cn/qw2index/2006hqjz/2006csrw/20071225oo16.htm.

Note: Data comes from a mainland website and so we can presume RMB, but it is not entirely clear.

considerable interest in poverty alleviation, although it is difficult to ascertain how hospitals located in the major cities have acted to realize such interest in practice.

Concurrent with the interest in donations to one's native place, there has been a countervailing trend in recent years toward greater institutionalization and specialization wherein ancestral place does not figure so prominently. An example of the trend toward specialization in Hong Kong and its subsequent impact on the China mainland is the Hong Kong Society for the Blind (HKSB). Founded in Hong Kong in 1955, the HKSB was for many years concerned with occupational training and rehabilitation for the blind in Hong Kong. In the 1980s, as reforms opened up the possibilities of occupational training, rehabilitation, surgery, and other services for the blind on the mainland, it expanded its operations there in collaboration with the CDPF. This collaboration has continued to the present day, including the raising of 1.8 million HKD for cataract operations on the mainland.

But the HKSB's activities were not limited to collaboration with the CDPF. In 1981, it played an active part in establishing the Asia Foundation for the Prevention of the Blind (AFPB); for many years, the HKSB's chief executive also served as chief executive of the AFPB. With support from the Lions Club of Happy Valley in Hong Kong, the HKSB launched the Sight Restoration Campaign in 1994, which led in 1996 to the joint establishment, with the Chinese University of Hong Kong and the Mid-America Eye Tissue Bank, of the Eye Bank at the Guangzhou Municipal No. 1 Hospital. Also in 1996, the HKSB and AFPB set up their first Mobile Eye Treatment Center, with complete facilities for offering cataract operations to patients in poor areas. Supported by donations from Hong Kong, the center briefly operated in Guangdong but eventually settled in Shaanxi Province. By 2011, 24 mobile eye treatment centers had been set up in as many provinces in China and had come to be run entirely by the AFPB, with continued funding from Hong Kong, the CDPF, and the Chinese Ministry of Health. Through 2011, the centers had performed 262,000 operations, including 49,000 from September 2010 through August 2011 alone. The broad and successful collaboration between the HKSB and the AFPB demonstrates the powerful effect a dedicated Hong Kong agency might have in terms of both catalyzing services and improving patient outcomes.

Table 13.3 sets out donations made in recent years, other than disaster relief from 2008 and 2010, that did not serve medical purposes. Aside from the aforementioned donation by the Hong Kong Jockey Club, the Hong Kong SAR government provided 1.5 billion RMB worth of medical relief and 260 million RMB worth of rehabilitation services. Ophthalmology again figures prominently in these efforts, with cataract operations being particularly well-supported. Presumably, donors sought certainty in treatment, and cataract sur-

Table 13.3. Personal and Institutional Donors without a Focus on Native Place

Donor	Activity
Hong Kong Society for the Blind	Mobile eye treatment centers, jointly with the Asian Foundation for the Prevention of Blindness; 90,000 operations from 1996 to 2007, 52 percent for free.
World Vision, Hong Kong	Immunization, health examination, nutrition programming, HIV and AIDS education, health education, medical training for village doctors and health care workers, provision of medical equipment, construction and renovation of clinics, and construction of toilets; 5.57 percent of 275 million RMB expenditure in 2010 spent on medical and health.
Hong Kong Jockey Club	Very substantial donations toward earthquake relief, of which 80 million RMB went into Mianyang City 3rd People's Hospital, and 53 million RMB went toward the Sichuan 8–1 Rehabilitation Center managed by the PLA.
Lifeline Express HK Foundation Ltd.	Cataract surgery, provision of 14 million HKD for 2009; 113,000 operations.
Project Vision	Cataract surgery from 10 local centers in poor areas, founded using a donation of 10 million HKD in 2007.
Chi Heng Foundation	Subsidizing HIV testing, aid to HIV victims and their families; received financial support from Hong Kong SAR Home Affairs Bureau, the Hong Kong AIDS Trust Fund, and other agencies. Project expenditures cited at 13 million HKD in 2010 accounts.
Gracious Glory (Buddhism) Foundation	Donations of medical equipment not only in Huizhou, but also in Hebei and Sichuan; focus on children with congenital heart problems in Hebei.
Liu Haoqing	Donation of four million Hong Kong dollars to Shanghai Ruijin Hospital (affiliated with Jiaotong University, formerly the Aurora University teaching hospital).

Kadoorie Charitable Foundation	Substantial donations on a broad front, including a rehabilitation program run by the CDPF in western China, health education and HIV prevention by the Shaanxi Research Association for Women and Families, and a collaborative research program on causes of premature death undertaken by Oxford University and the China Center for Disease Control.
Li Ka Shing Foundation	Aside from donations to Shantou, donations to Zhongren hospital in Shanghai (for geriatric care), provisions for cataract surgery with the China Disabled Persons' Foundation; to various hospices; to the Ministry of Civil Affairs for medical treatment of children in poor families; to the Cheung Kong New Milestone Plan, in collaboration with the CDPF, to provide artificial limbs, medical service, and training for disabled children in poor regions.
Peter KK Lee Care for Life Foundation	2010 donation of 15 million HKD for the Hong Kong–based Huaxia Foundation (largely focused on education) to provide treatment for children with congenital heart problems; 2011 donation of 10 million HKD to Huaxia for medical equipment and nurse training in Liaoning, Sichuan, Yunnan, Jiangxi, Hebei, and Zhejiang.
Chow Tai Fook (and Cheng Yu Tong)	Substantial donations are involved but precise figures are unavailable. The China Charity Foundation reports that the Chow Tai Fook Charity Foundation was started within the China Charity with a donation of 1.5 million RMB. It also donates via UNICEF. There was a substantial donation by Cheng Yu Tong to the Hong Kong University Faculty of Medicine to establish fellowships promoting training and exchange opportunities for mainland medical personnel at HKU. Also, a donation of 85 million RMB to Tsinghua University (Beijing) for the Cheng Yu Tung Medical Building.
HS Chau Foundation	Primarily provides education, but in 2006 donated 10 million RMB worth of equipment to the Shanghai Charity Federation for tumor examinations for women.

Table 13.3. *continued*

Donor	Activity
Ma Kam Ming	A member of a long-established Hong Kong family with a strong philanthropic record in Hong Kong. Has donated to the Ma Jinming Ophthalmology Department Center and the Obstetrics-Gynecology Department Center at the Beijing Shunyi Hospital.
Kerry Group Kuok Foundation	Active in village medical and health projects in Hunan Province, including cataract surgery, treatment of congenital heart problems and diabetes, rehabilitation, training of village health personnel, and health education.
S K Yee Medical Foundation	Donated one million Hong Kong dollars in 2008 toward medical treatments for children in Shenzhen; also made donations in Hebei Province in the same year.
China Soong Ching Ling Foundation and Chinachem Charitable Foundation	The establishment of the foundation was announced by Chinachem in 2010; the magnitude of its funding and direction are unclear.
Operation Concern	Charity organization (registered since 1994) comprising medical professionals and volunteers in Hong Kong who travel as medical teams to remote poverty-stricken rural areas in mainland China to treat the poor and the handicapped.
Asian Foundation for the Prevention of Blindness	Provides mobile eye treatment centers; see also the Hong Kong Society for the Blind.

Table 13.4. NGOs with International Connections

Organization	Activity
Médecins Sans Frontières (HK)	Has raised substantial sums through its its Hong Kong office (173 million HKD in 2009, and rising rapidly); allocation to China is very small in comparison (1 million HKD in 2009).
Christian Action	Hong Kong–based, donating largely to Qinghai and Tibet; mainly establishes rehabilitation centers and clinics.
Cedar Fund	Christian relief and development organization founded in Hong Kong in 1991; has implemented sanitation and health education in Hubei, HIV/AIDS prevention and education programming in Yunnan, community health programming in Gansu and Shanxi. Also supports staff dedicated to rehabilitating children with hearing impairments and cerebral palsy through the Jian Hua Foundation in Tianjin. Total of all its services (medical and health services being only a portion) in mainland China was seven hundred thousand U.S. dollars in FY 2009–2010.
Lions Club Hong Kong and Macau	The Lions Club International runs a very substantial international project under Sight First, providing treatment for blindness and prevention of blindness. Members of the club in Hong Kong have also donated to hospitals on the mainland, primarily in rural areas near Beijing. Lions Club Hong Kong websites include the Tam Wah Ching Hospital (Fanghan), the Wong Chung Ying Hospital (Daxing), the Hung Hin Shiu Hospital (Daxin zhuang in Beijing), and the Dai dong Yue Hospital (Miyun), among others.
Caritas Hong Kong	Active primarily in Hong Kong, but its Mainland Service Desk improved 20 village clinics and provided medical allowances for one hundred poor patients.

Table 13.4. *continued*

Organization	Activity
Hong Kong AIDS Association	Operates training, education, counseling, technical advising, and "microfinance" projects in Gansu, Shenyang, Yunnan, and Hubei.
Save the Children (HK)	Provides health education and health examination. China does not seem to be a major focus for the international organization.
Asia Compassionate Touch	An "international non-profit . . . foundation registered in Hong Kong" (Asia Compassionate Touch website, http://www.act-cn.org/en/) with a focus on children; has made some medical donations, including treatment of four cases of scoliosis and two of leukemia, and for AIDS education in a county in Henan.
Jianhua Foundation	"JHF is registered with the State Administration for Foreign Expert Affairs in Beijing as an approved overseas organization for recruiting professionals, and currently has 150 longer term expatriate associates from 17 nations serving together with local Chinese colleagues in several provinces across China" (Jianhua Foundation website, https://www.jhf-china.org /cms/index.php?id=about). Medical services include subsidized hernia operations for eight hundred children and subsidized medical care for the poor in Qinghai.
Heep Hong	Primarily focused on Hong Kong, but offering some exchanges and training for mainland medical personnel.
Richmond Fellowship of Hong Kong	"Established in 1984 as a non-profit making registered charity. It is affiliated with the Richmond fellowship International, a world-wide network of self-governing, non-profit organizations which shares the common aim of promoting good community care practice in the field of mental health" (Richmond Fellowship of Hong Kong website, http://www .richmond.org.hk/e/default_home.asp). Runs two rehabilitation centers in Shenzhen by agreement with the local disabled persons' federation.

gery—thanks to recent medical advances—now offers both clear objectives and unambiguous outcomes. The favoring of clear return on investment is probably at least part of the reason that hospitals are also well supported: philanthropy can readily be recognized when manifested in buildings. There is also a tendency for donors to work through established Chinese charities: both national and local CDPF agencies appear prominently on the list. Somewhat exceptional is Kadoorie's efforts to fund Oxford University and the China Center for Disease Control's collaborative research on premature death. The Chinachem Charitable Foundation, with its very substantial funds, appears to collaborate with the China Soong Ching Ling Foundation, which to date has been more focused on relations among Hong Kong, Macau, and Taiwan than on mainland charities. Little has been heard of their effort since early 2012, however, and much remains to be seen.

International NGOs are active in Hong Kong and China but many are engaged in activities that do not pertain to health care. Funds raised in Hong Kong, moreover, are not necessarily targeted at the mainland, as obviously Hong Kong donors have over the years developed a broad international outlook that matches that of international NGOs. Médecins Sans Frontières, for example, raised 226 million HKD in Hong Kong during 2010 but spent only 200,000 in China, while Oxfam raised 204 million HKD in FY 2010–2011 in Hong Kong and spent 124 million in China (Médecins Sans Frontières 2010, 26–27; Oxfam 2011, 36–37). A general summary of internationally connected NGO activity is presented here in table 13.4. The Lions Club's efforts are perhaps the most ambitious, part and parcel of the club's international mission of providing treatment for blindness. The other efforts are largely small-scale in comparison to those described in tables 13.2 and 13.3.

Conclusion

This brief chapter demonstrates that Hong Kong has proved to be a major source of donations for medical philanthropy on mainland China in recent years, and argues that with the institutionalization of personal connections to native place, this situation will likely persist. Hong Kong's domestic NGOs will also likely continue to raise money in Hong Kong for causes not only in China, but also—and in substantial quantities—in regions of need in other parts of the world. The coexistence of the China connection with an international outlook marks out Hong Kong's intermediary role, in medical philanthropy as well as in economic and social activity more broadly, as a catalyst for change within China and as a liaison for China with the world order.

Yet, some very marked contrasts can be noted between those charity funds raised and deployed in Hong Kong and those raised in Hong Kong and deployed in mainland China. First and foremost, it should be noted that the philanthropic scene in Hong Kong is strongly associated with a community orientation. Translated into the mainland context, attachment to native place has provided an incentive for major donations by the most successful businesspeople of Chinese descent in Hong Kong. Donations to the mainland have followed a pattern that has been observed in Hong Kong for a very long time; that is, Chinese people donate to their native places and people originating therefrom. In Hong Kong, donations to native places became institutionalized and developed into large-scale community involvement, through the efforts of institutions such as Tung Wah and Wong Tai Sin. On the mainland, with the exception of disaster relief, this has not happened. It is well known, if only anecdotally, that Hong Kong people frequently make smaller-scale donations to their native places outside the context of well-publicized campaigns by established mainland charities. There is considerable scope to raise funds in Hong Kong through high-profile media events, as disaster relief in recent years has demonstrated, and the community angle can moreover turn such events into regular funding sources even in the absence of disasters. Nevertheless, it should be noted that in the cases of philanthropic institutions such as Tung Wah and Wong Tai Sin, Hong Kong people have become accustomed not only to a very high standard of transparency and accountability, but also to such institutions possessing a high degree of independence from the government. It is Hong Kong's law that enables and requires independent audits, and permits the government to draw on the expertise and public support of such NGOs through participatory funding. The possibilities for fundraising in Hong Kong are very real, but so too is the need for institutional independence and openness.

It is hard to tell if Hong Kong's philanthropic culture will make much of an impact on the mainland, or if the Chinese government's treatment of philanthropic organizations will necessarily take into account practices established in Hong Kong. To be sure, Hong Kong adheres to an international standard that is widely shared in the developed world, and that could serve as a liaison between that philanthropic order and the mainland. Frequent contact between philanthropic interests in Hong Kong and the mainland leads to common concerns, but under the one-country two-systems rubric, major governmental decisions need be made before any easy convergence can be possible.

References

Chen, Ta. 1940. *Emigrant Communities in South China: A Study of Overseas Migration and Its Influence on Standards of Living and Social Change.* New York: Institute of Pacific Relations.

Deng Yusheng. 1910. *Quan Yue shehui shilu chugao* [Associations of All Guangdong]. Guangzhou: Diaocha Quan Yue shehui chu.

Ding Xinbao. 2010. *Shan yu ren tong, yu Xianggang tongbu chengzhang de Donghua sanyuan* [Charity is Virtue, the Tung Wah Group of Hospitals That Grows with Hong Kong] (1870–1997). Hong Kong: Sanlian.

Guldin, Gregory Eliyu. 1995. "Toward a Greater Guangdong: Hong Kong's Sociocultural Impact on the Pearl River Delta and Beyond." In *The Hong Kong-Guangdong Link: Partnership in Flux,* edited by Reginald Yin-Wang Kwok and Alvin Y. So, 89–118. Armonk, NY: M. E. Sharpe.

Internal Revenue Department. 2013. "List of Charitable Institutions and Trusts of a Public Character, Which Are Exempt from Tax under Section 88 of the Inland Revenue Ordinance." http://www.ird.gov.hk/eng/pdf/e_s881ist_emb.pdf.

Médecins Sans Frontières. 2010. *Hong Kong Activity Report.* Hong Kong: Médecins Sans Frontières.

Oxfam. 2011. *Oxfam Annual Report, 2010–2011.* Hong Kong: Oxfam.

Pok Oi Hospital. 2012. *Pok Oi Hospital Annual Report 2011–2012.* Hong Kong: Pok Oi Hospital.

Remer, C. F. 1968 [1933]. *Foreign Investments in China.* New York: Howard Fertig, 222.

Rogaski, Ruth. 2004. *Hygenic Modernity: Meanings of Health and Disease in Treaty-Port China,* Berkeley: University of California Press.

Sik Sik Yuen. 2012. *Sik Sik Yuen Annual Report 2011.* Hong Kong: Sik Sik Yuen.

Sinn, Elizabeth. 1989. *Power and Charity: The Early History of the Tung Wah Hospital, Hong Kong.* Hong Kong: Oxford University Press.

Su Quanyou, and Wang Hongying. 2010. "Minchu woguo jiuzai de zijin wenti pingshu" [Comments on the Sources of Capital for Disaster Relief in the Early Republic]. *Fangzai keji xueyuan xuebao* [Journal of the Institute of Disaster-Prevention Science and Technology] 12 (1): 288–292.

Tung Wah Group of Hospitals. 2012. *Tung Wah Group of Hospitals Annual Report 2011/2012,* Hong Kong: Tung Wah Group of Hospitals.

Wu Yanmin. 2012. "Nanjing guomin zhengfu shiqi jiuzai zijin laiyuan yu choumu zhi kaocha, yi 1927–1937 nian Henan sheng wei li" [Observations on the Sources of Capital and Fundraising in the Disaster-Relief Efforts of the Nanjing National Government: The Case Study of Henan Province in 1927–1937]. *Shandong shifan daxue xuebao (renwen shehui kexue ban)* [Journal of the Shandong Normal University (Humanities and Social Science Volume)] 57 (2): 109–116.

Yan Chai Hospital. 2012. *Yan Chai Hospital Annual Report 2011–2012.* Hong Kong: Yan Chai Hospital.

Young, Nick, and and June Shih. 2004. "Philanthropic Links between the Chinese Diaspora and the People's Republic of China." In *Diaspora Philanthropic and Equitable Development in China and India,* edited by Peter F. Geithner, Paula D. Johnson, and Lincoln C. Chen, 129–175. Cambridge, MA: Global Equity Initiative, Asia Center, Harvard University.

Zeng Ruiyan. 1988. *Huaqiao yu kang Ri zhanzheng* [The Overseas Chinese and the Anti-Japanese War]. Chengdu: Sichuan daxue chubanshe.

Zhuang Guotu. 2011. "Donations of Overseas Chinese to Xiamen since 1978." In *Rethinking Chinese Transnational Enterprises: Cultural Affinity and Business Strategies,* edited by Leo Douw, Cen Huang, and David Ip, 123–138. Richmond, UK: Curzon; Leiden: International Institute for Asian Studies.

14 Toward a Healthier Philanthropy

Reforming China's Philanthropic Sector

Xu Yongguang

Introduction

When Deng Xiaoping's Open Door policy reforms first began to be implemented, the Chinese economy was in a precarious state. In 1978 the national GDP amounted to the equivalent of $148 billion in current value. The next three decades witnessed a remarkable transformation as China progressed from economic stagnation to become the world's second-largest economy, with a GDP of $7.3 trillion by 2011 (World Bank 2013). This spectacular growth has frequently been hailed as "China's economic miracle," or "a miracle with Chinese characteristics" (Wu 2004). But it has not come without huge social upheaval, as the transition to a market economy also saw the disintegration of an already-strained state welfare system, most notably in rural areas, which had previously been organized under the Cooperative Medical System. Against a backdrop of limited state welfare provision and rising wealth inequality, the growth of modern Chinese philanthropy has been both heartening and necessary.

The burgeoning of modern philanthropy in China has received considerable media attention in recent years, and these reports have frequently focused on the role being played by the new "super rich," both highlighting philanthropic work already being done by certain wealthy individuals and also questioning the appetite for generosity among others (Koenig 2011; Wines 2010). A notable feature of China's economic growth in the three decades since the implementation of the Open Door reform program has been a concomitant rise in the number of these extremely wealthy mainland Chinese citizens. Various reforms since Deng Xiaoping famously declared in 1992, "Let a part of the population become rich first," have facilitated this process. In particular, there has been a dramatic acceleration in the accumulation of private wealth since the Chinese Communist Party (CCP) amended the Party Constitution in 2002 to accommodate private business owners and the government revised the State Constitution in 2004 to provide legal protection for private properties. As recently as 2002, there were no U.S.-dollar billionaires in China, yet by 2011, *Forbes* estimated the number at 115, a figure second only to the United States (Flannery 2012).[1] The number of mainland millionaires, meanwhile, has risen to a staggering 1.4 million (Neate 2012). The emergence of this broad stratum of highly affluent Chinese—particularly alongside an associated drastically widening national wealth gap—has understandably commanded the attention of the media and society at large. Yet while such individuals will likely be an increasingly key component in the growth of philanthropy, the reality is that the government has been, and remains, by far the primary agent in the development of modern Chinese philanthropy.

The prominence of the state is apparent in various chapters in this volume, from its role in the evolving legislative framework for philanthropy to its engagement with specific modern health challenges, and from its establishment of philanthropically oriented GONGOs (government-organized nongovernmental organizations) to its interactions with foreign foundations. For those involved in the philanthropic sector, a positive governmental approach that increasingly recognizes the significant beneficial role that philanthropy can play in society is to be welcomed. Further encouraging signs are evident in other chapters, including the development of private philanthropies focusing on underfunded and underresourced areas such as special health needs, the sustained involvement of major international foundations, and Hong Kong and Chinese diaspora charitable donations being stimulated by ancestral connections to mainland China.

As mentioned earlier, and as suggested in these different chapters, there is much that is heartening about the development of modern philanthropy in China. Yet enthusiasm for the progress being made must also be tempered with concerns about certain systemic issues that are hampering a greater realization of the positive potential of philanthropy. What follows is an overview of some of the most significant challenges facing the philanthropic sector, and an identification of certain key changes, which, if implemented, can help provide further opportunities for the sector to flourish. Central to this is the need for a diversification of the sector for the benefit of public welfare, a weakening of the state monopoly on charitable resources, and greater transparency across the field. If such improvements can be made, not only will state-run ventures operate more efficiently, but the productive capacity of grassroots initiatives will be unleashed. The potential of the aforementioned new "super rich" to direct their wealth toward projects for the greater good could thereby lead China toward a healthier and more impactful philanthropy.

Government Monopoly on Charity Resources

Before the Open Door reforms, the government was the sole entity managing the political, economic, and social rights and resources of the country: there was no free market or civil society of which to speak. With market liberalization also came the fragmentation of established social infrastructures such as the *danwei* system, presenting the state with new challenges in terms of providing education, health care, and social benefits to a population of over one billion people. Hence the government took the initiative in creating quasi-nongovernmental charitable vehicles (GONGOs) and mobilizing social resources in order to supplement its own fiscal investment. Starting in the 1980s, a group of charitable organizations supported by the government was created, such as the China Children and Teenagers' Fund in 1981—the first of all such foundations—as well as the China Charity Federation in 1994. Thirty years later, China had 2,732 national-level foundations and 1,932 charity associations at the county level or higher (CCDIC 2012).

Today there exist three forms of legally registered nonprofit organizations in China. Firstly, there are social organizations (*shehui tuanti*), which are what might be termed membership associations, including various professional and trade associations. Secondly, there is a category of nonprofit service providers, known as people-run non-enterprise organizations (*minban fei qiye danwei*). Finally, there are foundations (*jijinhui*), which can either be public foundations (entitled to engage in fundraising in public spaces, online, and through the media) or non-public fundraising foundations (typically referred to as private foundations and established through private or corporate wealth and unable to engage in public fundraising). These different organizations must register with the Ministry of Civil Affairs, and, additionally, some that also operate as for-profit businesses must register through the State Administration for Industry and Commerce. A further important category is that of quasi-governmental public institutions (*shiye danwei*), such as university and research institutes, public sports, and cultural bodies. A large number of these nonprofit entities—particularly social organizations and public foundations—were created by or are strongly linked to the government, and are known as GONGOs (ICNL 2013).

The formation of GONGOs became a pragmatic arrangement for different levels of government. Presently, 45 departments, including various ministries as well as worker, youth, and women's associations, have established 86 public fundraising foundations, which work in the same sector as their related managing department of the government, pursuing charitable projects and raising funds. Although these different public foundations have certainly engaged in valuable charitable work, their frequent deployment by the government as departmental financial supplements has not encouraged the best working practices. Although the Open Door reforms have seen China transition to a much more market-based economy, the social services sector, which incorporates these government-led foundations, has been prone to many of the drawbacks typically associated with a planned economy. Staff members of these national institutions have been able to rely on an "iron rice bowl"—"a stable, lifelong job with a regular salary whether the employee performs well or not" (Zhu 2013). A lack of competition and external monitoring has neither promoted efficient working practices nor encouraged the provision of the highest possible services, and at worst has given rise to avaricious and corrupt dealings.

Examples of inefficient, wasteful tendencies can be found in some cases of welfare projects for disabled people. For instance, 230 million RMB was invested in the first phase of the Dongguan Sports Center for the Disabled (*Dongguang Daily News* 2010), while 450 million RMB is to be invested in the construction of a service center for the handicapped in Qingdao, which will cover a land area of 9,900 to 13,200 square meters and extend over a gross floor area of 50,000 square meters (*Qilu Evening News* 2012). These facilities, along with the large numbers of institutional staff that must be allocated to them, have allowed the government to consume a great amount of resources. Yet there is little evidence that such grandiose facilities are actually required. It is likely they will be severely underutilized, providing employment for government staff but not serving the actual needs of local communities, who would likely benefit more from a wider range of smaller, well-targeted projects. There is a stark contrast here with certain more efficient, privately funded projects for the disabled, as discussed by Li Fan in chapter 12 of this volume.

Charitable activities and fundraising campaigns in China have at times been excessively mobilized by philanthropic organizations with a government background in order to supplement the government coffers. This has happened to the point where some local governments have used their administrative authority to "strongly encourage" companies or individuals to make "charity donations" (*Shaanxi Daily* 2010). For instance, after the Fugu provincial government in Shaanxi had collected 1.3 billion RMB in so-called "coal donations" from coal mine owners in 2010, the Shenmu provincial government did the same, collecting almost triple that amount—3.8 billion RMB (*21st Century Business Herald* 2011). Even putting aside the question of how the money raised from these enforced donations was ultimately spent, such practices clearly violate the free-will nature of charitable giving, negatively impacting people's attitudes toward charity, and likely depriving grassroots organizations of financial support they might otherwise obtain.

The term "grassroots" is worth considering at this point as it is frequently invoked in English-language discussions concerning philanthropy and civil society more broadly in contemporary China. Technically, the term applies to all organizations that are founded and run by people—that is, those organizations that have (largely) developed independent of government control. By that definition, large, privately endowed foundations are also grassroots organizations. But due to the scale and scope of the larger private foundations, they are typically regarded as a rather different category, with "grassroots" more commonly used to imply smaller, locally based initiatives. As such, when grassroots organizations are mentioned, it is often with reference to the huge number of unregistered nonprofit civil society organizations, which exist in addition to the different types of legally recognized nonprofit bodies already mentioned. Without registration, these grassroots organizations have no legal guarantees, or any prospect of favorable tax incentives. They retain their independence but are also subject to state discretion. But the current registration process is a double-edged sword: under the "dual management" system, organizations "must generally first obtain the sponsorship of a 'professional leading agency' such as a government ministry or provincial government agency, then seek registration and approval from the Ministry of Civil Affairs in Beijing or a local civil affairs bureau, and remain under the dual control of both agencies throughout their organizational life" (ICNL 2013). In practice, such sponsorship is not possible to obtain without strong government connections. Currently, therefore, unregistered grassroots organizations are in an unenviable position: either they retain independence but have no legal protection and very limited access to funding, or they manage to register only to abdicate that independence and become in thrall to the government agenda and the state's monopoly on the philanthropic sector. The scale of this monopoly is indicated by the fact that approximately 80 percent of the 76 billion RMB donated in the wake of the 2008 Wenchuan earthquake was deposited into government accounts for distribution to affected areas. A 2009 audit showed that only 4.7 percent of that money had so far been used (Deng 2009).

The implied corollary to an argument that the government should seek to end the state's monopoly on charitable infrastructure and move away from a planned economy model that still besets the provision of social services is that the promotion of people-led initiatives will be positive for the charitable sector. Well-targeted private foundations, independent from the government, are likely to be more financially prudent, innovative, and responsive to changing needs—with the caveat that they must of course be well-managed and governed by qualified boards of directors and subject to external scrutiny. This is particularly relevant with regard to the concept of philanthropy as a sustained and structured commitment to needy causes. Charitable funds closely aligned with and co-opted by government departments have certainly directed money to those in immediate need (e.g., those in extreme poverty or affected by natural disasters), but large proportions of these funds have also been absorbed and utilized by the government to supplement unrelated projects. Private and people-run institutions wishing to thrive in a competitive marketplace will have to not only provide immediate assistance to the needy but also stake out their own area of expertise and sustained commitment and pursue this with structured investment in long-term and worthwhile philanthropic projects. While such a scenario is desirable, it will not be realized simply by weakening the state's monopoly on the sector. It will also require fresh stimulus of the private sector and reform of the ways in which people-run non-enterprise organizations currently operate. The remainder of this chapter looks at the nature of these challenges and also identifies some of the success stories beginning to emerge.

Toward the Reformation of the Philanthropic Sector

In 2010, Wen Jiabao, then premier of China, explicitly identified the need for structural reform of social service provision and the state's management of charity resources: "China's reform of the social ventures sector is still lagging behind. The main problem lies in the fact that the government has shown ineffective management and has been too protective of its resources." He also recommended that "each social venture should be defined as 'fundamental' or 'non-fundamental.' The government should then make sure that within these 'non-fundamental' social undertakings, priority should be given according to social and market needs, their creative aspects and ability to satisfy these needs on different levels" (*Qiushi* 2010).

Exploring Wen Jiabao's statement more closely, it may be said that "fundamental" undertakings relate to services and products that are of such basic universal necessity (such as elementary and middle school education, and basic medical services from public hospitals) that they should be enjoyed by all and equally distributed, with the state taking responsibility. "Non-fundamental" services and goods are those which are not required by all, yet may be deeply needed by some (such as services for the disabled or orphans). These may be more effectively handled by people-run organizations, which can be more agile in meeting society's needs. The government may award contracts to such ventures, using funds to purchase services from these social organizations, but this would be contingent on the demonstration that the organizations are running efficiently and receiving positive evaluations from the public. So government contracts reward and strengthen already-effective organizations rather than propping up unproductive and wasteful ventures. There may also still be government-run providers of non-fundamental services, but these should be operating on a level playing field with the people-run social services, allowing for fair competition in the marketplace, and thus leading to a better overall standard of provision. Reform is needed to move toward that scenario, with steps taken to end the government monopoly that has already been described, increase the philanthropic involvement of the super rich, and foster the growth of civil non-enterprise organizations.

In order to moderate the government monopoly on charity infrastructure and more swiftly and effectively direct charitable resources to where there is the greatest social need, the following three measures would be advisable. Firstly, existing laws should be properly enforced in order to end the government's practice of using charity donations as a second source of income. According to the Public Welfare Donation Law, only provincial-level governments and above are allowed to receive donations in the event of a natural disaster and by request of the donors. Local governments pressuring for money in the name of charity are severely infringing on the private rights of donors and therefore should be stopped in accordance with the law. Secondly, public charity organizations which have obtained the right to publicly raise money should share resources with private charity organizations so as to support the development of public welfare. Thirdly, and most importantly, public foundations should themselves proactively revise and reform their development plans in order to attain the nature of private organizations and become the motivational force of public welfare development. The China Foundation for Poverty Alleviation has been a pioneer in this respect: ten years ago, it willingly shifted from governmental administration to a private and more suitable structure and became a "fund-type foundation" (Xu 2010). Alongside the China Foundation for Poverty Alleviation, successful structural transformations have also been achieved by the China Social Welfare Foundation and the China Youth Development Foundation. In addition, in recent years, several very significant new purely nonprofit, nongovernmental private foundations have also emerged, such as the Shanghai United Foundation, the China Beijing United Charity Foundation, the China Charities Aid for Children Foundation, and the Shenzhen One Foundation. These foundations are unusual because, although they are privately run, crucially they also have permission to engage in public fundraising. The success of the One Foundation, originally established by the actor Jet Li, may serve as a powerful example of both the fundraising potential of such entities and also the connection between this permission and public confidence in the greater transparency of such charitable initiatives.

Several recent incidents in China's charity sector have attracted severe public criticism due to fraudulent activities and low transparency with regard to the use of resources. August 2011 saw the China Charity Federation embroiled in a tax invoice scandal, as CCTV News aired an investigation into the tax affairs of Suntech Power Holdings. According to the report, Suntech had been provided with a receipt from the China Charity Federation claiming that the company had donated goods (mainly solar panels) worth a total of 17 million RMB to schools via the federation. The report alleged that the vast majority of these goods had not in fact been donated directly to schools, but rather sold for profit by the executor of Suntech's charity scheme, Beijing EduChina Education Corporation. A former EduChina employee furthermore stated that Suntech had been furnished with a receipt for 17 million RMB in exchange for a cash gift of 50,000 RMB. In effect, the report implicated the China Charity Federation in the sale of huge tax dodges in exchange for much smaller cash donations (Ji 2011).

That same year, the Henan Soong Ching Ling Foundation was accused of misusing funds and engaging in commercial activities for individuals' personal gain. Investigations revealed that much of the foundation's revenue had come from the sale of health insurance policies, and that such income had been used for profitable activities including real estate investment and the offering of illegal loans. Chinese charity regulations require that foundations use no less than 70 percent of their annual revenue for charitable purposes, yet of over 600 million RMB raised in 2009 only 140 million RMB was then spent on charitable projects. Furthermore, a children's activity center the foundation had pledged to build was only partially constructed before the project stalled, with capital shortages being cited as the reason. The land was then given over for the purpose of building residential structures, and acquired by a company in which some of the foundation's staff held shares (Zhang 2011).

The most infamous scandal of 2011, though, was the Guo Meimei affair. In June of that year images appeared on the microblogging site Sina Weibo of a 20-year-old woman flaunting her expensive lifestyle of business-class flights, designer clothing, and luxury cars. Guo identified herself as the general manager of the "Red Cross Chamber of Commerce," a company that allegedly oversaw advertising on Red Cross vehicles. The full details of the affair (including Guo's actual relationship to the Red Cross) remain somewhat opaque, and the amounts of money involved were seemingly not on a par with the two previously mentioned scandals. Nonetheless, the salacious nature of the incident, combined with the influence of new social media, resulted in a devastating blow to the reputation of one of the nation's oldest and most prestigious charitable organizations. Donations received by the Red Cross declined by almost 60 percent in 2011 compared to the previous year (CCDIC 2011).

If anything encouraging can be drawn from these various scandals, it is that the increasing prominence of social media and investigative journalism is helping to bring such cases to light. Clearly, though, there needs to be a stronger regulatory environment in place in order to prevent such instances from occurring in the first place, together with a determination that if scandals ever do arise, they are dealt with quickly and transparently in order to restore and sustain public confidence in the work of charitable organizations. It is notable that the three major scandals discussed above all relate to public foundations, closely linked to the government. This is not to suggest that privately endowed foundations are somehow immune from corruption. But when high-profile public organizations are implicated in malfeasance, the impact on public confidence may be more profound, as it suggests a problem beyond the bounds of a single organization and may be interpreted as something rotten in the state of philanthropy itself. Clearly such an interpretation is in the interests of neither the government nor the philanthropic sector, and yet the government monopoly on charity resources has frequently contributed to a lack of transparency. There is not yet a strong track record of such cases' being pursued through the courts, and the government will need to demonstrate greater determination in submitting these cases to fair and thorough investigation and, where appropriate, judicial process in order to restore public confidence.

One significant development did occur in August 2012 with the China Foundation Center's introduction of its Transparency Index. The index emerged from the need for people to better understand the operations of foundations with regard to revenues and expenses, project management, internal administration, and structural operations. Using 60 different transparency indicators, the index ranks all of China's more than 2,700 foundations "according to the level and quality of publicly disclosed information about their activities, finances and governance to meet growing demands for transparency in the digital age" (China Foundation Center 2013). These rankings will enable the public to make better-informed decisions with regard to donating money to charitable foundations, and should consequently stimulate greater transparency from these foundations and greater efficiency in their use of resources.

As mentioned earlier, the One Foundation is an example of a charitable organization that has reaped the benefits of positive public perceptions of its transparency. In the aftermath of the April 2013 Ya'an earthquake, the Red Cross Society of China struggled to attract donations following a string of scandals, most notably the Guo Meimei affair. In the first 24 hours after the earthquake, the Red Cross received only 142,000 RMB in individual donations. In a similar period, the One Foundation received 15 million RMB. Wang Shi, CEO of the One Foundation, was swift to emphasize that the Chinese public should not lose confidence in the Red Cross, but clearly there is currently far greater trust in Jet Li's privately run venture than in a large GONGO with a tarnished reputation. A report in the *Financial Times* quoted a typical comment from a Weibo user who had donated money: "I choose to trust One Foundation this time. I will never contribute to Guo Meimei's Maserati" (Zhu 2013).

The success of the One Foundation may prove a rallying cry for other super-wealthy Chinese to engage in philanthropy. In September 2010, after making a "philanthropic promise" at the American Federation, Bill Gates and Warren Buffet organized a dinner in Beijing—known as the "Bobby Charity Dinner"—to which more than 50 wealthy and influential Chinese were invited. The dinner was the focus of much media coverage, further exposing newly wealthy people to the field of philanthropy in China. The previous year, in October 2009, billionaire Chen Fashu, from Fujian, had announced that he would donate negotiable securities at a market value of 8.3 billion RMB to the newly established New Huadu

Foundation, which has registered capital of 100 million RMB. In May 2011, Cao Dewang, also from Fujian, donated shares in Fuyao Group valued at 3.5 billion RMB to the He Ren Charity Foundation, which is named after his father. In May 2012, the founder of the China Charity Foundation, Lu Dezhi, announced that his foundation will act as an umbrella organization to create more such foundations within 10 years. Bill Gates has predicted that such philanthropic gestures are only likely to increase, particularly due to the recent nature of these huge individual fortunes. In December 2011, he told a reporter at the Beijing office of his foundation that seeking donations from rich people in the United States is rather difficult as most of them are only inheritors of a fortune, whereas seeking donations from rich people in China is easier, as many of them are the very first generation of entrepreneurs who have built their own fortune and thus have the freedom to manage it the way they want (Narada Foundation 2011).

At present, though, private foundations are still in their initial development phase, with most still positioned as operational foundations. There are records of only some 30 private foundations (not even 3 percent of the national total) financially supporting smaller grassroots organizations. Private foundations positioned solely as financial-support providers are extremely scarce (Liu 2012). A more dynamic approach would see a shift toward more of a grant-making model, in which wealthy private foundations partner with local grassroots initiatives. The local partner would bring knowledge, staff, and contacts, while the private foundation would inject much-needed capital, paying for equipment and training, and providing other vital resources.

In order for such a partnership approach to flourish, further reform of the philanthropic sector will be required. In particular, the right of private foundations and people-run organizations to engage in public fundraising must be established in law. The One Foundation is a potent example of how effective this can be when allowed. If the long-delayed national Charity Law can be finalized, then progress may be made on this front. In order for grassroots initiatives to flourish there must also be changes to the current registration process, with its dual management model. In 2011, an agenda for solving the registration issue was submitted to the government. At the beginning of the year, the CCP Central Committee's general secretary Hu Jintao declared to all government bodies that they should "reinforce and renew social administration, fully stimulate social vitality, promote the self-creation of various social organizations and allow people's involvement in social administration" (Xinhua 2011). As a result, the minister of civil affairs, Li Liguo, requested in December 2011 that his department promote the actions taken by Guangdong Province in allowing social organizations to register directly through the local Ministry of Civil Affairs (Wei Ming 2011).

The Guangdong experiments have been the most high-profile of a range of trial reforms being explored in certain parts of China (significant policy experiments have also taken place in Shenzhen, Yunnan, and Jiangsu). Critically, in

January 2012 it was announced that by July of that year, the requirement that nonprofit organizations must first obtain sponsorship from a professional supervisory unit was to be eliminated. Allowing more than one trade association to operate per sector would foster competition, and the government purchase of services from social organizations is being encouraged. Finally, in May 2012, new fundraising regulations were put in place for the provincial capital of Guangzhou, whereby social organizations, civil non-enterprise units, and nonprofit public institutions will all be able to fundraise publicly. The positive response of the minister of civil affairs to these experimental reforms suggests they may form the blueprint for nationwide change, helping to break the monopoly that has existed on public fundraising in China (ICLN 2013).

It should be noted that the growth of grassroots NGOs in China as registration becomes easier will bring its own new challenges. With the emergence of more and more organizations servicing the lower strata of society, the lack of social investment and resources will become more obvious. The desire to help may exist, but the utility may be lacking. There will be a need for more organizations and philanthropists to act as social investors, and there will be an urgent need to train and attract a great number of qualified professionals, as it will be hard to find qualified personnel who understand the operational side of running such organizations.

Ultimately, though, the promotion of social services coordinated by civil society organizations, more independent from government, should foster a more effective utilization of financial resources and strengthen social capital. Funding comes not from taxation but instead from various revenue streams: donations, social investments, and service provision. The investment model is volunteer-based and open to competition. In order to flourish, these organizations will have to respond to the needs of the market, offering competitive services and targeted areas of expertise.

There is a pressing need for change to take place, particularly in the education and health care sectors in China, because public hospitals and schools opened by the government are not currently sufficient to meet people's needs. Furthermore, citizen pressure, prompted by a range of scandals involving public charitable organizations, is causing the issue of reform to emerge as a political imperative. Experimental reforms such as those being pioneered in Guangdong demonstrate the possibilities for, and the desire to achieve, a more dynamic, efficient, and effective linking of private-sector resources with social-welfare needs. High-profile scandals may have garnered much press coverage in recent years—and there is a need for such reporting in order to stimulate improvements—but if bold decisions can now be made, progressive policies put into place nationwide, and swift and effective action taken where wasteful and irresponsible practices are identified, then there is hope that the future can see positive moves away from the failings of a government-monopolized sector and toward a healthier state of philanthropy, one that brings with it social progress and increased well-being for Chinese society as a whole.

Note

1. In 2012 slower economic growth actually resulted in a decline in the number of billionaires for the first time in six years. However, at a total of 95, the figure remained high.

References

CCDIC (China Charity and Donation Information Center). 2011. *2011 China Charitable Donation Report*. http://news.sohu.com/20120628/n346770174.shtml.

———. 2012. *Report on the Development of Charitable Associations in China*. http://news .xinhuanet.com/politics/2012-07/15/c_123413494.htm.

China Foundation Center. 2013. "The Methodology of the Foundation Transparency Index." http://en.fti.org.cn/interpretation.html.

Deng Guosheng. 2009. *Responding to Wenchuan: China's Disaster Relief Mechanism*. Beijing: Beijing University Press.

Dongguan Daily News. 2010. "City Disabled Sports Center to Commence Early Next Year." December 27. http://jiaotong.zmt.dg.gov.cn/publicfiles/business/htmlfiles/cndg/ s332/201012/291929.htm.

Flannery, Russell. 2012. "China Leads the World in Billionaire Flame-Outs." *Forbes*, September 3. http://www.forbes.com/sites/russellflannery/2012/03/09/chinas-billionaire- boom-halts-country-leads-world-in-forbes-list-drops/.

ICNL (International Center for Not-for-Profit Law). 2013. "NGO Law Monitor: China." http:// www.icnl.org/research/monitor/china.html.

Ji Beibei. 2011. "State Charity Denies Tax Scam." *Global Times* (Beijing), August 18. http:// english.peopledaily.com.cn/90882/7572924.html.

Koenig, Neil. 2011. "Zhai Meiqing at the Forefront of Chinese Philanthropy." *BBC News*, December 1. http://www.bbc.co.uk/news/business-15980470.

Liu Zhouhong. 2012. "Private Foundations: Mission and Responsibility." In *Charity Blue Book* 137–159. Beijing: China Social Science Press.

Narada Foundation. 2011. "Bill Gates, Xu Yongguang and Wang Zhenyao Discuss Philanthropy." http://www.naradafoundation.org/sys/html/lm_22/2012-01-12/205108.htm.

Neate, Rupert. 2012. "China and India Swell Ranks of Millionaires in Global Rich List." *Guardian* (London), May 31. http://www.guardian.co.uk/business/2012/may/31/china -india-millionaires-global-rich-list.

Qilu Evening News. 2012. "Qingdao Invests 1.1 billon RMB in the Construction of 73 Facilities Servicing Disabled People." July 20. http://news.163.com/12/0720/06/ 86R9N8QH00014AED.html.

Qiushi. 2010. "Wen Jiabao: Issues Related to the Development of Social Enterprises and Improvement of People's Lives." *Qiushi*, April 1. http://news.xinhuanet.com/politics /2010-04/02/c_1211892.htm.

Shaanxi Daily. 2010. "The Story behind the 1.3 billion RMB in Donations from the Coal Mine Owners in Fugu." August 3. http://news.cnwest.com/content/2010-03/08 /content_2856659.htm.

21st Century Business Herald (Guangzhou). 2011. "The Truth Behind 'Forced Donations' from the Shenmu Coal Miners." April 26. http://finance.sina.com.cn/roll/20110426 /00399748570.shtml.

Wei Ming. 2011. "Ministry of Civil Affairs: Supporting the Registration of Charity Social Organizations." *Beijing News*, December 24. http://politics.people.com.cn/GB/16702999 .html.

World Bank. 2013. "GDP (Current US $)." UN Data. http://data.un.org/Data.aspx?q=china +gdp&d=WDI&f=Indicator_Code%3aNY.GDP.MKTP.CD%3bCountry_Code%3aCHN.

Wines, Michael. 2010. "Chinese Attitudes on Generosity Are Tested." *New York Times*, September 23. http://www.nytimes.com/2010/09/24/world/asia/24china .html?pagewanted=1.

Wu Yanrui. 2004. *China's Economic Growth: A Miracle with Chinese Characteristics*. London: RoutledgeCurzon.

Xinhua. 2011. "Hu Jintao: Improving Concretely and Scientifically the Level of Social Management." February 19. http://news.xinhuanet.com/politics/2011-02/19/c_121100198 .htm.

Xu Yongguang. 2010. "The Limitations and Innovations of the Transformations of Public Foundations." In *Charity Blue Book* 125–136. Beijing: China Social Science Press.

Zhang Dan. 2011. "Henan's Soong Ching Ling Foundation Accused of Misusing Funds." CCTV, September 6. http://english.cntv.cn/program/china24/20110906/103502.shtml.

Zhu, Julie. 2013. "China Earthquake: Donors Prefer Private Charities over Public." *Financial Times*, April 22. http://blogs.ft.com/beyond-brics/2013/04/22/china-earthquake -donors-prefer-private-charities-over-public/#axzz2TBWwNq45.

Glossary

benevolent societies 善堂 or 善会
civil non-enterprise units. *See* people-run non-enterprise units/organizations
competent business unit (supervisory unit, such as Ministry of Health) 业务主
    管单位
dual registration, dual management 双重登记, 双重管理
federations 联合会
foundations 基金会
fundraising 募集资金
governmental financial support 政府资助
government-organized nongovernmental organizations (GONGOs) 官办非政
    府组织 (政府部门发起成立的非营利性组织)
grassroots nonprofit organizations 草根非政府组织
health-related philanthropy 医疗慈善事业
industry/professional organizations 行业协会
medical assistance 医疗救助
Ministry of Civil Affairs 民政部
Ministry of Health (now the National Health and Family Planning Commis-
    sion) 卫生部 (国家卫生和计划生育委员会)
national NGO 全国性非政府组织
nongovernmental organizations 非政府组织
nonprofit public institutions 事业单位
not-for-profit organizations 非营利组织
people-run non-enterprise units/organizations 民办非企业单位
People's organizations 人民团体. *See also* government-organized nongovern-
    mental organizations
philanthropic organization 公益慈善机构
private foundation 私募基金会
private non-enterprise units. *See* people-run non-enterprise units/organizations
private (non-public fundraising) foundations 非公墓基金会
public fundraising foundation 公募基金会
registration administration (usually MoCA) 注册登记管理机关
registration reform 注册登记改革
social associations 社会团体
social organizations 社会团体
social welfare organization 社会福利机构
tax-exempt status 减免税资格

Significant Nonprofit Laws and Regulations in China (in chronological order)

1988
Measures for the Management of Foundations
基金会管理办法

1998
Regulations on the Registration and Management of Social Organizations
社会团体登记管理条例

1998
Interim Regulations on the Registration and Management of Civil Non-Enterprise Institutions
民办非企业单位登记管理暂行条例

1999
Public Welfare Donations Law
公益事业捐赠法

2004
Regulations on the Management of Foundations
基金会管理条例

2004
Charity Law (in draft)
慈善事业促进法 (草案)

GONGOs, NGOs, and Foreign Philanthropies in China referenced in book chapters

All-China Women's Federation 中华全国妇女联合会

Beijing Stars and Rain Autism Education Institute 北京星星雨自闭症教育研究所

Bill & Melinda Gates Foundation 比尔及梅林达·盖茨基金会

Cancer Foundation of China 中国癌症基金会

CanYou Group and the Zheng Weining Charity Foundation 残友集团和郑卫宁慈善基金会

Chi Heng Foundation 智行基金会

China Association for Disaster and Emergency Rescue Medicine 中国医学救援协会

China Association for the Blind 中国盲人协会

China Association for the Deaf 中国聋人协会

China Beijing United Charity Foundation 中国北京联益慈善基金会

China Charities Aid for Children Foundation 中华少年儿童慈善救助基金会

China Charity Federation 中华慈善总会
China Children and Teenagers' Fund 中国儿童少年基金会 (or 中国少年儿童
　基金会)
China-Dolls Care and Support Association 瓷娃娃关怀协会
China Foundation Center 中国基金会中心网 (registered as 北京恩玖非营利组
　织发展研究中心)
China Foundation for Poverty Alleviation 中国扶贫基金会
China Health Inspection Association 中国卫生监督协会
China Healthy Birth Science Association 中国优生科学协会
China Medical Board 美国中华医学基金会
China Rural Health Association 中国农村卫生协会
China Sexology Association 中国性学会
China Social Welfare Foundation 中国社会福利基金会
China's Women Medical Association 中国女医师协会
China Transplantation Development Foundation 中国器官移植发展基金会
China Youth Development Foundation 中国青少年发展基金会
Chinese Association of STD and AIDS Prevention and Control 中国性病艾滋
　病防治协会
Chinese Foundation for the Prevention of STDs and AIDS 中国预防性病艾滋
　病基金会
Chinese Medical Association 中华医学会
Chinese People's Relief Association 中国人民救济总会
Chinese Red Cross Foundation 中国红十字基金会
Chinese Red Cross Society 中国红十字协会
Chinese Rural Kids Care 中国农村儿童保健
Henan Soong Ching Ling Foundation 河南省宋庆龄基金会
He Ren Charity Foundation 河仁慈善基金会
Narada Foundation 南都公益基金会
New Huadu Foundation 福建新华都基金会
One Foundation 壹基金
One Foundation and Ocean Heaven Project 壹基金和海洋天堂项目
Red Cross Society of China 中国红十字会
Shanghai Puki Coordination Agency for Deaf People 小聋包聋人协力事务所
Shanghai United Foundation 上海公益事业发展基金会
Shenzhen One Foundation 壹基金, 深圳
Smile Angel Foundation 嫣然天使基金会
Soong Ching Ling Foundation 中国宋庆龄基金会v

Contributors

MARY BROWN BULLOCK is Executive Vice Chancellor of Duke Kunshan University and serves as Chair of the China Medical Board. Her previous positions include President of Agnes Scott College, Distinguished Professor of China Studies, Emory University, and Director of the Asia Program, the Woodrow Wilson Center, Washington, DC. She received her PhD in Chinese history from Stanford University.

MARY ANN BURRIS is Executive Director of the Trust for Indigenous Culture and Health (TICAH), a nonprofit trust based in Nairobi, Kenya. She left China in 1996 to lead the Ford Foundation's reproductive health and youth programs in Eastern Africa until 2003, when she founded TICAH.

BRONWYN CARTER is Research Associate at La Trobe University, Melbourne, Australia. She has been working in public health research and teaching at La Trobe University since 2008. Her publications include works relating to public health policy of local and global relevance.

LINCOLN C. CHEN is President of the China Medical Board, an independent American foundation endowed by the Rockefeller family for advancing health in China and Asia by strengthening medical education, research, and policies. He was the Founding Director of the Harvard Global Equity Initiative and the Taro Takemi Professor of International Health and Director of the Harvard Center for Population and Development Studies. Dr. Chen is Chair of the Board of BRAC USA and former Chair of the Board of CARE/USA.

DENG GUOSHENG is Professor at the Tsinghua University School of Public Policy and Management and Director of the Center for Innovation and Social Responsibility at Tsinghua University. He is the author of *NPO Performance Evaluation*.

DAVID FAURE is Wei Lun Professor of History at the Chinese University of Hong Kong. He is author of *Emperor and Ancestor: State and Lineage in South China* (Stanford University Press, 2007) and *China and Capitalism: A History of Business Enterprise in Modern China* (Hong Kong University Press, 2006).

SUSAN JOLLY currently leads the Ford Foundation's sexuality and reproductive health and rights grant-making program in China and is co-editor of *Women, Sexuality and the Political Power of Pleasure* (Zed Books, 2013).

JOAN KAUFMAN is Director of the Columbia Global Center East Asia and Senior Lecturer at the Mailman School of Public Health, Columbia University. She is the author of *A Billion and Counting: Family Planning Campaigns and Policies in the People's Republic of China* (1983) and lead co-editor of *AIDS and Social Policy in China* (2006). She served as the Ford Foundation Sexuality and Reproductive Health Program Officer for China from 1996 to 2001.

JEFFREY P. KOPLAN is Vice President of Global Health, Emory University, and Principal Investigator of the Emory Global Health Institute–China Tobacco Control Partnership.

EVE W. LEE is Senior Advisor for China Project, Pathfinder International. She served as the Ford Foundation Sexuality and Reproductive Health Program Officer for China from 2001 to 2010.

LI FAN is Co-founder and Executive Director of Global Links Initiative, a non-profit organization that aims to foster practical links among social entrepreneurs around the world. Fan is also chief editor and co-author of *A New Horizon: 10 Stories of Social Entrepreneurs in China* (2010) and *The Rising Civil Society in China* (2008).

VIVIAN LIN is Professor of Public Health at La Trobe University, Melbourne, Australia, and has been working in China with international organizations since the 1980s. Her recent books include *Health Policy in Transition: Of and For China* (Peking University Medical Press, 2010).

PAMELA REDMON is Executive Director of the Emory Global Health Institute–China Tobacco Control Partnership and immediate past Executive Director of the Tobacco Technical Assistance Consortium.

CAROLINE REEVES is an independent scholar affiliated with the Harvard Fairbank Center. She specializes in the history of Chinese philanthropy, and is known for her work on the history of the Red Cross Society.

JENNIFER RYAN is a Research Fellow at the China Medical Board. Her degree is from Harvard's Department of Regional Studies–East Asia, where her research focused on the history of medicine in China and the West.

TONY SAICH is Director of the Ash Center for Democratic Governance and Innovation and Daewoo Professor of International Affairs at Harvard Kennedy School. Saich is a trustee member of International Bridges to Justice and the China Medical Board.

MARK SIDEL is Doyle-Bascom Professor of Law and Public Affairs at the University of Wisconsin-Madison and consultant for China and Vietnam to the International Center for Not-for-Profit Law (ICNL). While serving at the Ford Foundation's Beijing office, Sidel and Peter Geithner began the foreign philanthropic community's work on nonprofits and philanthropy in China in 1987 with the Chinese Ministry of Civil Affairs.

DARWIN H. STAPLETON is Professor of History at the University of Massachusetts Boston, and Executive Director Emeritus of the Rockefeller Archive Center. He is co-editor of *Science, Health and the Modern State in Asia* (2012).

WANG ZHENYAO is Professor at Beijing Normal University China Philanthropy Research Institute. His notable accomplishments include developing the national minimum assistance benefits system, overseeing aid and reconstruction projects in the aftermath of the Wenchuan earthquake, and launching rural democratic elections. He was editor of the *2011 Annual China Philanthropy Sector Report*, the *2012 Annual Report of China's Charity Sector*, and *China's Nonprofit Sector: Progress and Challenges*.

XU YONGGUANG is Chairman of the Narada Foundation, Chairman of the China Foundation Center, and Vice Chairman of China Youth Development.

RAY YIP is Representative and Country Program Director for the Bill & Melinda Gates Foundation in China. He is a specialist in global health with specialized interest in program development and management in nutrition, maternal and child health, and infectious disease, particularly HIV/AIDS.

ZHANG LU holds a PhD in ancient Chinese history from Nankai University, where her research focused on medical charity institutions and midwifery reform in the nineteenth and twentieth centuries.

ZHANG XIULAN is Professor and Dean of the School of Social Development and Public Policy at Beijing Normal University. She is author of *Cigarette Smoking and Nursing Home Utilization in the United States*.

ZHAO XIAOPING is a Postdoctoral Fellow at the Center for Innovation and Social Responsibility at the Tsinghua University School of Public Policy and Management.

ZHAO YANHUI is a Senior Analyst in the Research Department at Beijing Normal University China Philanthropy Research Institute. She is co-author of the *2011 Annual China Philanthropy Sector Report* and the *2012 Annual Report of China's Charity Sector.*

ZI ZHONGYUN is Academician Emeritus of the Chinese Academy of Social Sciences (CASS) and Senior Fellow and former Director of the Institute of American Studies, CASS.

Index

commune system, dismantling of, 62
Convention on the Rights of Persons with Disabilities (CRPD), U.N., 235
Coolidge, Charles, 123
Cooperative Agreement on Advancing Integrated Reforms in Civil Affairs (Ministry of Civil Affairs), 48
Cooperative Medical System (CMS), 22, 24, 61
cooperative movement, 71–72
Country Coordination Mechanism of China, 33
CTFK (Campaign for Tobacco-Free Kids), 183–184
cultural diplomacy, international philanthropy as, 109
Cultural Revolution (1966–1976): dissolution of charities and relief agencies, 23; health impacts of, 22; Red Cross Society during, 226–227

DALYs (disability-adjusted life years), 58, 76n1
deafness, 246–247
demographic transition, as health challenge, 59–60, 72–73
Deng Fei, 208
Deng Pufang, 13, 235
Deng Xiaoping, 13, 23, 158, 235
Department for International Development (DFID), United Kingdom, 68, 70, 146–147, 160
Department of Social Welfare and Charity Promotion (Ministry of Civil Affairs), 27
development organizations, international, 26–27
differentiated management, 44–45
disability-adjusted life years (DALYs), 58, 76n1
Disabled People 101 (website), 244, 245
disabled persons (canji ren). See people with disabilities
disaster relief, 14, 205, 256
disease burden, 57, 58–59, 59
disease prevalence, 59–60
Disrupting Philanthropy: Technology and the Future of the Social Sector (Bernholz), 121
Doctors Without Borders. See Médecins Sans Frontières (MSF)/Doctors Without Borders
domestic violence, 164–166
Dong Biwu, 20
Dongguan Sports Center for the Disabled, 271
Du Yuesheng, 222, 224
Duchenne muscular dystrophy, 243
Dulles, Allen, 108
Dunant, Henri, 215–216

Economic Cooperative for Poverty Alleviation, 110
economy of China: growth in twenty-first century, 1; private wealth accumulation, 1, 24, 268–269, 279n1
education, medical. See medical schools
Emergency Relief Committee, 225
Emory Global Health Institute–China Tobacco Control Partnership (GHI-CTP), 187–188
employment of people with disabilities, 237
Enable Disability Studies Institute, 237
Environmental Defense Fund, 69
epidemiological transition, as health challenge, 58–59, 59, 72–73
European Organization for Rare Diseases (EURORDS), 244, 248n5
Eye Bank (Guangzhou Municipal No. 1 Hospital), 259

Fairbank, John K., 105, 108
Family Violence Prevention Network, 165
Fan Shixun, 96
Fang Hsien-chih, 125
"Father-Mother Officials" (fu-mu guan), 215
Faure, David, 13
Federation of Hong Kong Chiu Chow Community Organizations, 256
Federation of National Red Cross and Crescent Societies, 229
Fei Xiaotong, 105
Feng, L. C., 131
Feng Youlan, 105
FIC (John E. Fogarty International Center), 176, 179
Ford Foundation: autonomy and engagement in controversial areas, 160; case study, 107–111; domestic violence initiative, 164–166; establishing office in China, 26, 109, 158; focus on institution building, 107; HIV/AIDS initiatives, 162, 166; impact of funding on issues, 168–169; intersectoral and social science approaches, 162; joint advocacy with UNFPA for reproductive rights, 163–164; microloans, 110; outcome of engagement in China, 170–171; participation in policy debates, 108; reproductive and sexual health initiatives, 68, 110, 118n8, 155–156, 158, 161–163, 171n2; reproductive tract infections research, 168; sexuality and sex education initiatives, 166–168; shift in funding priorities, 110; support for China studies during Cold War, 107–108

CPSIA information can be obtained at www.ICGtesting.com
Printed in the USA
LVOW10s1915190914

404946LV00001B/68/P